Traumatic Childbirth

T0187910

Postpartum depression has become a more recognized mental illness over the past decade as a result of education and increased awareness. Traumatic childbirth, however, is still often overlooked, resulting in a scarcity of information for health professionals. This is in spite of up to 34% of new mothers reporting experiencing a traumatic childbirth and prevalence rates rising for high risk mothers, such as those who experience stillbirth or who have very low birth weight infants.

This groundbreaking book brings together an academic, a clinician, and a birth trauma activist. Each chapter discusses current research, women's stories, the common themes in the stories and the implications of these for practice, clinical case studies, and a clinician's insights and recommendations for care. Topics covered include:

- mothers' perspectives
- fathers' perspectives
- the impact on breastfeeding
- the impact on subsequent births
- PTSD after childbirth
- EMDR treatment for PTSD.

This book is a valuable resource for health professionals who come into contact with new mothers, providing the most current and accurate information on traumatic childbirth. It also presents mothers' experiences in a manner that is accessible to women, their partners, and families.

Cheryl Tatano Beck is Distinguished Professor at the School of Nursing, University of Connecticut, USA.

Jeanne Watson Driscoll is a board-certified clinical nurse specialist in adult psychiatric-mental health nursing. She maintains a private psychotherapy practice in Boston, Massachusetts specializing in the care of women experiencing mood and anxiety disorders during their reproductive years.

Sue Watson is co-founder of Trauma and Birth Stress (TABS), an organization dedicated to raising the profile of traumatic birth and the devastation it causes. She currently works as a childbirth educator in Auckland, New Zealand.

Traumatic Childbirth

Cheryl Tatano Beck,
Jeanne Watson Driscoll and
Sue Watson

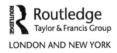
Routledge
Taylor & Francis Group

LONDON AND NEW YORK

First published 2013
by Routledge
2 Park Square, Milton Park, Abingdon, Oxon, OX14 4RN

Simultaneously published in the USA and Canada
by Routledge
711 Third Avenue, New York, NY 10017

Routledge is an imprint of the Taylor & Francis Group, an informa business

British Library Cataloguing in Publication Data
A catalogue record for this book is available from the British Library

Library of Congress Cataloging-in-Publication Data
Beck, Cheryl Tatano.
Traumatic childbirth / Cheryl Tatano Beck, Jeanne Driscoll, and Sue Watson.
p. ; cm.
Includes bibliographical references.
I. Driscoll, Jeanne. II. Watson, Sue, 1958– III. Title.
[DNLM: 1. Puerperal Disorders–psychology. 2. Stress Disorders, Post-Traumatic. 3. Parturition–psychology. 4. Postnatal Care–psychology. 5. Postpartum Period–psychology. WQ 500]
618.7'6–dc23
2012050443

ISBN13: 978-0-415-67809-4 (hbk)
ISBN13: 978-0-415-67810-0 (pbk)
ISBN13: 978-0-203-76669-9 (ebk)

Typeset in Bembo
by Keystroke, Station Road, Codsall, Wolverhampton

To the women who have shared their stories to give voice to their personal horrors to change the world!

Contents

Figures

Tables

1 Introduction

In the first chapter, the authors of this book introduce our readers to when and how each of us became involved with traumatic childbirth. For one of us, it was as a researcher, for another, it was as a clinician, and for another, it was as a mother who had suffered a traumatic childbirth.

Cheryl Tatano Beck

In the year 2001, I began my research into posttraumatic stress disorder (PTSD) after childbirth. Prior to this, I had been researching postpartum depression for 15 years. My clinical specialty is obstetrics and I am a certified nurse midwife. In my clinical practice I observed firsthand how devastating postpartum depression was for new mothers and their families. In the early 1980s not much at all was included in nursing or medical textbooks on postpartum depression. So in 1982 after receiving my doctoral degree from Boston University, I decided to focus my research program on postpartum depression.

From the very beginning of my research on postpartum depression I became aware of Jeanne Watson Driscoll, one of the prime mental health professionals in the field of postpartum mood and anxiety disorders. In 1993, at the annual convention of the Association of Women's Health, Obstetric, and Neonatal Nursing in Reno, Nevada, I finally had the privilege of meeting Jeanne in person. We were well aware of each other's experiences and accomplishments in women's health. This was the start of our long-term collaboration together. Jeanne likes to use the metaphor of a hand and glove saying that we have been a perfect fit—I as the researcher and she as the clinician.

During the 1990s, case study reports were beginning to be published in the literature on postpartum onset of panic disorder in new mothers. Some of the women who had participated in my postpartum depression studies recounted how they struggled with an incorrect diagnosis of postpartum depression after their latest birth. These women had suffered with postpartum depression after their previous births but they knew something was different this time. It was not postpartum depression even though that was the diagnosis the clinicians had given them. Eventually these women were given the correct diagnosis of postpartum onset of panic disorder, but only after they had suffered needlessly for months. In 1998, I conducted a qualitative study on mothers' experiences of postpartum onset of panic disorder in order to listen to the women's voices to help to differentiate their symptoms of this postpartum anxiety disorder from postpartum depression.

In 2001, I was asked to give a keynote address on perinatal anxiety disorders at the Australasian Marcé Society Biennial Scientific Meeting in Christchurch, New Zealand. The conference planning committee asked me to focus on the results of my research on postpartum panic disorder but to also address the range of anxiety disorders that can occur during pregnancy and the postpartum period. In preparing for this keynote address I reviewed the literature on perinatal anxiety disorders to make sure I was up to date on the current research. I came across a small number of studies on an anxiety disorder I had not heard of—PTSD due to childbirth. Of course, I knew about PTSD but never had connected this anxiety disorder to women as a result of their giving birth.

In delivering my keynote address I did include a little information on this new area of research on PTSD following traumatic childbirth. After I finished my keynote, the next presenter at the conference was a mother who powerfully spoke of her personal experience of PTSD following a traumatic childbirth. You could have heard a pin drop in this large auditorium as the attendees sat riveted to her story. This courageous woman was Sue Watson who had started a charitable trust in New Zealand called Trauma and Birth Stress (TABS) to support women who have experienced traumatic births (www.tabs.org.nz). At lunchtime that day Sue and I introduced ourselves to each other. We discussed the possibility of my doing some research with the mothers in TABS so that I could do for them what I had done for the mothers suffering with postpartum depression and postpartum panic disorder. I could use the findings of my study to help educate clinicians about traumatic childbirth and its resulting PTSD. So that very day Sue and I began our journey together, which has lasted for over a decade now. Sue has been instrumental in helping to recruit mothers from around the globe to participate in our research. Recruitment notices of our various studies were posted on TABS' website. Sue and I have now conducted seven qualitative studies on traumatic childbirth and PTSD following birth trauma in order to give voice to women's experiences. You will learn of our research findings throughout this book.

In 2006, Jeanne and I wrote our first book together, *Postpartum Mood and Anxiety Disorders: A Clinician's Guide.* It was given the American Journal of Nursing Book of the Year Award for 2006. Now we have come together again as authors to write this text, focusing specifically on traumatic childbirth and its resulting PTSD. For this book we have been extremely fortunate to add a third, very important perspective to the writings, that being the perspective of a mother, Sue Watson. Sue, who had experienced PTSD following a traumatic pregnancy and birth, not only survived it but went on to be a pioneer and a voice for women around the globe who have suffered from this postpartum anxiety disorder. In our book on traumatic childbirth as authors we now have a perfect triumvirate: researcher, clinician, and mother/consumer.

Jeanne Watson Driscoll

My interest in mental health issues related to pregnancy and postpartum began on a very personal note; I experienced what I now know to be postpartum obsessive thought disorder after the birth of my first child in 1976 and again after my second in 1978. At that time, no one spoke about these issues and although I had a master's degree in psychiatric nursing prior to the births of my children, I had not heard of an obsessive thought disorder related to having babies. My personal experiences and my own healing trajectory led me to study, learn, and question and I became a nurse expert in the field of perinatal psychiatry and mental health. I focused my energy on becoming a childbirth educator, lactation consultant, and a psychiatric clinical nurse specialist in an obstetrical nursing division prior to opening a private practice in psychotherapy. I was on a mission of educating women about the shadowy sides of pregnancy and postpartum with a non-judgmental, accepting attitude. I like to say I used my "creative rage" regarding what happened to me to try to change the experience for other women and their families and I continue this work today.

Through my clinical experiences in the hospital setting, I had had the privilege of being present, listening to women's stories of their birth experiences in the immediate time frame. When I moved to a private practice model of providing psychotherapy and pharmacotherapy for women who had experienced mood and anxiety disorders related to reproductive events, my clinical experiences changed. I was now honored to hear narratives and personal experiences that women had experienced and lived through. I was now able to work with them from initial assessment and diagnosis to their personal recoveries. It has been such a privilege to be part of their healing journeys, to bear witness to their experiences. I describe that what I do is promote, encourage, and facilitate a woman's sense of authenticity and self-esteem and to find her voice. I have had the most amazing career of reciprocity and mutuality with my patients and their families. It really hit me when I was beginning to see some of my patients' daughters that I knew I had become a crone. My patients have provided me with a wealth of clinical experience. They have been my teachers and I am honored to be invited into their healing journey.

As Cheryl shared with you, we met in the 1980s in Reno, Nevada, and it has been a truly unbelievable experience of evolving friendship and professional collaboration. Cheryl was my dissertation advisor during my doctoral work and was a guiding force on that journey for me. It has been a privilege and a pleasure to write this book and although I have never met Sue Watson, I feel like I know her through Cheryl. I welcome this amazing opportunity to collaborate with Cheryl, the researcher, and Sue, a healer in her own right.

Sue and Ralph Watson

This book has been a long-time dream for TABS. Each year I would ask, when can we write a book, Cheryl? And now here it is! The four of us (TABS Trustees) see this book as an extensive and in-depth study into the mental illness of posttraumatic stress disorder around childbirth. This book represents the progress of our endeavors since mid-1998.

What a privilege to be contributing as a voice of people who find themselves with posttraumatic stress disorder following pregnancy and childbirth! Together with the help of my husband, Ralph, we have been able to tell the story of TABS—Trauma and Birth Stress, www.tabs.org.nz. Since mid-1998 it has been my privilege to be one of the founders of TABS and more recently the main "face" of TABS. Throughout this time, Ralph has been an observer, an advisor, and in time the webmaster of the TABS website. So it has been only right that the two of us share in writing the TABS input into this book. Ralph brought his skills acquired in studying history to this project, ensuring more consistency than my enthusiasm alone could have achieved.

So we write, being ever so mindful that over the years we have heard the stories, seen the effect of PTSD and, yes, also the recovery of those who have been afflicted by it. We bring the voice of the mothers and fathers to this book. It all began in 1998 when five New Zealand mothers met after letters from two of us were published in a parenting magazine. We had all suffered PTSD due to traumatic pregnancies or childbirth experiences, and while still affected in various ways by the devastating and unpredictable symptoms of PTSD, we wanted to help others. We wanted to tell other mothers that help is at hand and that we can help by pointing the way to it. We also wanted to tell the health community that they must consider PTSD when helping emotionally charged mothers, to look for explanations other than postpartum depression.

As for me personally, I am motivated to challenge, inspire and to make a difference. I am simply a consumer, who wanted to tell my story and talk clearly about PTSD. My background is in horticulture, voluntary work, administration, and, lately, sales. Also, encouraged by one of the other TABS mothers, I trained as a Childbirth Educator and 11 years later am still doing this work that I enjoy so much. My approach in the classes, beside the usual curriculum, is to inspire people to ask questions, to think outside the square and be confident in their family-to-be! The story of TABS is clearly told in Chapter 16. Suffice it to say that, as a group of consumers, we never displayed anger or impatience, but rather we communicated gently and clearly but also passionately. I have of course moved on, and have recovered from PTSD, and yet the website remains our voice. It always amazed us how we opened doors and seized opportunities, and how one particular presentation truly opened the door. What a pleasure it has been to have done this work! Enjoy the book and know that mothers, fathers, and families can be well together. Regards, Sue and Ralph.

Overview of the book

The outline for the remaining 17 chapters is presented now to provide a sweeping overview of this book, written with both clinicians and mothers and their families in mind. In Chapter 2, traumatic childbirth and PTSD secondary to birth trauma are defined, to provide a common basis for the remainder of the book. The prevalence rates of traumatic childbirth and elevated post-traumatic stress symptoms in new mothers are described. Included in this literature review of research on this postpartum anxiety disorder are Cheryl's qualitative studies on mothers' experiences of birth trauma and also its resulting PTSD (Beck, 2004a; 2004b). A unique feature throughout this book entails a clinician's (Jeanne) reactions and a mother's (Sue) reactions to the narratives of the women who have participated in Cheryl and Sue's series of qualitative research studies.

In Chapter 3, Jeanne describes her introduction to PTSD secondary to a traumatic birth through her case study of Mrs. Robins, who was the first patient Jeanne ever cared for with this postpartum anxiety disorder.

A review of the literature on risk factors for postpartum posttraumatic stress response is the focus of Chapter 4. Risk factors are divided into two time periods: prenatal and intrapartum. After reading this chapter it will become apparent that elevated posttraumatic stress response in new mothers is an international phenomenon. Countries represented in this literature review include the United States (US), Canada, the United Kingdom (UK), Australia, Sweden, Switzerland, Italy, Germany, the Netherlands, Nigeria, and Israel.

In Chapter 5, the readers are privy to women's narratives of some of their specific risk factors for developing PTSD. These mothers were participants in Cheryl's research on women's experiences of PTSD following a traumatic childbirth (Beck, 2004b). Mothers' stories of the following risk factors are shared: increased medical intervention, pain, helplessness, postpartum hemorrhage, preeclampsia, perinatal loss, preterm birth, and childhood sexual abuse.

In Chapter 6, some of the neurophysiology is described that may be implicated in the process of the effects of trauma on the brain. With this information on brain biology as the basis, next the assessment and diagnosis of elevated posttraumatic stress symptoms in mothers are addressed. Jeanne's earthquake model for assessment is described in this chapter (Beck & Driscoll, 2006; Sichel & Driscoll, 1999).

A case study of Carol is presented in Chapter 7. Carol was one of Jeanne's patients in her private practice. This case study describes Carol's assessment, diagnosis, and treatment. Instruments available to screen for elevated post-traumatic stress symptoms in new mothers are reviewed in Chapter 8.

In Chapter 9, the impact of traumatic childbirth on breastfeeding is the focus. A literature review identifying factors that have been reported to impact mothers' breastfeeding experiences is presented. These factors include delivery type, labor stress, and postpartum mood and anxiety disorders. Cheryl and Sue's qualitative study on mothers' narratives of how their birth trauma impacted their breastfeeding experiences is highlighted (Beck & Watson, 2008). Experiences of two mothers from this study are shared to describe the struggles and triumph regarding their breastfeeding after their traumatic childbirths.

The focal point of Chapter 10 is the yearly anniversary of women's traumatic childbirth. Reports from research studies on anniversary reactions to different traumatic events, such as the World Trade Center terrorist attacks, have been published. The only study to date focusing on mothers' experiences of the anniversary of their birth trauma is Cheryl's research study (Beck, 2006). This chapter spotlights the mothers' narratives of their anniversaries which provide the readers a privileged insider's perspective of the yearly struggles these mothers endure.

In Chapter 11, the topic of focus is subsequent childbirth after a previous traumatic birth. Research is revealing the chronic nature of postpartum posttraumatic stress on women and their relationships with their infants and partners. Initial research on the long-term detrimental effects of traumatic childbirth is summarized in this chapter, along with a spotlight on Cheryl and Sue's qualitative study on women's experiences of their subsequent pregnancy and labor and delivery experiences following a previous birth trauma (Beck & Watson, 2010).

A case study of Anne is presented in Chapter 12. She was another one of Jeanne's patients and her case is described in detail from assessment through treatment.

In Chapter 13, treatment options for PTSD secondary to traumatic childbirth are discussed. Limited research has been conducted on treatments specific to PTSD when the trigger was traumatic childbirth. The treatments described in the chapter include debriefing, cognitive behavioral therapy, and eye movement desensitization reprocessing (EMDR). Narratives of mothers' experiences of EMDR treatment are shared from Cheryl and Sue's ongoing qualitative study. The chapter concludes with a case study of Jeanne's from her private clinical practice.

Chapter 14 focuses on the case study of Sheila. In this chapter, Jeanne describes her assessment, diagnosis, and subsequent treatment for Sheila.

Fathers now take center stage in Chapter 15. Attention is turned here to fathers' experiences being present at their partners' traumatic births. First a literature review of research on fathers and traumatic childbirth is reported. Next the narratives of some of the fathers who have participated in Cheryl and Sue's ongoing qualitative research are shared with the readers to provide a powerful and very private glimpse into the experiences of these men being present during birth trauma.

Chapter 16 spotlights the remarkable accomplishments of Trauma and Birth Stress (TABS), a charitable trust located in New Zealand, which Sue started, along with three other women. The chapter is written by Sue and her husband, Ralph, who also was instrumental in creating and maintaining the TABS' website and in providing his expert guidance. The readers are given a rare behind-the-scenes account of the stages that TABS has undergone, starting with its beginnings and finishing with its stepping back. The information in this chapter is invaluable for anyone interested in starting a self-help group.

Up to this point the chapters in this book have concentrated on traumatic childbirth and its potential to develop into PTSD in new mothers and fathers. Now in Chapter 17 attention is directed to the impact that being present at traumatic births can have on labor and delivery staff. An understudied aspect of PTSD is secondary traumatic stress, which can be described as the "cost of caring" for clinicians with traumatized patients. Research is reviewed on secondary traumatic stress in health care providers, such as mental health professionals, social workers, pediatric clinicians, emergency department nurses, oncology nurses, and obstetrical nurses. In this literature review, instruments used to screen health care providers for secondary traumatic stress symptoms are described. The chapter concludes with experiences of five obstetrical nurses selected from a mixed methods study conducted by Cheryl on secondary traumatic stress in labor and delivery nurses (Beck & Gable, 2012).

The final chapter, Chapter 18, is the epilogue, and concludes with recommendations for health care providers to help prevent or at least minimize traumatic childbirth and its resulting PTSD. These recommendations span the childbearing phases: antepartum, intrapartum, and postpartum.

References

Beck, C. T. (2004a). Birth trauma: In the eye of the beholder. *Nursing Research, 53,* 28–35.

—— (2004b). PTSD due to childbirth: The aftermath. *Nursing Research, 53,* 216–224.

—— (2006). The anniversary of birth trauma: Failure to rescue. *Nursing Research, 55,* 381–390.

Beck, C. T., & Driscoll. J. W. (2006). *Postpartum mood and anxiety disorders: A clinician's guide.* Sudbury, MA: Jones & Bartlett Publishers.

Beck, C. T., & Gable, R. K. (2012). A mixed methods study of secondary traumatic stress in labor and delivery nurses. *Journal of Obstetric, Gynecologic, and Neonatal Nursing, 41,* 747–760.

Beck, C. T., & Watson, S. (2008). Impact of birth trauma on breast-feeding: A tale of two pathways. *Nursing Research, 57,* 228–236.

Beck, C. T. & Watson, S. (2010). Subsequent childbirth after a previous traumatic birth. *Nursing Research, 59,* 241–249.

Sichel, D., & Driscoll, J. W. (1999). *Women's moods.* New York: HarperCollins.

2 What Is Traumatic Birth and Posttraumatic Stress Due to Childbirth?

In this chapter research on traumatic childbirth and its resulting posttraumatic stress is reviewed. Also included in this chapter is the story of Jill's birth trauma. Jill was one of the mothers who participated in Cheryl's first study of traumatic childbirth (Beck, 2004a). The chapter ends with a new area of research on posttraumatic growth as a possible positive outcome of experiencing a traumatic childbirth.

"Beauty is in the eye of the beholder" was first penned by Margaret Wolfe Hungerford in her 1878 novel, *Molly Bawn*. Beauty, however, is not the only phenomenon or quality that lies in the eye of the beholder. Traumatic childbirth also does. What one woman perceives as a traumatic birth may be viewed quite differently through the eyes of labor and delivery staff who may see it as a routine birth.

Birth trauma is defined as "an event occurring during the labor and delivery process that involves actual or threatened serious injury or death to the mother or her infant. The birthing woman experiences intense fear, helplessness, loss of control, and horror" (Beck, 2004a, p. 28). After completing her series of research studies on traumatic childbirth, Cheryl has now revised this definition of birth trauma to also include an event occurring during labor and delivery where the woman perceives she is stripped of her dignity.

Research is revealing that between 33–45% of women perceive their births to be traumatic. In Australia, Creedy, Shochet, and Horsfall (2000) reported that 33% (n = 164) of a community sample of 499 mothers between four–six weeks postpartum had experienced a traumatic childbirth. Out of a sample of 103 women four weeks postpartum in the US, Soet, Brack, and Dilorio (2003) found that 34% of this sample perceived that childbirth experience as traumatic. In 2009, Sawyer and Ayers reported that 37.2% of their Internet sample of 219 women within 36 months postpartum (mean = 11 months) viewed their childbirth as traumatic. In Australia, 45.5% (n = 394) of the community sample of women four–six weeks postpartum reported birth trauma (Alcorn, O'Donovan, Patrick, Creedy, & Devilly, 2010). In the most recent study Sawyer, Ayers, Young, Bradley, and Smith (2012) found that 23% of the mothers perceived their childbirth to be traumatic. Not all women, however, who perceive their childbirth to be traumatic, go on to develop PTSD. Risk factors related to PTSD secondary to birth trauma are reviewed in Chapter 4.

What are the essential elements of labor and delivery that are perceived as so traumatic by women? In Beck's (2004a) qualitative study of birth trauma with 40 mothers, what became apparent was that women were systematically stripped of protective layers of caring. This was why one mother could, for instance, have experienced postpartum hemorrhage and be fine while another mother perceived this same event as a traumatic birth. Women frequently portrayed traumatic childbirth as being raped on the delivery table with everyone watching and no one offering to help. During her labor and delivery, one mother "felt like a piece of meat on the bed. After, I was afraid to look at myself in the mirror. I was afraid to look myself in the eyes. I felt like my soul had died." What happened to make this mother believe her soul had died?

The four themes that emerged from the stories of mothers' traumatic births in Beck's (2004a) study revealed the answer. The first theme was "To care for me: Was that too much to ask?" Women did not feel cared for. They felt stripped of their dignity, alone and abandoned. Women described the care they had received from labor and delivery staff as "arrogant," "mechanical," and that it lacked any sense of empathy. One young woman who had moved from Puerto Rico to the US shared that during her labor:

> They had me in all kinds of positions (including all fours) to hear the heartbeat with a stethoscope, and about 20 students came in the room without my permission. All I heard them saying was that I was now $7^1/_2$ dilated. By the way, while I was on all fours, I was trying to cover my bottom by holding the gown, and a nurse took my hands from the gown. So, I felt raped and my dignity was taken from me.
>
> (Beck, 2004a, p. 32)

Theme 2 was entitled "To communicate with me: Why was this neglected?" Obstetric care providers failed to communicate with the laboring women. The mothers revealed that they felt invisible as clinicians talked to each other as if the laboring woman were not there. For example, one primipara recounted:

> After an hour trying to deliver the baby with a vacuum extractor, the obstetrician said it was too late for an emergency cesarean. The baby was truly stuck. By now the doctors are acting like I'm not there. The attending physician was saying: "We may have lost this bloody baby." The hospital staff discussed my baby's possible death in front of me and argued in front of me just as if I weren't there.
>
> (Beck, 2004a, pp. 32–33)

For the third theme, "To provide safe care: You betrayed my trust and I felt powerless," women shared that they perceived they received unsafe care, and feared for their own safety and that of their infants. As one mother shared:

> I remember believing that the labor and delivery team would know what was right and would be there should things go wrong. That was my first

mistake. They didn't and they weren't! I strongly believe my PTSD was caused by feelings of powerlessness and loss of control of what people did to my body.

(Beck, 2004a, p. 33)

The fourth theme, "The end justifies the means: At whose expense? At what price?" highlighted how women perceived that what they had to endure during their traumatic births was pushed into the background as clinicians, family, and friends celebrated the delivery of a healthy baby. A successful birth was defined only by the outcome of the baby. Mothers, who perceived their births as traumatic, viewed labor and delivery as a battlefield where they had engaged in battle without any protective armor, stripped of protective layers of caring leaving themselves exposed. As this woman recalled,

I was congratulated for how "quickly and easily" the baby came out and that he scored a perfect 10! The worst thing was that nobody acknowledged that I had a bad time. Everyone was so pleased it had gone so well! I felt as if I had been raped!

(Beck, 2004a, p. 34)

Thomson and Downe (2008) conducted a phenomenological study in the United Kingdom (UK) with 14 mothers who had experienced a traumatic birth. Analysis of in-depth interviews revealed that these women described their childbirth as abuse, torture, and violence. Three themes emerged: being disconnected, being helpless, and being isolated. Traumatized women felt disconnected with their health care providers during labor and delivery. Interactions with the staff were portrayed as cold, lacking support or personal regard for women as individuals. At times, women dissociated to cope with their birth trauma. A complete sense of helplessness permeated their labor and delivery. Women felt isolated as their voices were disregarded. They were devalued and felt like a slab of meat on the delivery table, leading to a dehumanizing birth.

A synthesis of 10 qualitative studies on women's experiences of traumatic childbirth revealed six major repetitive themes (Elmir, Schmied, Wilkes, & Jackson, 2010). First, women felt invisible and out of control during their birthing. Women were ignored and not considered as individuals. They shared that they had a sense of powerlessness and vulnerability. Second, women vividly described their labor and delivery care as degrading and inhumane. Third, after delivery, they had distressing recurring nightmares of their traumatic births. The fourth theme focused on the rollercoaster of emotions mothers endured after their traumatic births, such as panic, depression, anger, and suicidal thoughts. In the fifth theme, the effects traumatic births had on women's relationships with their infants and partners were highlighted. Mothers felt disconnected from their infants. Their disrupted relationships with their partners centered on feeling their traumatic birthing experiences were not acknowledged and understood by their partners. Women avoided sexual intimacy because it was a constant reminder of their birth trauma. The sixth theme spoke to breastfeeding as a way for some mothers to help overcome their traumatic births and prove themselves as successful mothers.

Beck (2011) integrated the findings from six qualitative studies on birth trauma and its resulting PTSD she conducted in her program of research. Noblit and Hare's (1988) method for synthesizing the findings of qualitative studies was used. This metasynthesis provided a wide-angle lens to view the far-reaching, stinging tentacles of traumatic childbirth. Bring privy to the findings of all six studies revealed the destructive domino effects of birth trauma on various aspects of motherhood which took the form of amplifying causal looping. In amplifying causal looping "as consequences become continually causes and causes continually consequences one sees either worsening or improving progressions or escalating severity" (Glaser, 2005, p. 9).

In causal looping, feedback occurs which can effect further changes that can either intensify or oppose the original change. Causal loops can be classified as either a balancing loop or a reinforcing loop. A balancing loop occurs when feedback decreases the impact of a change. When feedback increases the impact of a change, this is classified as a reinforcing loop. The terms positive or negative can also be applied to the direction of causal looping. In a positive direction the changes are reinforced. Positive does not necessarily imply that the effects are good. A negative direction indicates that the effects are resisted but it does not necessarily imply the changes are bad.

The metasynthesis of Beck's six qualitative studies unearthed a series of amplifying causal loops (Beck, 2011). Traumatic childbirth was the original trigger which sets in motion six amplifying loops (Figure 2.1). Four of these loops were reinforcing (positive direction) and two were balancing loops (negative direction). The detrimental impact that birth trauma can have on women's breastfeeding experiences is the focus of Reinforcing Loop #1. As a result of traumatic childbirth, intruding flashbacks, disturbing detachment with their infants, feeling violated, enduring physical pain, and insufficient milk supply all contributed to the positive (reinforcing) effect which created a vicious cycle of trauma and increased posttraumatic stress symptoms. Balancing Loop #1 also focused on the feedback between posttraumatic stress symptoms resulting from birth trauma and breastfeeding. In this balancing loop the original effects of the posttraumatic stress due to traumatic birth were opposed and helped to decrease these distressing symptoms. Women shared that proving themselves as mothers after their birth trauma, atoning to their infants for the traumatic way they were brought into the world, and helping the mothers heal mentally contributed to the negative direction of this feedback loop.

Reinforcing Loop #2 involved the detrimental effects of traumatic childbirth on mother–infant interaction. The disturbing detachment of mothers from their infants led to this positive amplifying loop. The anniversary of a mother's traumatic childbirth intensified their posttraumatic stress symptoms and was the focus of Reinforcing Loop #3. The fourth reinforcing loop was a balancing loop which concentrated on subsequent childbirth following a previous traumatic

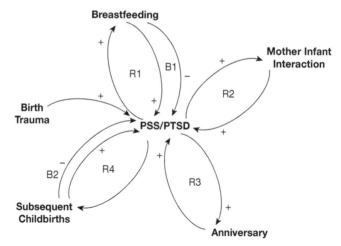

Figure 2.1 Causal looping

Source: Reprinted with permission from Beck (2011 p. 307).

birth. In Reinforcing Loop #4 the amplifying feedback loop was reinforced (positive direction) as some women did not experience their longed-for healing birth. For other women they were indeed fortunate and described their subsequent childbirth as a healing experience. This balancing loop involved an opposing effect to the feedback loop and helped decrease posttraumatic stress symptoms in these mothers.

This panoramic view permitted by this metasynthesis provides clinicians with an insider's glimpse of the repetitive, reinforcing amplifying causal loops that haunted mothers as they endured the long-term consequences of traumatic childbirth. Leverage points can be located where pressure applied to the amplifying causal loops can yield desired outcomes that can break the feedback loop where necessary. Leverage points can target the four reinforcing feedback loops that increase mothers' posttraumatic stress symptoms. We as clinicians fail to rescue these mothers time and time again. We fail to rescue women during the initial target trauma of childbirth and afterwards as they struggle to successfully breastfeed, as they interact with their infants, during the anniversary of their traumatic births, and in subsequent childbirth.

Some leverage points that clinicians can employ include, for example, with Reinforcing Loop #3 at children's yearly well child checkups. These yearly physical exams provide a perfect opportunity for clinicians to determine if mothers are struggling with memories of their traumatic births around their yearly anniversary. Another example of a leverage point, this time for Reinforcing Loop #1, would involve providing intensive one-on-one support for traumatized mothers as they initiate their breastfeeding attempts.

In this next section of the chapter, one mother's story is presented from Cheryl's qualitative study on the experience of birth trauma (Beck, 2004a).

Jill's Story

Jill's story of her being "raped and robbed" during the birth of her first baby vividly illustrates the essential elements of a traumatic childbirth. After laboring for 48 hours at home, Jill was told by her nurse midwife that the baby was "stuck" and she needed to be transported to the hospital by ambulance. The remainder of Jill's story is in her own words:

> Why did we have to come through the ER entrance? The message is birth is a medical emergency. Don't trust yourself, don't trust your body, your body doesn't work, you are a failure so just trust us and sign away your human dignity on the "informed consent" line. The gross misuse of "informed consent" is occurring without my knowledge as my husband signs away my rights. Later there will be no discussion of a treatment plan or course of action. There will be no discussion of my birth plan despite my handing it to several nurses for them and the doctor to review. There will be no discussion of risks and benefits of any treatment. I am aware of most of the risks of an epidural, which is why I clearly stated in the birth plan well in advance that I would not be choosing an epidural under any circumstances. I never deviate from this discussion. I am unaware that the decision has been made for me over the phone before I arrive. The doctor believes she is saving me from discomfort that I have not complained of, to "get me comfortable," to let me "rest." My belief system is overthrown before I even arrive. No one has authority to make this decision for anyone for any reason. This is an elective procedure, not necessary and charged with risks and emotions. It means the end of participating with the birth of your child. It means your birth is a mere medical procedure incapable of doing it yourself any longer. It is now managed and controlled by strangers. My body belongs to them before I arrive. They seize full control of my body, my birth, before I arrive. I am unaware of this all. I am not in pain since I haven't had a contraction for about 45 minutes and they had been so weak and very manageable compared to earlier. I never requested any pain relief and no one ever asks me if I am in pain or if I would like drugs of any kind. So, I think I am safe from drug-managed labor. I am completely unaware that they have given me a very high dose of pain medication.
>
> A nondescript-looking woman who was a complete stranger with glasses comes in stoically and announces that I can have a vaginal birth. I am not aware that she has put her hand inside me and examined me. I am puzzled that she has determined this. I said that the midwife said the baby was stuck. She says sarcastically that he is not "stuck" any more. I am elated that I will not be given drugs or a caesarean. She says to the nurse but not to me directly "Let's get her comfortable." I believe this means she will be lowering the lights and getting me a blanket, and some much needed food and water. There is talk of a fever. That's all I can make out. No one is speaking to me. I take two pills for the fever. I am unaware of an IV or anything going into it. My husband is not in my vision. A man comes in

and coldly announces that he is there to give me an epidural. I panic in my mind. I feel trapped, terrified, confused, helpless, powerless to protest. I say I don't want to hear what he has to say. The midwife and my husband and a nurse begin coercing me and baby talking me to turn over and lie down in the fetal position. I began to dissociate. I can only conclude that I am having a caesarean and I've been lied to or there is a turn of events that I am not aware of. Why else would they be doing this to me? I don't want this. Above all, I do not want this. I do not need this. They are making me watch the caesarean. I requested general anesthesia if I was to have a surgical procedure or I need nothing to birth my child vaginally. My mind cannot process this. I can't speak. I can't protest. I want to scream and run. I am terrified. I have no advocate. I am not safe. My fears were real. I am completely powerless to stop this. I leave my body and see myself from a bird's eye view. I am horrified. I return to my body when I feel the most invasive painful sensation from my lower back. I whine and cry and grit my teeth. I plead for it to be over. I cry and I get more baby talk. The nurse midwife tells me to curl up more. It continues. They aren't stopping. I can't take the pain anymore. I am being tortured by those who I trusted. No one is responding to my pain. My anguish is ignored. It takes an eternity. I am sobbing and want death. The pain is relentless. It won't stop and I know that no one cares and no one will save me. I learn later that I have four compressed vertebras and that they were hitting a major nerve. My cries should have been an indication to the anesthesiologist that he was in the wrong place. Why didn't anyone ask me if I wanted this? I cannot feel my legs now. I cannot move my legs. I am completely incapacitated. There are straps/monitors tightly around my waist. I am miserable. I am shaking uncontrollably and falling out of the bed. I push a button that was placed in my hand to call the nurse, someone to help me from falling out of the bed.

My husband is asleep, I am too afraid to wake him. I am all alone. There are nurses in the hall talking and laughing in the open door. No one responds to the call button. I meekly call out for help. An annoyed woman lifts me back to a safer position. I am embarrassed that I need help and that I am shaking. I say the straps are putting so much pressure on my abdomen, can she loosen them? A nurse lifts my gown without asking or telling me and she announces that my bladder is full. I am completely unaware that a stranger has spread my labia and inserted a tube in my urethra. I am again confused as to how she knows this since I didn't feel like I had to pee. I believe still at this time that I will be getting a C-section at any time. I believe that my only mode of survival is obedience and politeness. My fright–flight response is in overdrive and I cannot move. My brain is in extreme distress. I have no means of defense other than full surrender to these cold, annoyed people. I feel ashamed to ask them for anything. There is rarely anyone next to me. They come into check the machines and never once look at me or touch me kindly or say any kind words. I am apologetic about any request. I attempt nervous small talk in attempt to make my torturers more compassionate towards me. I am desperately alone and afraid. I receive no information about the baby or me ever. I call for a nurse again as I have been pushing that button forever and I am still shaking and falling out of bed again. I have never been able to not move my legs or any part of my body. I am very distressed by this and having no consistent human being that I can trust will help me. I have never in my life felt so vulnerable and helpless and made to feel so much shame for being dependent on total strangers. I did hate to bother them. I did feel ashamed for my discomfort and fear. I tried to smile at them when they came to check the monitors. I got no response. I just wanted to hear that I would be okay and that nothing would happen to me without my knowledge but it was way too late for that. They had already drugged me with a narcotic, rendered me paralyzed, and stolen my birth, all for my own good, according to them. What is "my own good?" "Our own good" will truly be protected when western-trained medical professionals learn to trust the laboring women as they trust themselves and honor their decisions, i.e. their birth plan. The straps were still the main focus of discomfort. I believed that if I can feel this I would feel being cut open. The button I had been pushing for a nurse was actually the self-medication delivery device for the catheter that was in my spine. I was told this by the same anesthesiologist when I told them that I could still feel my abdomen. I pinched it and could feel it. I politely asked for help. He was annoyed and seemed confused. He said to push the button that I had been pushing for over an hour. They must have thought I wanted no sensation during the birth of my child. Because I had been forced to have an epidural without my consent and against my will.

No communication creates chaos and terror in a vulnerable state. Lack of information allows for worst-case scenarios to be firmly accepted realities in times of vulnerability and trauma. PTSD is making itself at home in my body where it will remain for a lifetime acutely or residually. Please, someone, talk to me. Look at me. Hold my hand. Compassionately ask me how I am doing. No one ever asks this question. Establish trust with me. I need human contact desperately. A little goes a long way. This is the birth of my child and I am feeling like a prisoner of war waiting for another rape. This is psychological abuse. Just say something kind to me and I can give this another name other than traumatic maybe. I may be able to heal from this if I am given an ounce of empowerment. Let me do my job. Let me birth my child. I know I can do it but I've been through too much under my incarceration. I need your support. Don't take this from me. It's not too late. Obedience was my only survival but I was in survival mode since they had shown no mercy during the epidural; it wouldn't be a far stretch for them to cut me open with ineffective anesthesia.

During this time, however, I am so far removed from the birthing process. I am transitioning and missing it. I am dilating fully and my baby is descending. I am missing it. I no longer have a dialogue with him. He is on his own and completely alone too. What are the drugs doing to him as well? What is he experiencing, disconnected from my body, my heart? Is he experiencing the fear and terror that I am? Are the stress hormones passing to him? I am no longer there for him. I am a passive bystander in the entire birthing process. I am being raped and robbed. All I can do is survive by submission. My body is currently being riveted by superhuman unnatural contractions. From a drug, pitocin, that I am not aware is pumping through me even though I requested that pitocin be administered only with discussion according to my birth plan. Of course, there is no discussion or information on the risks and benefits, no informed consent again. I know in advance that pitocin has never been approved by the FDA for routine use, although it is standard in hospitals in this country. What is my baby feeling as a result? I am unaware of his torment. There is no mind–body connection. The guilt is still overwhelming me as I write. Mommy is so sorry, baby! No one is caring for us.

Neglect is abuse. I remember feeling so ashamed and embarrassed and vulnerable when strange nurses begin opening my legs and exposing my vagina that is crusted with blood and pubic hair. I am so ashamed. They haven't told or asked me if they could or would be opening my legs for pushing. They look around indifferently and proceed to expose me. Again I am immobile and have no control. Kind communication and permission would have gone a long way in empowering me just one iota through this whole ordeal. I was nothing more than a human body not a human being. After a while I could not feel anything more than an object as well. The feeling has never left me in three years postpartum. I have not reconnected with my body. It's so violated that I want nothing to do with it. The nurse and the midwife quickly and obediently hold my legs back up parallel to my chest and begin barking orders to push again and to "get angry." I am terrified that I have to push my guts out to please these women. I am a burden, after all. I am a nuisance and a failure. I am preventing another poor woman from emergency care. I could not feel more worthless and ashamed for being in labor at this time and in this hospital. My body is not performing to their standards and I have no right to ask for anything more. I obediently push blue in the face style for several more hours. A vacuum is mentioned but I have no information as to why. I ask them not to use it. I'm told to get angry again and push. My eyes feel as though they are bugging out and they are. I have an oxygen mask on and feel more and more detached. I know that I can't quit yet. I forget I am giving birth completely. I'm just trying to please them and avoid torment. I forget everything I know out of fear. They tell me to look at a mirror and touch the baby's head. I don't want to. I'm too frightened. The OB says something I can't under-stand about a vacuum. But no one tells me why she is saying it. The baby is being strongly extracted out and I don't even realize that I'm now giving birth to my son. It's an extraction not a birth. I feel awful tugging and shock. I can't close my eyes. They're too swollen. I'm frozen stiff. My child was born without me feeling or knowing it. I didn't know he was out of my body because there was no sound. Nothing. I see something purple and bloody rushed across the room in strangers' arms. My husband ran too. The baby wasn't moving or breathing. I felt nothing. Many minutes went by. No word. I had no connection with him whatsoever. Several strangers saw and touched him before I even laid eyes on him. Another total stranger put him on me. I could barely hold him. Large eyes. Long fingers. I took off his hat. Huge purple bruises on his head. I'm being sewn back up and I can feel it.

A hopeless numbness had set in that still resides and dominates this life that does not feel like mine. I remained bed-ridden for weeks and months to come. Little healing and terrible complications began rearing their ugly heads well past the period of postpartum state health insurance coverage, not to mention an ongoing overwhelming psychological illness (PTSD). A brief summary of medical complications include obturator nerve damage, motor skills impairment, femoral neuropathy, weakness in both legs, leg buckling, noticeable muscle atrophy, inability to bend down, walk properly without appearing intoxicated, inability to run, ride a bike, or dance, all of which I loved to do, both hip abductors and any and all muscles and ligaments were torn from having my legs pulled beyond my head for an extended period of time by two different people, PTSD, which I have mentioned, insomnia, depression, self-destructive behavior, no libido, painful sex still after three years, inability to relate to humans again, social isolation, completely shot pelvic floor muscles from the vacuum, painful second degree and perineum tears that still cause problems.

Clinician's Reaction

As I read and re-read this above story, my heart is breaking that this experience had to occur at all. Where were the nurses? Why was this woman left alone? Why were major assumptions made that she knew how to use the patient control anesthesia pump or the pain medication pump? In so many ways what jumps out at me is the fact that all too often health care providers assume too much. A woman who enters the hospital system does not know the rules. She is in essence a stranger in a strange land. She is already vulnerable to the experience of birthing a baby and for this woman her desire for a home birth, and the respect for a birth plan, which I am sure she spent hours developing, was devalued and dismissed. In her words, you get to experience what it was like for her to lie in that bed and the continual impact of this experience for over three years since the birth. This is emotional, physical, and verbal abuse by a health delivery system and its providers. Would you like to be taken care of that way?

When I became a nurse, I vowed that I would treat patients the way that I would want my family to be treated: with dignity and respect. Now I do know that there are two sides to every story and this narrative is the woman's perception, but if we take it step by step and look at potential interventions that may have helped along the way, it becomes clear that the primary intervention that was missing here is an advocate for her: who took care of her? She does not share that anyone introduced themselves, but remembers scary people coming to her and doing things to her without permission. Her husband, one would imagine, was just as scared in that he too was a stranger in a strange land dependent on the people who worked there to take care of his wife, baby and, yes, him.

The rates of occurrence are high and global. The stories have a theme of a woman feeling that she has been raped. Many of the women who have taken part in Cheryl and Sue's research do NOT have a history of physical, emotional, and/or sexual abuse so this birth precipitated, as this woman shared, "the loss of her soul."

Mother's Reaction

In listening to Jill's story, my first question would be, "Tell me about the elements of support that were there for you during your birth." I would be saying, "Oh, my goodness, this was not your fault, you are not alone and this is not in your imagination. Your telling the story is the beginning of your recovery. Anyone who had gone through this would be just as you are. Telling this can mean that one less person might be treated as you were." A birthing woman is never a patient. Yes, things might vary from the usual, yet communication and support must be prominent parts of her care, or must be established as soon as the situation may permit. Being introduced to the health professional and knowing his or her role is empowering for the woman (and support people/father). Speaking directly to the mother is imperative; a mother is not a slab of meat or an imbecile. Even if the woman is not vocally communicative, she is taking everything in and so eye-to-eye contact is normal. I could say so much more.

Prevalence of Elevated Posttraumatic Stress Symptoms

As can be seen in Table 2.1, the prevalence of women suffering with elevated posttraumatic stress symptoms ranges from 1.25% (Cigoli, Gilli, & Saita, 2006) to 41.2% (Anderson, 2010). Contributing to this wide range of prevalence rates are the varying times postpartum that women were assessed and the instruments used to measure posttraumatic stress symptoms. Ten different instruments were used in the studies included in Table 2.1. The time after birth when posttraumatic stress symptoms were assessed was as short as 72 hours to as long as six years postpartum. The sample with the highest prevalence was Latina adolescents in the US at 72 hours after birth (Anderson, 2010).

What is readily apparent from these studies in Table 2.1 is that posttraumatic stress secondary to traumatic childbirth is an international phenomenon. Studies took place in the US, Canada, the UK, Sweden, Australia, Italy, Switzerland, the Netherlands, Nigeria, and Israel. Ayers and Pickering (2001) was the only study that measured PTSD in pregnancy and then removed those women from their analysis after delivery. Their reported incidence rate was 2.8% at 6 weeks and 1.5% at 6 months.

In addition to assessing the level of mothers' posttraumatic stress symptoms, in Canada Verreault et al. (2012) interviewed women at 1, 3, and 6 months

Table 2.1 Prevalence of elevated posttraumatic stress symptoms

Study/country	Sample	Data collection	Instruments	Prevalence (%)
Menage (1993)/UK	102	Mean = 4.6 yr postpartum	PTSD-I	29
Wijma et al. (1997)/Sweden	1640	First 1 yr postpartum	TES	1.7
Ryding et al. (1998)/Sweden	326	2 days and 1 yr postpartum	IES	2.2–5.6
Creedy et al. (2000)/UK	499	4–6 wks postpartum	PSS-SR	5.6
Czarnocka & Slade (2000)/UK	264	6 wks postpartum	PTSD-I	3
Turton et al. (2001)/UK	66	1 yr postpartum	PTSD-I	20
Soet et al. (2003)/US	103	4 wks postpartum	TES	1.9
Cigoli et al. (2006)/Italy	160	3–6 mos postpartum	PTSD-Q	1.25
Maggioni et al. (2006)/Italy	93	3–6 mos postpartum	PTSD-Q	2.4
Onoye et al. (2009)/US	54	4–8 postpartum	TLEQ	21
Soderquist et al. (2006)/Sweden	1224	1–11 mos postpartum	TES	3
Adewuya et al. (2006)/Nigeria	876	6 wks postpartum	MINI	5.9
Zaers et al. (2008)/Switzerland	47	6 wks & 6 mos postpartum	PDS	6/14.9
Ayers et al. (2009)/UK	502 (community)	10 mos postpartum	PDS	2.5
	921 (Internet)	12 mos postpartum		21
Sawyer & Ayers (2009)/UK	219 (Internet)	Up to 36 mos postpartum (mean = 11 mos postpartum)	PDS	12.4
Anderson (2010)/US	85	72 hours postpartum	IES	41.2
Beck et al. (2011)/US	903	7–18 mos postpartum	PSS-SR	9
McDonald et al. (2011)/UK	81	2 yrs postpartum	IES	17.3
Stramrood et al. (2011)/the Netherlands	137	6 wks & 15 mos postpartum	PSS-SR	11 PE/17 PPROM
Polachek et al. (2012)/Israel	89	1 mos postpartum	PDS	25.9
Verreault et al. (2012)/Canada	308	1, 3, 6 mos postpartum	MPSS-SR	7.6, 6.1, 4

Notes: PTSD-I = PTSD Interview; TES = Traumatic Event Scale; IES = Impact of Event Scale; PSS-SR = Posttraumatic Stress Disorder Symptom Scale-Self Report; PTSD-Q = PTSD Questionnaire; TLEQ = Traumatic Life Events Questionnaire; MINI = Mini International Neuropsychiatric Interview; PDS = Posttraumatic Stress Diagnostic Scale; PE = preeclampsia; PPROM = preterm premature rupture of membranes; MPSS-SR = Modified PTSD Symptom Scale-Self Report.

postpartum using the Structured Clinical Interview for DSM-IV (SCIDS) in order to be able to diagnosis PTSD where the traumatizing event was childbirth (Table 2.2). Verreault and colleagues reported that at 1 month postpartum 1.1% (n = 3) and at 3 months postpartum, 0.8% (n = 2) of the Canadian sample met the diagnostic criteria for full PTSD. None of the women met these criteria at 6 months postpartum.

Mothers' Voices of Living with PTSD

Beck (2004b) examined mothers' experiences living with PTSD following childbirth. In this qualitative study 38 mothers participated from New Zealand, the United States, Australia, and the United Kingdom. Women sent their stories describing their PTSD due to their traumatic births via the Internet. Five themes captured the essential components of their PTSD.

Theme 1. *Going to the Movies, Please Don't Make Me Go*

Women described how they felt like in their minds a video tape was replaying nonstop of their traumatic births and it left loop tracks in their brains. Mothers had no control over this "video tape" or terrifying nightmares and flashbacks of their birth trauma. The following quote explains further this theme:

> My vaginal delivery resulted in severe physical damage to me i.e., birth injuries referred to as third world birth injuries, namely, pelvic floor injuries, urine incontinence, loss of part of my labia majora, and rectal sphincter damage leaving me with fecal incontinence. I had repair surgeries which will need redoing. My daughter was flat at delivery and was resuscitated. Her apgars were 2, 4, 4. Her head was very severely bruised and very swollen. She had a cut on the outer left eye which has left a scar. No matter how hard I try I cannot get these images to stop replaying over and over again in my mind.

Theme 2. *A Shadow of Myself: Too Numb to Try and Change*

Women frequently used the image of losing their souls during their labor and delivery. Nothing was left but an empty shell of their former selves. "Numbness" and "detachment" were words often used by women to describe their relationship with their infants, family, and friends.

Theme 3. *Seeking to Have Questions Answered and Wanting to Talk, Talk, Talk*

What had gone so wrong with their giving birth that left women with the feeling of just having been raped on the delivery table? Women were tenacious in their questioning of the persons who were present at their childbirth. What were the missing details of their labor and delivery that women could not completely remember? After a while the mothers painfully discovered that

Table 2.2 Diagnostic criteria for posttraumatic stress disorder

A. The person has been exposed to a traumatic event in which both of the following were present:
  (1) the person experienced, witnessed, or was confronted with an event or events that involved actual or threatened death or serious injury, or a threat to the physical integrity of self or others.
  (2) the person's response involved intense fear, helplessness, or horror

B. The traumatic event is persistently reexperienced in one (or more) of the following ways:
  (1) recurrent and intrusive distressing recollections of the event, including images, thoughts, or perceptions
  (2) recurrent distressing dreams of the event
  (3) acting or feeling as if the traumatic event were recurring (includes a sense of reliving the experience, illusions, hallucinations and dissociative flashback episodes, including those that occur on awakening or when intoxicated)
  (4) intense psychological distress at exposure to internal or external cues that symbolize or resemble an aspect of the traumatic event
  (5) physiological reactivity on exposure to internal or external cues that symbolize or resemble an aspect of the traumatic event

C. Persistent avoidance of stimuli associated with the trauma and numbing of general responsiveness (not present before the trauma), as indicated by three (or more) of the following:
  (1) efforts to avoid thoughts, feelings, or conversations associated with the trauma
  (2) efforts to avoid activities, places, or people that arouse recollections of the trauma
  (3) inability to recall an important aspect of the trauma
  (4) markedly diminished interest or participation in significant activities
  (5) feeling of detachment or estrangement from others
  (6) restricted range of affect
  (7) sense of a foreshortened future

D. Persistent symptoms of increased arousal (not present before the trauma), as indicated by two (or more) of the following:
  (1) difficulty falling or staying asleep
  (2) irritability or outbursts of anger
  (3) difficulty concentrating
  (4) hypervigilance
  (5) exaggerated startle response

E. Duration of the disturbance (symptoms in Criteria B, C, and D) is more than 1 month

F. The disturbance causes clinically significant distress or impairment in social, occupational, or other important areas of functioning.

Source: Reprinted with permission from American Psychiatric Association (2000, pp. 467–468).

clinicians and family were tired of listening to this. As one women shared whose traumatic birth involved the delivery of her twins:

> I was so devastated at people's lack of empathy. I told myself what a bad person I was for needing to talk. I felt like the ancient Mariner doomed to forever be plucking at people's sleeves and trying to tell them my story which they didn't want to hear.
>
> (Beck, 2004b, p. 221)

Theme 4: The Dangerous Trio of Anger, Anxiety, and Depression: Spiraling Downward

Mothers lived on a daily basis filled with these distressing emotions. There was no room left for any positive emotions. Women felt like a volcano filled with anger ready to explode. Anger regarding their birth trauma was directed at clinicians, their family members who were present at the birth, and the women themselves for allowing the trauma to occur. This mother provided a glimpse of an insider's view of her anger:

> Powerful seething anger would overwhelm me without warning. To manage it I would go still and quiet, then eventually "come to", realizing that one or all of the children were crying and I had no idea for how long!
>
> (Beck, 2004b, p. 221)

Women's heightened level of anxiety often escalated to panic attacks. Struggling to survive their PTSD while trying to cope with the constant demands of new motherhood led some mothers to a severe enough depression that they started to consider ending their own lives to end their living nightmare.

Theme 5: Isolation from the World of Motherhood: Dreams Shattered

This is a very disturbing theme which has significant implications for not only mother–infant bonding but also infant cognitive and emotional development. Anyone with PTSD, no matter what the traumatic event, tries to avoid triggers of the traumatic event to prevent terrifying flashbacks. For women whose traumatic event was childbirth, their infants are constant reminders of their birth trauma. Much to the distress of mothers, their PTSD did result in distancing themselves from their children. An example from one mother whose child is now three years old vividly brings home this point:

> My child turned 3 years old a few weeks ago. I suppose the pain was not so acute this time. I actually made him a birthday cake and was grateful that I could go to work and not think about the significance of the day. The pain was less, but it was replaced by a numbness that still worries me. I hope that as time passes I can forge some kind of real closeness with this child. I am still unable to tell him I love him, but I can now hold him and have times when I am proud of him. I have come a long, long way.
>
> (Beck, 2004b, p. 222)

Women's thoughts and emotions during traumatic birth were explored by Ayers (2007) with 25 mothers with posttraumatic stress symptoms and 25 mothers without such symptoms. Women with posttraumatic stress symptoms experienced more mental defeat, thoughts of death, and dissociation during labor and delivery than women with no symptoms. Following birth, compared to mothers with no symptoms, women with posttraumatic stress symptoms reported experiencing more painful and intrusive memories and rumination regarding their labor and delivery. More negative emotions such as pain, anger, aggression, annoyance, and irritability were experienced in women with posttraumatic stress symptoms.

Nicholls and Ayers (2007) in the UK examined the effect of childbirth-related posttraumatic stress disorder in six couples. Women and their partners were interviewed separately. Analysis revealed four themes. Birth factors, the first theme, included pain and inadequate pain relief; negative emotions in labor such as feeling helpless, humiliated, violated, and dehumanized; perceived lack of control; lack of choice or involvement in decision-making, and unmet expectations. The second theme of quality of care involved poor communication on the part of clinicians; negative staff attitudes such as disparaging comments; lack of continuity of care, and an unpleasant physical environment of lack of privacy and poor hygiene. The third theme focused on perceived effects on the relationship with their partners. Traumatic birth affected their physical relationship, mainly avoidance of sex. Their communication with each other was also impacted as couples avoided discussing the birth. Negative emotions within the relationship were maintained, such as women feeling abandoned by their partners and men feeling rejected by their partners. The perceived effect of the traumatic birth on their relationship with their child was the fourth theme. Parents recognized their poor bonds with their child and tried to compensate for this by different bonding styles. The two main bonding styles were overprotective/anxious bonds and avoidance/rejecting bonds.

Posttraumatic Growth

Researchers have paid much less attention to the possibility that traumatic events can lead to some positive outcomes. Tedeschi, Park, and Calhoun (1998) defined posttraumatic growth as a positive change in a person's beliefs or ability to function due to struggling with an extremely challenging life event. These positive outcomes can occur in a person's relationships with others, their self-perception, and their philosophy of life (Tedeschi & Calhoun, 1995). In order to begin to measure these positive outcomes to traumatic events, Tedeschi and Calhoun (1996) developed the Posttraumatic Growth Inventory (PTGI). This is a self-report scale, consisting of 21 items which measure five factors: new possibilities, relating to others, personal strength, spiritual change, and appreciation of life. Respondents indicate the degree of change that occurred in their lives as a result of a crisis using the following Likert response range from $0 =$ no change to $4 =$ great degree.

To date, two studies have been located that assessed posttraumatic growth in women after traumatic childbirth using the PTGI in the UK. Sawyer and Ayers (2009) assessed posttraumatic growth and also posttraumatic stress which was measured using the Posttraumatic Stress Diagnostic Scale (Foa, Cashman, Jaycox, & Perry, 1997). Their Internet sample consisted of 219 women who had given birth within the past 36 months. The average time since birth and when the mothers completed the questionnaires was 11 months. Fifty percent of the sample reported at least a moderate amount of positive change after childbirth. Age was the only demographic variable that was significantly associated with posttraumatic growth ($r = -.21$). Younger women reported more posttraumatic growth. In the sample, 37% of the mothers fulfilled the PTSD stressor criterion A (see Table 2.2) and 12% met all the criteria for diagnosis of PTSD secondary to childbirth. No significant relationships were found between posttraumatic growth and posttraumatic stress symptoms. Women endorsed the appreciation of life factor on the PTGI most frequently.

Using a prospective, longitudinal design, 125 women were followed from their third trimester of pregnancy through 8 weeks postpartum (Sawyer, Ayers, Young, Bradley, & Smith, 2012). These mothers completed the Impact of Event Scale-Revised (Weiss & Marmar, 1997) during pregnancy and the PTGI (Tedeschi & Calhoun, 1996) and the Posttraumatic Stress Disorder Symptom Scale-Self Report (Foa, Riggs, Dancu, & Rothbaum, 1993) after birth. A total of 23% of the mothers fulfilled the PTSD stressor criterion A. In this sample, 48% of the women reported at least a small amount of posttraumatic growth. Appreciation of life was the factor on the PTGI that mothers endorsed most often. As in Sawyer and Ayers' (2009) study, age was the only demographic variable significantly related to posttraumatic growth ($r = -.24$). Again younger women experienced more posttraumatic growth. Posttraumatic stress symptoms related to childbirth were not related to posttraumatic growth. Analysis of the data revealed that the strongest predictors of posttraumatic growth after birth were operative delivery and posttraumatic stress symptoms in pregnancy.

Conclusion

In this chapter a review of published research on birth trauma and its resulting posttraumatic stress disorder and posttraumatic growth has been described to lay a foundation for the rest of the book. In Chapter 3, Jeanne describes a general case study of traumatic childbirth and PTSD secondary to birth trauma from her own clinical practice.

References

Adewuya, A. O., Ologun, Y. A., & Ibigbami, O. S. (2006). Post-traumatic stress disorder after childbirth in Nigerian women: Prevalence and risk factors. *BJOG, 113,* 284–288.

Alcorn, K. L., O'Donovan, A., Patrick, J. C., Creedy, D., & Devilly, G. J. (2010). A prospective longitudinal study of the prevalence of post-traumatic stress disorder resulting from childbirth events. *Psychological Medicine, 40,* 1849–1859.

American Psychiatric Association (2000). *Diagnostic and statistical manual of mental disorders.* Washington, DC: American Psychiatric Association.

Anderson, C. (2010). Impact of traumatic birth experience on Latina adolescent mothers. *Issues in Mental Health Nursing, 31,* 700–707.

Ayers, S. (2007). Thoughts and emotions during traumatic birth: A qualitative study. *Birth, 34,* 253–263.

Ayers, S., & Pickering, A. (2001). Do women get posttraumatic stress disorder as a result of childbirth? A prospective study of incidence. *Birth, 28,* 111–118.

Ayers, S., Harris, R., Sawyer, A., Parfitt, Y., & Ford, E. (2009). Post-traumatic stress disorder after childbirth: Analysis of symptom presentation and sampling. *Journal of Affective Disorders, 119,* 200–204.

Beck, C. T. (2004a). Birth trauma: In the eye of the beholder. *Nursing Research, 53,* 28–35.

—— (2004b). PTSD due to childbirth: The aftermath. *Nursing Research, 53,* 216–224.

—— (2011). A meta-ethnography of traumatic childbirth and its aftermath: Amplifying causal looping. *Qualitative Health Research, 21,* 301–311.

Beck, C. T., Gable, R. K., Sakala, C., & Declercq, E. R. (2011). Posttraumatic stress disorder in new mothers: Results from a two-stage U.S. national survey. *Birth, 38,* 216–227.

Cigoli, V., Gilli, G., & Saita, E. (2006). Relational factors in psychopathological responses to childbirth. *Journal of Psychosomatic Obstetrics & Gynaecology, 27,* 91–97.

Creedy, D. K., Shochet, I. M., & Horsfall, J. (2000). Childbirth and the development of acute trauma symptoms: Incidence and contributing factors. *Birth, 27,* 104–111.

Czarnocka, J., & Slade, P. (2000). Prevalence and predictors of posttraumatic stress symptoms following childbirth. *British Journal of Clinical Psychology, 39,* 35–51.

Elmir, R., Schmied, V., Wilkes, L., & Jackson, D. (2010). Women's perceptions and experiences of a traumatic birth: A meta-ethnography. *Journal of Advanced Nursing, 66,* 2142–2153.

Foa, E., Cashman, L., Jaycox, L., & Perry, K. (1997). The validation of a self-report measure of posttraumatic stress disorder: The Posttraumatic Stress Diagnostic Scale. *Psychological Assessment, 9,* 445–451.

Foa, E., Riggs, D. S., Dancu, C. V., & Rothbaum, B. O. (1993). Reliability and validity of a brief instrument for assessing post-traumatic stress disorder. *Journal of Traumatic Stress, 6,* 459–473.

Glaser, B. G. (2005). *The grounded theory perspective III: Theoretical coding.* Mill Valley, CA: Sociology Press.

Hungerford, M. W. (1878). *Molly Bawn.* London: Smith, Elder, and Company.

Maggioni, C., Margola, D., & Filippi, F. (2006). PTSD, risk factors, and expectations among women having a baby: A two-wave longitudinal study. *Journal of Psychosomatic Obstetrics and Gynaecology, 27,* 81–90.

McDonald, S., Slade, P., Spiby, H., & Iles, J. (2011). Post-traumatic stress symptoms, parenting stress and mother–child relationships following childbirth and at 2 years postpartum. *Journal of Psychosomatic Obstetrics & Gynecology, 32,* 141–146.

Menage, J. (1993). Post-traumatic stress disorder in women who have undergone obstetric or gynecological procedures. *Journal of Reproductive Infant Psychology, 11,* 221–228.

Nicholls, K., & Ayers, S. (2007). Childbirth related post-traumatic stress disorder in couples: A qualitative study. *British Journal of Health Psychology, 12,* 490–509.

Noblit, G. W., & Hare, R. D. (1988). *Meta-ethnography: Synthesizing qualitative studies.* Newbury Park, CA: Sage Publications.

Onoye, J.M., Goebert, D., Morland, L., Matsu, C., & Wright, T. (2009). PTSD and postpartum mental health in a sample of Caucasian, Asian, and Pacific Islander women. *Archives of Women's Mental Health, 12,* 393–400.

Polachek, I. S., Harari, L. H., Baum, M., & Strous, R. D. (2012). Postpartum post-traumatic stress disorder symptoms: The uninvited birth companion. *Israeli Medical Association Journal*, *14*, 347–353.

Ryding, E. L., Wijma, B., & Wijma, K. (1998). Experiences of emergency cesarean section: A phenomenological study of 53 women. *Birth*, *25*, 246–251.

Sawyer, A., & Ayers, S. (2009). Posttraumatic growth in women after childbirth. *Psychology and Health*, *24*, 457–471.

Sawyer, A., Ayers, S., Young, D., Bradley, R., & Smith, H. (2012). Posttraumatic growth after childbirth: A prospective study. *Psychology and Health*, *27*, 362–377.

Sheehan, D. V., Lecrubier, Y., Harnett-Sheehan, K., Amorim, P., Janavs, J., Weiller, E., et al. (1998). The Mini International Neuropsychiatric Interview (M.I.N.I.): The development and validation of a structured diagnostic psychiatric interview. *Journal of Clinical Psychiatry*, *59*, (Suppl. 20), 22–33.

Soderquist, J., Wijma, B., & Wijma, K. (2006). The longitudinal course of post-traumatic stress after childbirth. *Journal of Psychosomatic Obstetrics and Gynaecology*, *27*, 113–119.

Soet, J.E., Brack, G.A., & Dilorio, C. (2003). Prevalence and predictors of women's experience of psychological trauma during childbirth. *Birth*, *30*, 36–46.

Stramrood, C. A., Wessel, I., Doornbos, B., Aarnoudse, J. G., van der Berg, P. P., Weijmar Schultz, W. C., & van Pampus, M. G. (2011). Posttraumatic stress disorder following preeclampsia and PPROM: A prospective study with 15 months follow-up. *Reproductive Sciences*, *18*, 645–653.

Tedeschi, R., & Calhoun, L. (1995). *Trauma and transformation: Growing in the aftermath of suffering*. Thousand Oaks, CA: Sage Publications.

—— (1996). The Posttraumatic Growth Inventory: Measuring the positive legacy of trauma. *Journal of Traumatic Stress*, *9*, 455–472.

Tedeschi, R., Park, C., & Calhoun, L. (1998). *Posttraumatic growth: Positive changes in the aftermath of crisis*. Mahwah, NJ: Erlbaum.

Thomson, G., & Downe, S. (2008). Widening the trauma discourse: The link between childbirth and experiences of abuse. *Journal of Psychosomatic Obstetrics and Gynaecology*, *29*, 268–273.

Turton, P., Hughes, P., Evans, C. D., & Fainman, D. (2001). Incidence, correlates and predictors of post-traumatic stress disorder in the pregnancy after stillbirth. *British Journal of Psychiatry*, *178*, 556–560.

Verreault, N., DaCosta, D., Marchand, A., Ireland, K., Banack, H., Dritsa, M., & Khalife, S. (2012). PTSD following childbirth: A prospective study of incidence and risk factors in Canadian women. *Journal of Psychosomatic Research*, *73*, 257–263.

Weathers, F. W., & Litz, B. T. (1994). Psychometric properties of the Clinician-Administered PTSD Scale, CAPS-1. *Archives of Women's Mental Health*, *5*, 2–6.

Weiss, D. S., & Marmar, C. R. (1997). The Impact of Event Scale-Revised. In J. P. Wilson, & T. M. Keane (Eds.). *Assessing psychological trauma and PTSD: A handbook for practitioners* (pp. 399–411). New York: Guilford.

Wijma, K., Soderquist, M. A., & Wijma, B. (1997). Posttraumatic stress disorder after childbirth: A cross sectional study. *Journal of Anxiety Disorders*, *11*, 587–597.

Zaers, S., Waschke, M., & Ehlert, U. (2008). Depressive symptoms and symptoms of posttraumatic stress disorder in women after childbirth. *Journal of Psychosomatic Obstetrics and Gynaecology*, *29*, 61–71.

3 Jeanne's Introduction to Posttraumatic Stress Disorder Secondary to Birth Trauma

About 30 years ago, it was an eye-opening experience for me when I met a woman in my private practice whose symptom presentation led me to formulate the posttraumatic stress disorder secondary to birth trauma, not sexual, physical or emotional abuse. The symptoms the woman shared with me at the time could only fit into that diagnostic criteria, yet I had never heard of PTSD secondary to a birth experience.

In the late 1970s and early 1980s, the focus of the childbirth movement was on "natural childbirth" and father attendance at birth. There was what appeared to me significant focus on the pregnant women feeling empowered and knowledgeable regarding birthing her baby. The trend in obstetrics was to involve the woman and her partner in the "natural and normal" process of birthing a baby. Over the past 30 years, however, there has been a significant increase in the use of technology in the "normal birth experience": the use of fetal ultrasound, fetal monitoring, dopplers have replaced fetascopes, vacuum extraction versus forceps use, and epidural anesthesia for labor experiences. Has this move toward technological assisted birth experiences altered the interpersonal aspects of pregnancy, labor and delivery? Has this increase encouraged the perceived traumatic experience of women regarding their birth experience or is it just that as a society we are acknowledging issues that affect women's mental health? We do have a somewhat increased awareness of pregnancy and postpartum mood and anxiety disorders being diagnosed and treated at a higher frequency over the past years. However, has the increased use of technology in the pregnancy and birth experience taken away the personal interactions, the basic need for human interaction and care and concern? We may not have that answer for a long time but what is very clear is that we have an increase in the diagnosis of posttraumatic stress disorders related to birth trauma and women's postpartum and parenting experiences are being impacted by this increasing trend. As I said, it was over 30 years ago that I "formally" diagnosed a woman in my private practice with posttraumatic stress disorder secondary to birth experience. The following is a narrative of that case study presented from my memory and some help from the old chart; the woman's name and any identifying information have been changed to protect her privacy.

Mrs. Robins left a voice-mail message describing that she had been having "horrific nightmares" and was "extremely anxious." She was contemplating a second pregnancy. She had a 2-year-old, but she was having a difficult time and needed some help. I returned her call and we set up an appointment for an evaluation and consultation meeting at my office for the next week. My private practice was then and continues today to be exclusive to the psychiatric care (psychotherapy and pharmacotherapy) of women experiencing mood and anxiety disorders through the childbearing years. This woman's case still clearly stays in my memory and it was long before Cheryl had met Sue Watson and begun her research journey of exploring the phenomenon of posttraumatic stress disorder secondary to birth trauma. This woman taught me so much about the impact of experience upon the brain and embedded memories; I will never forget her and the honor of working with her on her healing journey.

When I met Mrs. Robins, she was a petite, neatly dressed woman, in her early thirties. Married with a 2-year-old son, she was a stay-at-home mother and shared with me, "my life is good, so I am not sure why this is happening."

She had been referred to me by her friend who had heard me speak on postpartum depression (PPD) at a professional meeting and her friend had thought that she might have PPD. Mrs. Robins could not understand that connection in that she was two years postpartum but "I did have a horrible birth experience and the early weeks after my son was born were just awful, I thought all that was behind me." She sat across from me and shyly began to tell me her story.

She and her husband had recently begun to talk about having another baby, and

> almost immediately I felt like I was going to jump out of my skin. I started to shake and felt like I was going to throw up. My husband got scared and told me we didn't have to have any more children if it made me feel like that just beginning the conversation . . . I had no idea what came over me.

She went on to describe that since that discussion with her husband she had experienced "a lot of anxiety and nightmares." I asked her to describe the nightmares if she could remember them. She proceeded to tell me that the dream was repetitive. She is "lying on a table and I see a table saw coming up onto my belly from between my legs and I wake up with a startle, shaking and sweating, I wake my husband and he just holds me while I sob." This dream is recurrent about two to three times per week. "I do not understand what is happening to me. My life is good. I love my husband and son. I have a great life, and it is so scary."

I remember feeling a bit unsure myself as to what was going on so I proceeded with the evaluation. This was before the development of the Earthquake Assessment Model that Deborah Sichel and I evolved based on our clinical practice in 1999 (Sichel & Driscoll, 1999).

Mrs. Robins described that both her parents were alive and did not have any significant issues with mood and/or anxiety issues. "My mom can get a little anxious but she talks about it and can calm herself down. She does not take any medication." Her siblings, one brother and one sister, did not have any mood and/or anxiety histories that she knew of.

> I am sure they would tell me if they did. They have been very supportive to me over the past few weeks, fortunately, they live nearby and are able to come over and help me when I am really feeling like I am a mess and my husband is not around. I am so afraid that this can hurt my son, my anxiety, you know.

Mrs. Robins had had what she described as a "normal" childhood, nothing significant that she could remember. She had grown up in the same house, had good experiences in school, still had friends from high school that she felt very connected to and close to. "A few of us have children the same age so we get together as families." Her life history seemed uneventful; she denied any history of sexual, physical and/or emotional abuse. She again restated "I was fine until the past few weeks since we have begun to think about having another baby."

Mrs. Robins had her first period when she was 12 years old and did not recall any problems with headaches, stomach aches, anxiety, irritability, nor sleep pattern changes with her menstrual cycle. She informed me that she had been on oral contraceptives for about five years prior to conceiving her son and had not gone back on them after his birth. "We have been using condoms. I didn't want to mess with my hormones as I knew that we wanted more children." She denied any mood changes or physical problems with taking the pill. She and her husband had planned their first pregnancy. "I had gone off the pill for about four months before we really actively began to try to conceive. It took about 4 months after that so it was about 8 months after I stopped the pill."

Mrs. Robins' pregnancy was welcome and described as uneventful. She was working as an administrative assistant for a local school and did not remember missing any work. She described that she just remembered "feeling excited that I was pregnant. We were so ready to have a baby." She described some nausea, mostly early evening, "lots of fatigue. I wanted to sleep all the time in the first trimester." As she moved into the second trimester, she felt physically better and was thrilled once she started feeling the baby move. "We did not know the sex of our son until he was born, so I would just talk to the baby all the time and loved feeling the movements." The third trimester went along smoothly, according to her description. "We attended childbirth classes at the hospital, and we were prepared and excited." She then began to describe, what I considered at that time, a most violent birth experience followed by significant traumatic experiences.

When she was about 39 weeks pregnant, she woke in the middle of the night with a major contraction. She remembers waking up, going to the bathroom and just getting excited. I was so ready to have the baby. I labored until the early morning hours. My husband was timing the contractions which continued after that abrupt wakening. I was able to breathe through them and we were doing well at home so I did not rush to call the doctor.

It was about nine in the morning that she started to feel "really uncomfortable, so I called the doctor and was told to head over to the hospital. It was only about 15 minutes away so I wasn't worried about not getting there in time." She describes that when they got to the hospital she was about 4 centimeters dilated and her membranes were intact. She and her husband walked around the labor floor, found the breathing techniques helpful and felt things were moving along as they had been told would happen. After about 12 hours since she had woken up abruptly with that first contraction, it was noted that the baby's heart rate was dropping significantly during contractions.

The nurses said there was nothing to worry about as long as the rate returned to baseline and that they would keep watching . . . a few minutes later though, all hell broke loose. I didn't know what was wrong. They kept telling me to roll over on my left side and put the oxygen mask on my face and then they said that they had to take the baby and the next thing I know I was being rushed to the operating room for a c-section. I have no idea where my husband went. All I remember is thinking my baby was going to die and I had no idea what I would do.

She recalled the ride on the bed from the labor room to the transfer to the operating table and the anesthesiologist coming to her head. She still did not know where her husband was, "but it was very crazy in there, they were rushing around to get me ready for the operation." At this point, in front of my eyes, Mrs. Robins' breathing began to change. She pulled herself up into a small ball. Her hands were in fists and her whole demeanor changed.

I felt this severe burning, pressure and excruciating pain to my abdomen and then nothing. When I woke up, all I remember is that I had such pain and I wasn't sure what happened to my baby. I just started crying and then my husband told me the baby was a boy and he was fine that everything was alright . . . I remember just crying and feeling like I couldn't stop shaking. Everyone told me that that was normal and that everything was okay but I didn't feel like everything was okay at all. I told them that I remembered feeling a searing pain and that I was panicked regarding pain. The doctor told me that I couldn't have felt anything because of the general anesthesia and that they gave me something that also causes amnesia. I didn't understand and they kept telling me that I could not have felt anything, yet why did I have this intense memory of that searing pain? Where did that come from?

She then began to sob as she continued to be rolled up on the couch.

I sat quietly in my chair and my mind was spinning, primarily with my own frustration that too often health care providers dismiss patients' feelings and emotions if they don't fit into the providers' scope of reality, and how she could indeed begin to feel like she was crazy if all of these "professionals" were telling her that she didn't feel the incision. I was reminded of how often women are silenced from their experience and set up to doubt what they are feeling (Jordan, Kaplan, Miller, Stiver & Surrey, 1991; Jack, 1991; Jordan, 1997). I wanted to hear more of her story and provide a safe environment for her to be heard and held in her memories and her realities. I validated her memories, using reassurance and empathic connection. I shared with her that what she remembered was indeed her reality and that it must have been so hard for her to have that experience. It was interesting that as Cheryl analyzed the data from her first qualitative study she used the quote "beauty is in the eye of the beholder" as a segue to the concept of perceptive reality and women's birth experiences in 2004 and I met Mrs. Robins in 1982.

I know that we each perceive our own reality based on our history and our past. I wanted to hear more about her experience. I did not, however, want to do anything to further traumatize her so I stayed quiet and let her cry on the couch. I had some sense of the "why now?" to her symptom presentation: as she began to consider another pregnancy she was triggered to the experience of the past which as she described was not validated by others when she was going through it.

Mrs. Robins continued her story:

> Postpartum was very hard for me. I felt as though I had had an out-of-body experience and in many ways I thought I was crazy. Everyone in the hospital told me I could not have felt anything and that the baby was fine and so was I. So what was wrong with me?

She described feeling invalidated in her truth and that no one really wanted to just listen. "They all told me I would be fine when I got home to my own house and focused on taking care of my incision and my baby." So after a while, she felt she just put it all away, inside her mind, and moved on with the work of postpartum: recovering from the labor and delivery experience, the cesarean incision, and learning to become a mother to her son.

> I was very tired postpartum and cried if you looked at me cross-eyed. Fortunately, my husband is a fantastic man and he took excellent care of me and our son. My mom and dad were available whenever I needed them as were my sibs. I had all the help in the world but there was this low grade sadness/depression that I felt. I began to believe everyone else that I didn't feel the incision and it was just my imagination and my fear.

She went on to describe that eventually, "time heals all wounds" and she moved on to being a stay-at-home Mom who absolutely loved caring for her son and her husband. However, when the idea of having another baby became a reality, her embedded memories of the first birth experience began to surge and her body, which remembers everything, began to want to be heard. The thought of having another baby was a trigger to the resurgence of the feelings and she was re-traumatized.

Mrs. Robins shared with me that she remembered that she had spoken with her obstetrician after the birth about her feelings and that her doctor told her that she was given some medicine with the general anesthesia that caused amnesia, so they had no idea how she could remember what the incision felt like. Again she describes feeling "not heard," and getting the sense that he knew better than her and that she had best move on. Perhaps this is what Miller and Stiver mean by the "central relational paradox" that women have described, when the relationship is more important than what they are feeling (Miller and Stiver, 1997, p. 155). Mrs. Robins was in a situation where she, in essence, denied her own reality, and believed that someone else knew better.

As was previously stated, it was the discussion of the potential of another baby that triggered the reaction of panic, anxiety, nightmares and other physical symptoms. She began having the recurrent nightmare, "I feel as though I am on a table and a huge table saw is coming at me, I am screaming but no one shuts it off." She felt as though this altered sleep had affected her activities of daily living, "I just feel nervous, like something bad is going to happen. It is that 'what if worst scenario' that keeps playing in my brain." This led to further assessment of her mental and physical status. She described that her nutrition was good and that she exercised regularly. "I have a 2-year-old who loves to run." She also used the treadmill regularly in addition to chasing after a 2-year-old. She did feel that her sleep had significantly been affected by the recurrent nightmare. "I am a bit afraid to go to sleep. It is such a horrific dream and I just don't want to be in that sleep state." She continued to describe that she felt "down" at times and has been telling herself to "just shake it off . . . my husband told me that he is fine with one child if this is going to happen to me . . . he is scared . . . I can tell, as am I. I really want to have more than one child but I am not sure I can handle this if it keeps on."

I validated Mrs. Robins' experience, helping her to understand that what she felt was indeed her truth and that she had a right to those thoughts and feelings. I apologized to her for her experience of not feeling heard by the people she had put her trust into, her health care providers. We talked about how each person sees the world through their own lenses and how sometimes people tend to automatically believe that what they see is the truth, although the reality is really somewhere in between what we each see and experience. We spoke about what might help in the immediate future, which was to help to calm the anxiety feelings, get her to sleep through the night again without waking with panic and terror. When her biology was a bit quieter, we could begin the work of planning strategies to help her with the decision-making regarding another pregnancy.

I felt that Mrs. Robins' immediate physiological need was to get her to sleep solidly through the night to allow her brain to replenish itself physiologically. So we went over a basic nursing care plan. Our goals were to promote restful sleep and then process the birth experience in a more controlled way. We discussed sleep hygiene aspects of regular bedtimes and went over the environment in her bedroom. She did not have a television in her bedroom and did not use any form of ambient noise to help her sleep. She was familiar with breathing strategies as she had taken childbirth classes and we went over the key one "cleansing breath followed by regular inhalations and exhalations." We discussed the short-term use of a long-acting benzodiazepine, clonazepam, to help quiet the anxiety/panic and perhaps help her to sleep uninterrupted. We went over her nutrition, exercise, and our continued work together to process the birth experience and work on the new experience of planning, conceiving and birthing the second child. I gave her a prescription for low dose clonazepam (0.25–0.50 mg.) at bedtime, as needed. She was encouraged to keep a journal of whatever came into her mind as a method of moving the emotional material out of her brain and onto the paper. We set up an appointment for the next week.

When I met with Mrs. Robins a week later, she described that she had been feeling better. She had used the clonazepam at bedtime and that helped her sleep all night with no nightmares or night waking. We continued to process the memories of the birth experience and began to strategize ways for her to feel empowered and to have a "voice" in her next birth experience. Over the weeks, she described that she felt less anxious; she decided that she wanted to secure a new team of health care providers and birth at a different hospital setting as she felt going back to where her son was born would be too stressful. We developed a list of questions to ask the new members of her team and practiced responses so that she felt authentic in the relationship and felt that she was in charge. She made appointments and interviewed obstetricians, sharing her story with them and, in the end, pulled together a team that felt supportive and nurturing to her. Happily she conceived her second baby a few months after we began meeting. Her pregnancy was uneventful; we continued our sessions every other week during her pregnancy. She had stopped the clonazepam prior to pregnancy as she felt that she did not need it anymore. "I feel so much more in control now."

Mrs. Robins had a planned caesarean birth with her second child with a spinal anesthesia. She chose this birth method so that she had more control and felt it would give her less worry to have a birth plan that she was part of. She met with the anesthesiologist, shared her story of her first birth and described that the anesthesiologist was supportive and played an active role in providing emotional support to her during the whole birth experience. She had a baby boy and her postpartum experience was normal and balanced. We terminated our relationship about one year postpartum.

It was that experience, 30 years ago, that set the stage for my expansion of the mental/emotional responses to childbirth for women. In the early 1980s, there was a surge of articles regarding "repressed memories" of sexual abuse/trauma and whether they were real or imagined, as well as more being published regarding PTSD. Most of the literature was about the memories of victims of childhood sexual abuse.

Mrs. Robins' story did not include a history of sexual trauma but her experience of birth trauma precipitated similar symptoms and presentation as the PTSD from abuse and war. Her experience left an indelible mark on her life, her memory and her body. Fortunately, she was able to have a corrective experience and process events in an integrated, healing manner.

References

Jack, D. C. (1991). *Silencing the self: Women and depression.* Cambridge, MA: Harvard University Press.

Jordan, J. V. (Ed.). (1997). *Women's growth in diversity: More writings from the Stone Center.* New York: Guilford Press.

Jordan, J. V., Kaplan, A. G., Miller, J. B., Stiver, I. P., & Surrey, J. L. (1991). *Women's growth in connection: Writings from the Stone Center.* New York: Guilford Press.

Miller, J. B. & Stiver, I. P. (1997). *The healing connection: How women form relationships in therapy and in life.* Boston: Beacon Press.

Sichel, D. & Driscoll, J. W. (1999). *Women's moods.* New York: HarperCollins.

4 Review of Literature on Risk Factors for Postpartum Posttraumatic Stress Response

Research investigating risk factors for posttraumatic stress response in new mothers due to childbirth is the focus of this chapter. This research is categorized into two time periods: prenatal (Table 4.1) and intrapartum (Table 4.2). As can be seen in these tables, elevated posttraumatic stress response in new mothers is an international phenomenon. Countries represented include the United States (USA), Canada, the United Kingdom (UK), Australia, Sweden, Italy, Germany, the Netherlands, Nigeria, Switzerland, and Israel.

Prenatal Risk Factors

As one reflects on Table 4.1, what becomes clear is that it is our most fragile and vulnerable women who are at most risk of perceiving their labor and delivery as so traumatic as to lead to elevated posttraumatic stress symptoms. In the research to date, what is being confirmed is that prenatal depression, prenatal anxiety, prenatal PTSD, a history of psychiatric problems, and prior trauma, especially childhood sexual abuse, are the leading predictors of posttraumatic stress response following childbirth.

Demographic variables have not been found to date to be in the forefront as significant predictors of posttraumatic stress response due to childbirth. Socioeconomic status is the one demographic characteristic reported to be a risk factor; however, these studies found opposite findings. Lyons (1998) in the UK reported that pregnant women with low socioeconomic status were at risk, but in Canada Cohen et al. (2004) reported that higher income was the predictor of posttraumatic stress after childbirth. Having your first baby was found in two studies to be a predictor. One study was conducted in Italy (Cigoli et al., 2006) and one in Sweden (Wijma et al., 1997).

History of Psychiatric Problems

Having a history of psychological problems is a definite risk factor for development of posttraumatic stress response to childbirth. In Italy, Cigoli et al. (2006) and Stramrood, Paarlberg et al. (2011) and Stramrood, Wessel et al. (2011) in the Netherlands reported that a history of depression was a significant

Table 4.1 Prenatal risk factors for posttraumatic stress symptoms after childbirth

Study/country	Sample	Data collection	Instruments	Prevalence (%)	Risk factors
Wijma et al. (1997)/Sweden	1640	First 12 mos postpartum	TES	1.70	History of psychiatric counseling. Negative cognitive appraisal of post delivery, Primigravida
Lyons (1998)/UK	42	1 mos postpartum	IES		Low socioeconomic status
Czarnocka & Slade (2000)/UK	264	6 wks postpartum	PTSD-I	3	History of mental health difficulties Trait anxiety
Turton et al. (2001)/UK	66 previous pregnancies ended in stillbirth	1 yr postpartum	PTSD-I	20	Pregnancy after stillbirth
Keogh et al. (2002)/UK	40	36 weeks postpartum 2 wks postpartum	IES		Prenatal anxiety, depressive symptoms
Soet et al. (2003)/US	103	4 wks postpartum	TES	1.9	Sexual trauma history Trait anxiety, Low social support during pregnancy
Cohen et al. (2004)/Canada	200	8–10 wks postpartum	DTS		Prenatal depression Prior traumatic life events Higher income
Cigoli et al. (2006)/Italy	160	3–6 mos postpartum	PTSD-Q	1.25	Primigravida, History of psychiatric problems
Maggioni et al. (2006)/Italy Soderquist et al. (2006)/Sweden Feirbrother & Woody (2007)/Canada	93 1224 127	3–6 mos postpartum 1–11 mos postpartum	PTSD-Q TES PSS-SR	2.4 3	Prenatal depression
Zaers et al. (2008)/Switzerland	47	6 wks and 6 mos postpartum	PDS	6, 14.9	Anxiety/psychiatric symptoms late pregnancy

Table 4.1 (Continued)

Study/country	Sample	Data collection	Instruments	Prevalence (%)	Risk factors
Lev-Wiesel et al. (2009)/Israel	837	Midpregnancy, 2 and 6 mos postpartum	PSS-I		Childhood sexual abuse
Onoye et al. (2009)/US	54	4–8 wks postpartum	TLEQ PSS-I	21	Prenatal PTSD
Lev-Wiesel et al. (2009)/Israel	1071 Jewish	Midpregnancy, 1 and 6 mos postpartum	TEQ		Prenatal posttraumatic stress Prenatal depression
Ayers et al. (2009)/UK	502 community sample 921 Internet sample	10 mos postpartum	PDS	2.5	Sexual trauma
Lev-Wiesel & Daphna-Tekoah (2010)/Israel	1003 Jewish women	12 mos postpartum 18–24 wks pregnant and 2 mos postpartum	PSS–SR TEQ	21 9	Primipara Childhood sexual abuse Prenatal PTSD Prenatal depression
Beck et al. (2011)/US	903	7–18 mos postpartum	PSS–SR	9	Unplanned pregnancy No private health insurance
Stramrood, Paarlberg et al. (2011)/ The Netherlands	428	2–6 mos postpartum	TES	1.2	History of depression
Stramrood, Wessel et al. (2011)/ The Netherlands	137 PE or PROM	Pregnancy, 6 wks and 15 mos postpartum	PSS–SR	11 PE 17 PROM	History of depression Prenatal depression Previous traumatic birth History of psychiatric treatment Fear of childbirth
Polacheck et al. (2012)/Israel	89	1 mos postpartum	PDS	25.9	
Verreault et al. (2012)/Canada	308	24–40 wks gestation, 1, 3, & 6 mos postpartum	MPSS-SR	4.9–7.6	Sexual trauma history Anxiety sensitivity

Notes:
PTSD-I = PTSD Interview; TES = Traumatic Event Scale; IES = Impact of Event Scale; DTS = Davidson Trauma Scale; PSS-SR = Posttraumatic Stress Disorder Symptom Scale-Self Report; PTSD-Q = PTSD Questionnaire; TLEQ = Traumatic Life Events Questionnaire; PDS = Posttraumatic Stress Diagnostic Scale; PSS-I = Posttraumatic Stress Disorder Symptom Scale Interview; TEQ = Trauma Events Questionnaire; PE = preeclampsia; PPROM = preterm premature rupture of membranes; MPSS-SR = Modified PTSD Symptom Scale-Self Report.

risk factor for women to develop a posttraumatic stress response to childbirth. In Sweden, previous psychological problems also were pre-birth predictors of women going on to report experiencing posttraumatic stress symptoms after birth (Wijma et al., 1997; Soderquist et al., 2006). In the UK, a history of mental health problems was again confirmed as a significant risk factor for women (Czarnocka & Slade, 2000). In Israel, Polachek, Harari, Baum, and Strous (2012) also reported a significant association between a previous history of psychiatric treatment and elevated posttraumatic stress symptoms.

Prenatal Anxiety

Anxiety and depression during pregnancy have reportedly been confirmed as pre-birth predictors of posttraumatic stress symptoms following labor and delivery. Trait anxiety was a significant risk factor identified in the UK (Czarnocka & Slade, 2000) and the USA (Soet et al., 2003). Elevated anxiety during pregnancy was examined in the UK (Keogh, Ayers, & Francis, 2002), Switzerland (Zaers et al., 2008), and Canada (Feirbrother & Woody, 2007) as a predictor of PTSD following childbirth. Also in Canada, Verreault et al. (2012) reported that higher anxiety sensitivity in pregnancy was a significant risk factor for developing PTSD following childbirth. All these studies confirmed that prenatal anxiety was a significant risk factor that needs to be addressed during pregnancy.

PTSD and associated prenatal behavioral risk factors were investigated in a sample of Caucasian, Asian, and Pacific Islander women (Onoye, Goebert, Morland, Matsu, & Wright, 2009). Fifty-four mothers were interviewed at their postpartum clinic visit using the PTSD Checklist Civilian-Version (PCL-C; Weathers & Litz, 1994). Of these women, 21% screened positive for postpartum PTSD or subclinical PTSD. There were no significant differences, however, by ethnicity. Women with prenatal PTSD were three times more likely to have postpartum PTSD than mothers without prenatal PTSD, and women who experienced interpersonal violence were twice as likely to have postpartum PTSD as women who had not experienced interpersonal violence. Mothers with PTSD or subclinical PTSD during the postpartum period were significantly more likely to also have elevated depressive symptoms.

Prenatal Depression

Prenatal depression has also been repeatedly confirmed as a significant predictor of posttraumatic stress response to childbirth. For example, in the UK (Keogh et al., 2002), in Israel (Lev-Wiesel et al., 2009), in Sweden (Soderquist et al., 2006), in Canada (Cohen et al., 2004), and in the Netherlands (Stramrood, Paarlberg et al., 2011; Stramrood, Wessel et al., 2011), prenatal depression was found to be a significant risk factor for mothers to develop a posttraumatic stress response due to traumatic childbirth.

Two studies, one in the USA (Onoye et al., 2009) and one in Israel (Lev-Wiesel & Daphna-Tekoah, 2010) reported that pregnant women with elevated posttraumatic stress symptoms were at risk of experiencing these heightened distressing symptoms after labor and delivery.

Prior Trauma

Having experienced trauma prior to childbirth sets the perfect stage for women to be prone to be retraumatized during labor and delivery, especially women who are survivors of childhood sexual abuse. In the USA, prior history of sexual trauma was a significant predictor of women's experience of psychological trauma during childbirth (Soet et al., 2003). Mothers in Israel had significantly higher levels of posttraumatic stress symptoms if they were survivors of childhood sexual abuse compared to mothers without such a history (Lev-Wiesel & Daphna-Tekoah, 2010). History of sexual trauma was also found to be a significant risk factor in Canadian women (Verreault et al., 2012).

For survivors of childhood sexual abuse, typical interventions or events that occur during labor and delivery may act as triggers to their abuse. These women may have exaggerated or inappropriate reactions to these seemingly normal procedures, such as a vaginal examination to determine the progress of dilatation of the cervix in labor. Simkin and Klaus categorize these triggers into intrinsic and extrinsic triggers. Intrinsic triggers "come with the spontaneous, uncontrollable process of labor, and are evoked by previous negative experiences involving the same parts of the body" (2004, p. 73). For example, the feeling of the infant in her vagina can result in a woman's conscious or unconscious memories of her childhood sexual abuse. Extrinsic triggers are not caused by the labor and delivery process itself. The hospital environment, medical interventions, and labor and delivery staff are examples of extrinsic triggers that may evoke feelings of helplessness, distrust, fear, and danger. Genitals being exposed, lack of respect for a woman's modesty, catheterization, vaginal examinations, and being attached to a fetal monitor are all examples of such triggers as well as interpersonal conflicts and lack of perceived respect.

Simpkin and Klaus warn labor and delivery clinicians that phrases such as "open your legs," "relax your bottom," "this will hurt only a little," and "relax and it won't hurt so much" (2004, p. 74) can be interpreted negatively by childhood sexual abuse survivors. Even though the clinician meant to help with these phrases, the very same words may have been uttered time and again by the laboring woman's abuser. Simpkin and Klaus also warn that to a laboring woman phrase such as "trust your body" and "do what your body tells you to do" (2004, p. 74) may be frightening to a survivor of childhood sexual abuse who perceives her body as a source of shame, as for most of her life she may have been trying to disconnect from her damaged body.

Having some control in labor is not only important for women but is paramount for women who are survivors of childhood sexual abuse. Often, women who have suffered such abuse may equate powerlessness, helplessness, and loss of control with being abused. For some women even though the use of narcotics may help bring pain relief from their contractions, the side effects such as grogginess may increase their feelings of being out of control. Also, pain-relieving medication may not erase the emotional distress as women may still feel violated by feeling trapped with their legs spread apart and fully clothed clinicians staring at their exposed genitals.

During childbirth the usual boundaries of a body are typically invaded. Labor and delivery staff may take this invasion for granted but not survivors of childhood sexual abuse. Kitzinger warns:

> The experiences of women who have been sexually abused represent in microcosm those of all women who feel degraded and abused by what is done to them in pregnancy and childbirth. When birth is conducted with no personal consideration and respect, when management is crude and insensitive, it is itself a form of sexual abuse.
>
> (2006, p. 69)

Sperlich and Seng (2008) warn that for women who are survivors of sexual abuse trusting in their bodies during childbirth is not easy since their bodies have been violated and have been "unsafe territory" in the past. Labor and delivery care can be re-traumatizing for survivors of sexual abuse if they perceive it as uncaring and incompetent. Sperlich and Seng wonder if re-traumatization taking place at one of the most important events in a woman's life increases the negative power of this trauma. If, however, a woman feels she has received caring, competent support and care from labor and delivery staff and she has successfully met the challenges of birthing her infant, she can experience an increased empowerment.

Not only sexual abuse but also emotional abuse were significant risk factors for high levels of posttraumatic stress symptoms in a Canadian study (Cohen et al., 2004). In this study, having experienced two or more traumatic events was a significant predictor of women experiencing posttraumatic symptoms. Having experienced a stillbirth with a previous pregnancy was an example of a specific prior traumatic event that was significantly related to British women with elevated posttraumatic stress symptoms in their subsequent childbirth (Turton, Hughes, Evans, & Fainman, 2001).

In Israel, Polachek et al. (2012) reported that women who had experienced a previous traumatic birth were at significant risk of developing elevated posttraumatic stress symptoms.

Intrapartum Risk Factors

From the research listed in Table 4.2, the risk factors that were repeatedly reported provide a profile of women most vulnerable to perceiving their labor and delivery as traumatic and experiencing a posttraumatic stress response. These predictors include medical interventions, powerlessness, pain/long labor, uncaring labor and delivery staff, and lack of support. Increased medical intervention during the birthing process included: such procedures as induction,

Table 4.2 Significant intrapartum risk factors for elevated posttraumatic stress symptoms after childbirth

Author/country	Sample	Data collection	Instruments	Prevalence (%)	Risk factor
Menage (1993)/UK	102	Mean = 4.6 yr postpartum	PTSD-I	29	Powerlessness in labor Lack of information Increased physical pain Clinicians' unsympathetic attitude
Wijma et al. (1997)/ Sweden	1640	First 12 mos postpartum	TES	1.7	Negative rating of contact with delivery staff
Ryding et al. (1998)/ Sweden	326	2 days and 1 mos postpartum	IES	5/6 emergency c/s group; 2.2 in vacuum extraction/ forceps group	Emergency c/s Vacuum extraction/forceps
Lyons (1998)/UK	42	1 mos postpartum	IES		Loss of control during delivery Increased neuroticism, difficult pregnancy Induction, epidural Increased depressive symptoms
Czarnocka and Slade (2000)/UK	264	6 wks postpartum	PTSD-I	3	Low levels of support from partner and staff Low perceived control in labor Patterns of blame
Creedy et al. (2000)/ Australia	499	4–6 wks postpartum	PSS-SR	5.6	Obstetric intervention Inadequate intrapartum care Partner support
MacLean et al. (2000)/ UK	40	6 wks postpartum	IES		Instrumental delivery (forceps and episiotomy)
Soet et al. (2003)/US	103	4 wks postpartum	TES	1.9	Pain Low levels of social support Feeling powerlessness Medical intervention

continued

Table 4.2 (Continued)

Author/country	Sample	Data collection	Instruments	Prevalence (%)	Risk factor
Adewuya et al. (2006)/ Nigeria	876	6 wks postpartum	MINI	5.9	Lack of control during childbirth Mode of delivery
Cigoli et al. (2006)/Italy	160	3–6 mos postpartum	PTSD-Q	1.25	Low levels of support from family and medical personnel
Lev-Wiesel et al. (2009)/ Israel	1071	midpregnancy, 1 and 6 mos postpartum	PSS-I TES		Pain
Sawyer & Ayers (2009)/UK	219	Mean = 11mos postpartum	PDS	12.4	Pain Cesarean birth
Stramrood, Paarlberg et al. (2011)/the Netherlands	428	2–6 mos postpartum	TES	1.2	Unplanned cesarean Severe labor pain Poor coping skills
Verreault et al. (2012)/ Canada	308	1, 3, & 6 mos postpartum	MPSS-SR	4.9–7.6	Low levels of support

Notes: PTSD-I = PTSD Interview; TES = Traumatic Event Scale; IES = Impact of Event Scale; PSS-SR = Posttraumatic Stress Disorder Symptom Scale–Self Report; PTSD-Q = PTSD Questionnaire; MINI = Mini International Neuropsychiatric Interview; PDS = Posttraumatic Stress Diagnostic Scale; PSS-I = Posttraumatic Stress Disorder Symptom Scale Interview; MPSS-SR = Modified PTSD Symptom Scale–Self Report.

forceps and vacuum extractions, and emergency cesareans. These procedures can be viewed as contributing factors to women who developed elevated post-traumatic stress symptoms following childbirth. This was reported to be a significant predictor in such countries as the USA (Soet et al., 2003), Sweden (Ryding et al., 1998), Australia (Creedy et al., 2000), the UK (MacLean, McDermott, & May, 2000), and Nigeria (Adewuya et al., 2006).

Loss of control and feeling powerless during labor and delivery contributed to the vulnerability of women and the probability that they would experience a posttraumatic stress response following childbirth. Lyons (1998) in the UK, Adewuya et al. (2006) and Soet et al. (2003) in the USA all found that this was a significant risk factor.

PTSD after childbirth was examined in Nigerian women (Adewuya et al., 2006). At 6 weeks postpartum, 876 women were assessed for PTSD with the MINI International Neuropsychiatric Interview (Sheehan et al., 1998). In this sample 5.9% (n = 52) of the mothers fulfilled the DSM-IV criteria for PTSD. Four predictors of PTSD in the postpartum period were identified: pregnancy-related hospital admission, mode of delivery, mode of delivery of placenta, and mothers' experiences of control during childbirth. These four variables accounted for 45% of the variance in PTSD in Nigerian postpartum women.

An uncaring, unsympathetic attitude on the part of clinicians during labor and delivery and perceptions by the women of inadequate support and care were repeatedly confirmed as other risk factors. Stripped of a protective layer of feeling cared for and not respected by obstetrical staff left women at risk of a post-traumatic stress response. As can be seen in Table 4.2, this predictor occurred in the UK (Menage, 1993), Italy (Cigoli et al., 2006), Australia (Creedy et al., 2000), Sweden (Wijma et al., 1997), and the USA (Soet et al., 2003). In addition to lack of support from clinicians, low levels of support from family members during the childbirth process were a predictor of elevated posttraumatic stress symptoms in mothers (Creedy et al., 2000; Czarnocka & Slade, 2000; Cigoli et al., 2006). One study conducted in Israel did not report a significant relationship between support during labor by a significant other and elevated posttraumatic stress symptoms (Polachek et al., 2012).

Pain in childbirth played a significant role in women developing posttraumatic stress symptoms. In Israel, Lev-Wiesel et al. (2009) reported that high levels of subjective pain during labor and delivery accounted for postpartum posttraumatic stress symptoms. Menage (1993) in the UK, Soet et al. (2003) in the USA, and Sawyer and Ayers in the UK (2009), also reported increased pain as a risk factor.

Cesarean Birth

Seven studies were located in which posttraumatic stress symptoms were examined in women who had cesarean births. The majority of these studies were conducted in Sweden.

In 1995, the first case study was reported of a 32-year-old woman in the UK who developed PTSD after having an emergency cesarean birth under epidural anesthesia which was not fully effective (Ballard, Stanley, & Brockington, 1995).

> She experienced excruciating pain during an operation which took 10 minutes. She was screaming, shouting, and struggling to get off the operating table during the procedure, and was held down by attendants . . . Afterwards, she experienced recurrent images of her experience. She would stand at the kitchen sink and relive the operation again and again, feeling protracted terror as well as sweating and trembling
>
> (Ballard et al., 1995, pp. 525–526)

In Sweden, Ryding, Wijma, and Wijma conducted a study to answer the following question: "Do women experience any posttraumatic stress reactions or even posttraumatic stress disorder 1 to 2 months after emergency cesarean section?" (1997, p. 856). Twenty-five women underwent a diagnostic interview according to DSM III-R criteria. In this sample, 19 (76%) of the women reported these cesarean births as a traumatic event. Eight mothers (33%) experienced posttraumatic stress reactions. None of these women met all the diagnostic criteria for PTSD.

In Sweden, 53 women were interviewed 1 to 2 days after emergency cesarean births to determine whether this mode of delivery met the stressor criteria of PTSD (Ryding, Wijma, & Wijma, 1998). Fifty-five percent of these mothers reported experiencing intense fear for their own life and/or that of their infant. They fulfilled the stressor criteria of DSM IV. Thirteen percent (n = 7) of the sample had a loss of contact with reality in a very frightening manner.

Mothers' posttraumatic stress symptoms three months after having undergone an emergency cesarean birth were assessed in Sweden (Tham, Christensson, & Ryding, 2007). The sample of 122 new mothers completed the Impact of Event Scale (IES-15; Horowitz, Wilner, & Alvarez, 1979). Twenty-five percent of these mothers reported a moderate level of posttraumatic stress symptoms and 9% more had a high level of these symptoms indicative of possible PTSD.

In the UK, Sawyer and Ayers (2009) conducted an Internet study with 219 women within 36 months after birth (Mean = 11 months postpartum). The Posttraumatic Stress Diagnostic Scale (PDS; Foa et al., 1997) was completed by the mothers. Women who had cesarean births reported significantly higher posttraumatic stress symptom levels than either mothers who had an instrumental or a normal birth.

Experiences of support were compared among 42 women with and 42 women without posttraumatic stress symptoms following emergency cesarean births in Sweden (Tham, Ryding, & Christensson, 2010). These women were interviewed by telephone 6–7 months postpartum. Compared to mothers without posttraumatic stress symptoms, mothers experiencing posttraumatic symptoms described their midwives as unprofessional, nervous, or non-interested. Mothers with posttraumatic stress symptoms shared their intense fear and shame during these emergency cesarean births. These women also reported a lack of postpartum follow-up, fatigue after childbirth, and inadequate support from their husbands as influencing factors for their posttraumatic stress symptoms.

In the Netherlands, Stramrood, Paarlberg et al. (2011) examined the prevalence of PTSD following childbirth in homelike versus hospital settings. Within 2 to 6 months after birth, 428 women completed the Traumatic Event Scale-B (Wijma et al., 1997). In this sample of Dutch women, 1.2% was determined to have PTSD due to childbirth and 9.1% experienced their childbirth as traumatic. No differences in PTSD were reported after controlling for complications and interventions. Unplanned cesarean births, poor coping skills, and severe labor pain were associated with higher levels of posttraumatic stress symptoms.

Preeclampsia/HELLP

Van Pampus et al. (2004) brought attention to women who can develop PTSD after pregnancies complicated by either severe preeclampsia or HELLP syndrome. Preeclampsia is a syndrome women can experience after the 20th week of pregnancy. It consists of increased blood pressure and protein in their urine. HELLP syndrome is a type of preeclampsia. H stands for hemolysis (breakdown of red blood cells). EL stands for elevated liver enzyme and LP for low platelet count. In the Netherlands Stramrood, Wessel et al. (2011) reported a prevalence rate for PTSD of 11% in women who had preeclampsia.

Pregnancy Loss

Two studies were located in which the focus was PTSD in women following pregnancy loss. In the Netherlands, Engelhard, van den Hout, and Arntz (2001) conducted a study of PTSD after pregnancy loss. At 1 month and 4 months after their pregnancy loss women completed the Posttraumatic Symptom Scale-Self-Report (PSS-SR; Foa, Riggs, Dancu, & Rothbaum, 1993). At one month after miscarriage 25% of the women met the criteria for PTSD diagnosis and at 4 months 4% of the sample. Women who met the criteria for PTSD had an increased risk of depression. An example of the intrusive recollections women had of their pregnancy loss is illustrated by the following quote from a mother who had a stillbirth in her 32nd week:

> At the moment of birth, I saw Sara's head come out of me. I held her, and she was red, her skin was torn. One of her eyes was open. I looked to see if it was a girl. Her belly was dark-red. She had beautiful ears. A very white nose. Blood was running from her nose. Her legs looked broken.
>
> (Engelhard et al., 2001, p. 65)

In Germany, the long-term posttraumatic stress response 2–7 years after termination of pregnancy due to fetal malformation was examined (Kerstin et al., 2004). The Impact of Event Scale-Revised (IES-R) (Horowitz et al., 1979) was used to assess posttraumatic stress symptoms and compare levels among the 83 women who had terminated their pregnancy 2–7 years earlier, 60 women who had experienced a termination of pregnancy 14 days earlier, and 65 women who had a spontaneous birth of a healthy infant. Women at 14 days and 2–7 years post termination had similar levels of elevated posttraumatic stress symptoms. The mothers who had delivered healthy newborns reported a significantly lower level of posttraumatic stress symptoms than the two groups of women who had a termination of pregnancy.

Spontaneous abortion has been described as one of the worst traumatic events in a woman's lifetime (Hamama, Rauch, Sperlich, Defever, & Seng, 2010). Women exposed to uncaring clinicians during their miscarriage are at an even higher risk of developing PTSD. Often women experience miscarriage at home and often get little care from clinicians, depending on weeks of gestation, so this variable is a high risk factor that needs to be included in the history/assessment aspects of the initial interview.

Preterm Birth

Seven studies were located in which posttraumatic stress symptoms were investigated in mothers of infants in the NICU (Neonatal Intensive Care Unit). The majority of these studies focused on preterm infants. Findings from all these studies confirmed that mothers of infants in the NICU had significantly higher levels of posttraumatic symptoms than mothers whose infants were not in the NICU.

The first study examining PTSD in mothers of high risk infants was conducted by DeMier, Hynan, Harris, and Manniello (1996). The sample consisted of 142 mothers who were primarily white, middle-class women. The sample was divided into three categories: mothers of premature infants, mothers of full-term infants in the NICU, and mothers of healthy full-term infants. Women completed the Perinatal PTSD Questionnaire via a mailed questionnaire. Women whose infants were premature and those whose term infants were in the NICU reported significantly more posttraumatic stress symptoms than mothers of healthy, full-term infants. Data analysis revealed that the severity of postnatal infant complications, gestational age, and length of NICU stay explained 35% of the variability in posttraumatic stress symptom scores in the sample.

Parental posttraumatic stress reactions to a premature birth were investigated in Switzerland using two groups: 55 parents of a preterm infant and 25 parents of a full-term infant (Pierrehumbert, Nicole, Muller-Nix, Forcada-Guex, & Ansermet, 2003). When the children were 18 months old, parents completed the Perinatal PTSD Questionnaire (PPQ: Quinnell & Hynan, 1999). Parents of premature infants had significantly higher posttraumatic stress scores than parents of full-term infants. Parents of preterm infants were subdivided into low and high risk groups depending on the severity of the perinatal stress. Using the cutoff of six or more positive responses on the PPQ, 4% of mothers in the low risk group compared to 26% of mothers in the high risk group met the DSM criteria for PTSD reactions.

Thirty mothers of preterm infants were interviewed when their infants were 6 months old (Holditch-Davis, Bartlett, Blickman, & Miles, 2003). The data from the interviews were analyzed for the three major symptom clusters of PTSD: re-experiencing, avoidance, and hyperarousal. All 30 mothers reported at least one posttraumatic stress symptom. Twelve mothers had two symptoms and 16 had all three symptoms. Avoidance and re-experiencing were each described by 24 women while 26 women reported hyperarousal symptoms.

Kersting et al. (2004) were the first to conduct a longitudinal study of posttraumatic stress in mothers of very low birth weight (VLBW) infants who weigh less than 1500 grams. Fifty women of VLBW infants and 30 women of healthy term infants completed the Impact of Event Scale (IES-R; Horowitz et al., 1979) at four points in time: 1–3 days after birth, 14 days postpartum, 6 months and 14 months postpartum. At all four points in time, mothers of VLBW infants experienced significantly higher levels of posttraumatic stress symptoms than mothers of full-term, healthy infants.

In France, 21 mothers of preterm infants underwent a semistructured interview given by a psychologist at 2 months and again at 1 year after birth (Garel, Dardennes, & Blondel, 2006). Eight women (38%) reported the preterm birth had been a traumatic event. They experienced posttraumatic stress symptoms such as avoidance and re-experiencing the traumatic births.

Acute posttraumatic stress symptoms within the first week postpartum were compared in 59 mothers of infants in the NICU and 60 mothers of infants in the well baby nursery (Vanderbilt, Bushley, Young, & Frank, 2009). Women completed the Perinatal PTSD Questionnaire (PPQ) (Quinnell & Hynan, 1999). Women whose infants were in the NICU reported significantly more acute posttraumatic stress symptoms than mothers of infants in the well baby nursery. Using the screening criteria on the PPQ for risk of PTSD, 24% of NICU infants' mothers compared to 3% of well baby nursery infants' mothers met the criteria. When statistically removing the effects for depressive symptoms and prior lifetime history of traumatic events, having an infant in the NICU was significantly associated with mothers' posttraumatic stress symptoms scores.

At 30 days or more post admission to the NICU, parents completed the PTSD Symptom Checklist (PCL; Weathers & Ford, 1996) (Lefkowitz, Baxt, & Evans, 2010). Nine mothers (15%) and two fathers (8%) met criteria for a diagnosis of PTSD with an additional 11.7% (n = 7) of the mothers and 4% (n = 1) of the fathers with subsyndromal PTSD.

Most recently, posttraumatic stress symptoms in mothers of late preterm infants have been studied. Late preterm infants are infants born between 34 and 36 completed weeks of gestation. Using the PPQ (DeMier et al., 1996), Brandon et al. (2011) reported that mothers of late preterm infants had significantly higher levels of posttraumatic stress symptoms than mothers of full term infants.

Conclusion

As evidenced by the studies presented in this chapter, researchers have identified numerous risk factors of women perceiving their labor and delivery as traumatic. Research is needed, however, that investigates the diagnosis of PTSD and not just the severity of posttraumatic stress symptoms. Research is also needed into the etiology of why some women, and not others, develop PTSD secondary to traumatic childbirth. Treatment methodologies also need to be researched to determine the most effective strategies for new mothers suffering with PTSD due to birth trauma.

In order to add mothers' voices to the risk factors for PTSD discussed in this chapter, Chapter 5 highlights mothers' narratives of the following risk factors: increased medical intervention, pain, helplessness, postpartum hemorrhage, preeclampsia, perinatal loss, preterm birth, and childhood sexual abuse.

References

Adewuya, A. O., Ologun, Y. A., & Ibigbami, O. S. (2006). Post-traumatic stress disorder after childbirth in Nigerian women: Prevalence and risk factors. *BJOG, 113,* 284–288.

Ayers, S., Harris, R., Sawyer, A., Parfitt, Y., & Ford, E. (2009). Post-traumatic stress disorder after childbirth: Analysis of symptom presentation and sampling. *Journal of Affective Disorders, 119,* 200–204.

Ballard, C. G., Stanley, A. K., & Brockington, I. F. (1995). Post-traumatic stress disorder (PTSD) after childbirth. *British Journal of Psychiatry, 166,* 525–528.

Beck, C. T., Gable, R. K., Sakala, C., & Declercq, E. R. (2011). Posttraumatic stress disorder in new mothers: Results from a two-stage U.S. national survey. *Birth, 38,* 216–227.

Brandon, D. H., Tully, K. P., Silva, S. G., Malcolm, W. F., Murtha, A. P., Turner, B. S., & Holditch-Davis, D. (2011). Emotional responses of mothers of late-preterm and term infants. *Journal of Obstetric, Gynecologic, and Neonatal Nursing, 40,* 719–731.

Cigoli, V., Gilli, G., & Saita, E. (2006). Relational factors in psychopathological responses to childbirth. *Journal of Psychosomatic Obstetrics & Gynaecology, 27,* 91–97.

Cohen, M. M., Ansara, D., Schei, B., Stuckless, N., & Stewart, D. E. (2004). Posttraumatic stress disorder after pregnancy, labor, and delivery. *Journal of Women's Health, 13,* 315–324.

Creedy, D. K., Shochet, I. M., & Horsfall, J. (2000). Childbirth and the development of acute trauma symptoms: Incidence and contributing factors. *Birth, 27,* 104–111.

Czarnocka, J., & Slade, P. (2000). Prevalence and predictors of posttraumatic stress symptoms following childbirth. *British Journal of Clinical Psychology, 39,* 35–51.

DeMier, R. L., Hynan, M. T., Harris, H. B., & Manniello, R. L. (1996). Perinatal stressors as predictors of symptoms of posttraumatic stress in mothers of infants at high risk. *Journal of Perinatology, 16,* 276–280.

Engelhard, I. M., van den Hout, M. A., & Arntz, A. (2001). Posttraumatic stress disorder after pregnancy loss. *General Hospital Psychiatry, 23,* 62–66.

Feirbrother, N., & Woody, S. R. (2007). Fear of childbirth and obstetrical events as predictors of postnatal symptoms of depression and posttraumatic stress disorder. *Journal of Psychosomatic Obstetrics and Gynaecology, 28,* 239–242.

Foa, E. B., Cashman, L., Jaycox, L., & Perry, K. (1997). The validation of a self-report measure of posttraumatic stress disorder: The Posttraumatic Stress Diagnostic Scale. *Psychological Assessment, 9,* 445–451.

Foa, E. B., Riggs, D. S., Dancu, C. V., & Rothbaum, B. O. (1993). Reliability and validity of a brief instrument for assessing post-traumatic stress disorder. *Journal of Trauma Stress, 6,* 459–473.

Garel, M., Dardennes, M., & Blondel, B. (2006). Mothers' psychological distress 1 year after very preterm childbirth. Results of a epipage qualitative study. *Child: Care, Health and Development, 33,* 137–143.

Hamama, L., Rauch, S. A. M., Sperlich, M., Defever, E., & Seng, J. S. (2010). Previous experience of spontaneous or elective abortion and risk for posttraumatic stress and depression during subsequent pregnancy. *Depression and Anxiety, 27,* 699–707.

Holditch-Davis, D., Bartlett, T. R., Blickman, A. L., & Miles, M. S. (2003). Posttraumatic stress symptoms in mothers of premature infants. *Journal of Obstetric, Gynecologic, and Neonatal Nursing, 32,* 161–171.

Horowitz, M. J., Wilner, N., & Alvarez, W. (1979). Impact of Event Scale: A measure of subjective stress. *Psychosomatic Medicine, 41,* 209–221.

Iles, J., Slade, P., & Spiby, H. (2011). Posttraumatic stress symptoms and postpartum depression in couples after childbirth: The role of partner support and attachment. *Journal of Anxiety Disorders, 25,* 520–530.

Keogh, E., Ayers, S., & Francis, H. (2002). Does anxiety sensitivity predict post-traumatic stress symptoms following childbirth? A preliminary report. *Cognitive Behavior Therapy, 31,* 145–155.

Kersting, A., Dorsch, M., Wesselmann, U., Ludorff, K., Witthaut, J., Ohrmann, P., Hornig-Franz, I., Klockenbusch, W., Harms, E., & Arolt, V. (2004). Maternal posttraumatic stress response after the birth of a very low birth weight infant. *Journal of Psychosomatic Research, 57,* 473–476.

Kitzinger, S. (2006). *Birth crisis.* New York: Routledge.

Lefkowitz, D. S., Baxt, C., & Evans, J. R. (2010). Prevalence and correlates of posttraumatic stress and postpartum depression in parents of infants in the neonatal intensive care unit (NICU). *Journal of Clinical Psychology in Medical Settings* (DOI 10.1007/s10880-010-9202-7).

Lev-Wiesel, R., & Daphna-Tekoah, S. (2010). The role of peripartum dissociation as a predictor of posttraumatic stress symptoms following childbirth in Israeli Jewish women. *Journal of Trauma and Dissociation, 11,* 266–283.

Lev-Wiesel, R., Daphna-Tekoah, S., & Hallak, M. (2009). Childhood sexual abuse as a predictor of birth-related posttraumatic stress and postpartum posttraumatic stress. *Child Abuse Neglect, 33,* 877–887.

Lev-Wiesel, R., Chen, R., Daphna-Tekoah, S., & Hod, M. (2009). Past traumatic events: are they a risk factor for high-risk pregnancy, delivery complications, and postpartum posttraumatic symptoms? *Journal of Women's Health, 18,* 119–125.

Lyons, S. (1998). A prospective study of post-traumatic stress symptoms 1 month following childbirth in a group of 42 first-time mothers. *Journal of Reproductive & Infant Psychology, 16,* 91–105.

MacLean, L. I., McDermott, M. R., & May, C. P. (2000). Method of delivery and subjective distress: Women's emotional responses to childbirth practices. *Journal of Reproductive and Infant Psychology, 18,* 153–162.

Maggioni, C., Margola, D., & Filippi, F. (2006). PTSD, risk factors, and expectations among women having a baby: A two-wave longitudinal study. *Journal of Psychosomatic Obstetrics and Gynaecology, 27,* 81–90.

Menage, J. (1993). Post-traumatic stress disorder in women who have undergone obstetric or gynecological procedures. *Journal of Reproductive Infant Psychology, 11,* 221–228.

Olde, E., Van der Hart, O., Kleber, R. J., Van Son, M. J. M., Wijnen, H. A. A., & Pop, V. J. M. (2005). Peritraumatic dissociation and emotions as predictors of PTSD symptoms following childbirth. *Journal of Trauma and Dissociation, 6,* 125–142.

Onoye, J. M., Goebert, D., Morland, L., Matsu, C., & Wright, T. (2009). PTSD and postpartum mental health in a sample of Caucasian, Asian, and Pacific Islander women. *Archives of Women's Mental Health, 12,* 393–400.

Pierrehumbert, B., Nicole, A., Muller-Nix, C., Forcada-Guex, M., & Ansermet, F. (2003). Parental post-traumatic reactions after premature birth: Implications for sleeping and eating problems in the infant. *Archives of Diseases in Childhood-Fetal Neonatal Edition, 88,* F400–F404.

Polachek, I. S., Harari, L. H., Baum, M., & Strous, R. D. (2012). Postpartum post-traumatic stress disorder symptoms: The uninvited birth companion. *Israeli Medical Association Journal, 14,* 347–353.

Quinnell, F. A., & Hynan, M. T. (1999). Convergent and discriminant validity of the Perinatal PTSD Questionnaire (PPQ): A preliminary study. *Journal of Traumatic Stress, 12,* 193–199.

Ryding, E. L., Wijma, B., & Wijma, K. (1997). Posttraumatic stress reactions after emergency cesarean section. *Acta Obstetricia et Gynecologica Scandinavica, 76,* 856–861.

—— (1998). Experiences of emergency cesarean section: A phenomenological study of 53 women. *Birth, 25,* 246–251.

Sawyer, A., & Ayers, S. (2009). Post-traumatic growth in women after childbirth. *Psychology and Health, 24,* 457–471.

Sheehan, D. V., Lecrubier, Y., Harnett-Sheehan, K., Amorim, P., Janavs, J., & Weiller, E. et al. (1998). The Mini International Neuropsychiatric Interview (M.I.N.I.): The development and validation of a structured diagnostic psychiatric interview. *Journal of Clinical Psychiatry, 59* (Suppl. 20), 22–33.

Simpkin, P., & Klaus, P. (2004). *When survivors give birth: Understanding and healing the effects of early sexual abuse on childbearing women.* Seattle, WA: Classic Day Publishing.

Soderquist, J., Wijma, B., & Wijma, K. (2006). The longitudinal course of post-traumatic stress after childbirth. *Journal of Psychosomatic Obstetrics and Gynaecology, 27,* 113–119.

Soet, J. E., Brack, G. A., & Dilorio, C. (2003). Prevalence and predictors of women's experience of psychological trauma during childbirth. *Birth, 30,* 36–46.

Sperlich, M., & Seng, J. S. (2008). *Survivor moms: Women's stories of birthing, mothering, and healing after sexual abuse.* Eugene, OR: Motherbaby Press.

Stramrood, C. A., Paarlberg, K. M., Huis In't Veld, E. M., Berger, L. W., Vingerhoets, A. J., Weijmar Schultz, W. C., & Van Pampus, M. G. (2011). Posttraumatic stress following childbirth in homelike- and hospital settings. *Journal of Psychosomatic Obstetrics & Gynecology, 32,* 88–97.

Stramrood, C. A., Wessel, I., Doornbos, B., Aarnoudse, J. G., van der Berg, P. P., Weijmar Schultz, W. C., & van Pampus, M. G. (2011). Posttraumatic stress disorder following preeclampsia and PPROM: A prospective study with 15 months follow-up. *Reproductive Sciences, 18,* 645–653.

Tham, V., Christensson, K., & Ryding, E. L. (2007). Sense of coherence and symptoms of post-traumatic stress after emergency caesarean section. *Acta Obstetricia et Gynecologica, 86,* 1090–1096.

Tham, V., Ryding, E. L., & Christensson, K. (2010). Experience of support among mothers with and without post-traumatic stress symptoms following emergency cesarean section. *Sexual and Reproductive Healthcare, 1,* 175–180.

Turton, P., Hughes, P., Evans, C. D., & Fainman, D. (2001). Incidence, correlates and predictors of post-traumatic stress disorder in the pregnancy after stillbirth. *British Journal of Psychiatry, 178,* 556–560.

Vanderbilt, D., Bushley, T., Young, R., & Frank, D. A. (2009). Acute posttraumatic stress symptoms among urban mothers with newborns in the neonatal intensive care unit: A preliminary study. *Journal of Developmental and Behavioral Pediatrics, 30,* 50–56.

Van Pampus, M. G., Wolf, H., Weijmar Schultz, W. C. M., Neeleman, J., & Aarnoudse, J. G. (2004). Posttraumatic stress disorder following preeclampsia and HELLP syndrome. *Journal of Psychosomatic Obstetrics and Gynecology, 25,* 183–187.

Verreault, N., Da Costa, D., Marchand, A., Ireland, K., Banack, H., Dritsa, M., & Khalife, S. (2012). PTSD following childbirth: A prospective study of incidence and risk factors in Canadian women. *Journal of Psychosomatic Research, 73,* 257–263.

Weathers, F., & Ford, J. (1996). Psychometric properties of the PTSD Checklist (PCL-C, PCL-S, PCL-M, PCL-PR). In B. H. Stamm (Ed.). *Measurement of stress, trauma, & adaptation.* Lutherville, MD: Sidran Press.

Weathers, F. W., & Litz, B. T. (1994). Psychometric properties of the Clinician-Administered PTSD Scale (CAPS-1). *PTSD Research Quarterly, 5,* 2–6.

Wijma, K., Soderquist, M. A., & Wijma, B. (1997). Posttraumatic stress disorder after childbirth: A cross sectional study. *Journal of Anxiety Disorders, 11,* 587–597.

Zaers, S., Waschke, M., & Ehlert, U. (2008). Depressive symptoms and symptoms of posttraumatic stress disorder in women after childbirth. *Journal of Psychosomatic Obstetrics and Gynaecology, 29,* 61–71.

5 Women's Narratives of Risk Factors for Posttraumatic Stress Response

In this chapter, women's stories of the following risk factors for posttraumatic stress response are shared: increased medical intervention, pain, helplessness, postpartum hemorrhage, preeclampsia, perinatal loss, preterm birth, and childhood sexual abuse. These women shared their stories with Cheryl as part of her research (Beck, 2004a; 2004b) and wanted others to hear their narratives.

Medical Intervention (Janice's Story)

Janice shared her terrifying experience of unnecessary medical intervention that occurred over 25 years ago. After suffering the after effects of her traumatic birth for 20 years, Janice finally was diagnosed with PTSD 5 years ago. In her own words:

> I was pregnant with twins. I had a regular appointment that morning but was too tired to go because my sister had been visiting with her twins (aged 9 months) and I had really done too much and was so tired I could hardly get out of bed. I called my husband and told him I did not want to go to my appointment because I was too tired and he was very upset. He wanted me to go because he felt I had been doing too much and he wanted me to go to make sure everything was okay. I reluctantly agreed.
>
> When I arrived at the doctor's office, my favorite doctor had opened up his own practice out of town, and had been replaced by another physician. I had never seen him before. He took one look at me (I must have looked awful) and he asked if I had had any symptoms. I said my back had hurt on Wednesday (this was Friday). He rolled his eyes and said he needed to examine me. He did and said I needed to go to the hospital immediately that I had dilated to 4 cm!! I remember asking, Are you sure? 4 cm? and he said yes, and he would meet me at the hospital. When he examined me, it felt like he swiped my cervix which was very painful, and when I went to the bathroom before I left, there was some blood and it concerned me. I sat in my car for a long time because I could not figure out how I could have dilated to 4 cm when there was nothing wrong with me. I called my husband and told him what the doctor had said. He said he would wrap things up at work and meet me at the hospital.

When I arrived at the hospital, the nurse was waiting for me. She told me to put on a gown which I did. I remember resting (sleeping) and later she came in and shaved me. Then I went right back to sleep. I remember my husband arriving and the doctor. He told me he wanted me to go to the Medical Center. I said okay. He hooked me up to a labor machine and a few minutes later examined me again, it felt like he swiped my cervix and I noticed what was a straight line on the machine was now this HUGE labor contraction!! The doctor went to another room and called a doctor at the Medical Center. My husband and I could not hear what was being said because he was talking in another room. The nurse obviously heard, and she came over to me and examined me and said, you have not dilated to 4 cm!!!

I remember telling him that when the time was right, I wanted an epidural. I was terrified of natural childbirth. He said okay. I knew it would be a while, though, because I knew that I was not in labor!! Everything seemed crazy and out of control. The nurse is continually saying, You have not dilated to 4 cm!! The doctor says I will be accepted only at the Medical Center if I agree to be a resident's first patient. I said okay, I do not mind being a resident's first patient. The nurse just glares at the doctor and walks off. I am immediately put in an ambulance to go to University Medical Center. I truly thought the doctor was a quack/idiot and I wanted to get away from him. I thought that a true expert would agree with the nurse and I would be observed and sent home. That was what my husband was hoping for, too. I was not worried in the least.

I remember the ambulance ride was bumpy and so unnecessary. My husband followed in his car with the flashers on. When I arrived, I was taken to a room with no one in it. I looked up and saw a doctor and the resident. The doctor has a look of, "Great, here she is," like I had been pawned off on him. He says something to the resident and the resident walks off. He comes over and examines me. He does not say anything. He feels my stomach. He acts like he does not know what to do with me. He examines me again and feels my stomach. He says it feels like both twins weigh the same. I found that to be very interesting. He does not ask me anything and I am very, very comfortable because he is examining me without killing me. He sits down and says some doctors worry that one twin might weigh more that the other twin. Then, it was like a light bulb went off in his head. The way he acted was, my doctor was making way too big a deal about twins and he was trying not to die laughing. This is when I became concerned. I realized that the doctor did not know when my due date was and probably did not know anything about me. I did not say anything. I just knew that there would be no babies born because I was not in labor. Then he said, Go lay down on that table over there. I notice there is a table with what seems like a HUGE towel lying across it. I do what he says, wondering what is going on. The doctor disappears and I remember looking up and seeing him in the doorway hiding something behind his back. I remember trying to see what he is hiding, but he does not want me to see it. He walks carefully to the end of my bed. He does something. Then he says, "You will be swimming for a while" and he is grinning from ear to ear. And he walks out still hiding what he has in his hand. I sit up wondering what is going on. I notice that my gown is wet and the towel is wet and it dawns on me what he did. He broke my water!! I was in total shock, not knowing why in the world he would do such a thing. I sat there all by myself. I remember getting very cold, my teeth were chattering. There was no one around. It seemed like I was in there forever. I would lay down and then sit back up. I did not know what to do. I could not believe what just happened!!

In the meantime, the doctor goes and introduces himself to my husband. He says that the twins will be born tonight. My husband says, "Say that again." The doctor said that he broke my water and the twins will be born tonight. My husband says, "What do you mean you broke her water? Didn't you know she is only 7½ months pregnant?" The doctor became very apologetic and put all the blame on our original doctor. He said he can only go by what my doctor has told him. He thought I was full term and was being sent there for low birth weight twins, not premature twins. He said he was so sorry. My husband said it took a while to convince the doctor that I was only 7-½ months' pregnant. The doctor said he was truly sorry but that the twins had to come no matter what. My husband said he managed to say okay. The doctor left and that was the last time my husband talked to him.

After what seemed like an eternity, the doctor comes back in the room. Someone has knocked that stupid smile right off his face. He now looked concerned and told me that the twins were going to be born, that they would be just fine. Small, but fine. Dummy me believed him. I was not happy with it but if my twins were going to be fine, then I could deal with that. I then was taken to another room where the resident came in and told me to bend over as far as possible. He said I would feel a bee sting and to let him know if I felt pain. I felt the bee sting and felt pain. I told him I felt pain. He repeated the procedure. I felt the bee sting and told him I felt pain. He tried one more time. I felt the bee sting and told him I felt pain. He said in a rather irritated voice, "Are you sure it is not just pressure you feel?" I told him I felt pain. I guess three strikes and you are out because that is when the doctor came in and gave the epidural to me. (The damage was done, though. I had pain down my right leg and walked with a limp for about ten years.) Then I was taken to another room.

I remember the next two or three hours as a blur. I just wanted to sleep. I did not see anyone except the doctor. Eventually, the doctor came in and said I was going to delivery. I could not believe what was happening. I asked for my husband. He said my husband was not allowed back there especially in delivery. I felt totally helpless. I told him I was thirsty and he told me I could not drink because I might throw up. He said he would give me a few ice cubes.

Before I knew it, I was in the delivery room. I saw two nurses come in, one young and one older. The older nurse came in and her mouth was open and she looked in shock. She took my hand and started to say something. She looked up and saw the doctor who was standing behind me. There were no words exchanged, only looks. The nurse decided not to say anything and let go of my hand and walks to the side of the room. I have wondered for almost 30 years what she was going to say to me. My guess is that she knew that what was about to happen was so wrong!!! . . .

The doctor gives the anesthesiologist the first nod and he gives me the first drug though the epidural. Right then and there, my bowels let loose and some of it actually got on the resident's shoes. If I thought I had any dignity at all, it was certainly gone at this moment. The resident gives me a dirty look (just like I did it on purpose) and then I feel tremendous pain. I call it the "slash of revenge." (I guess to get back at me) and I can feel it and I say out loud, I can feel that!! I look up (there is a huge mirror that everyone can see) and I see the slash. It is not straight up and down like an episiotomy would be but to the left towards my thigh. The doctor says, "Give her more, give her more." I receive more deadening medicine.

I pushed for what seems like an eternity. The first twin is born. I really think she was asleep. She came out and did not do anything for about a minute and then she started crying. They immediately took her away. The second twin got up as high as she could go after the first twin was born. I pushed and pushed, but she did not want to come. Finally, the doctor put his hand up there and said, "I feel a forehead, I believe." The second twin was born almost 30 minutes after the first and that was after the doctor said, "Give her more. Give her more." She did NOT want to come but finally did. The next day, her forehead was black with the bruise the doctor gave trying to find her. I also got a bad kidney infection and was not allowed to see my twins for three days because of high fever—no doubt in my mind from my body not being ready to go through the birthing process and/or the amount of drugs used to force them out of my body.

I remember being taken back to my room. I never knew anything was wrong or that my twins were fighting for their lives. It was not until the next morning when I saw them in intensive care with their heads shaved and IVs in their heads did I realize that they were very, very sick. They were not just fine. I was heartbroken. I could not talk about what had happened to me. They were fed with a tube down their throats. My daughter had jaundice and they thought she had a heart defect. Both of them had hyaline membrane disease.

The next few weeks are heartbreaking with everything that I saw in the NICU. I had never seen a preemie in trouble. The only preemie I had ever seen was my little cousin who was born three weeks early and he was fine. That is what I thought would happen to my twins, too. They would be born early but would be fine. That is what I was told. I had no idea the torture that preemies have to go through in order to save their lives. I was totally unprepared for that. And to think that I was not even in labor. I never had one labor pain whatsoever!! I felt really stupid and responsible because I "let" the doctors do that to me.

I told myself that the twins were finally well and that I should get on with my life but I would still think about it every now and then. I still dealt with depression and anxiety for a long time. It was not until about 20 years later when I was working as a medical transcriptionist that it all came back in a sudden memory, that is, the severity of it all. I typed reports for premature babies and I would have nightmares on a regular basis (just re-living what had happened to me). One night, I woke up in a sweat after one of the flashbacks and realized I could no longer handle it on my own. I made an appointment with a counselor.

What really bothers me is the way the doctor induced labor. That is where my nightmares and flashbacks lie. Him standing in the doorway hiding something behind his back. That is what I relive. I am convinced it will haunt me until the day I die.

Clinician's Reaction

As I read Janice's story, I am struck by how her memories are so clear even though her twins were born over 25 years ago. This is another testament to the way the traumatic events are embedded into the memory and the body. The major theme in Janice's story is ruptured trust and lack of collaborative communication. She describes how she was surprised that the doctor whom she really liked had left the practice and a new person that she did not know had replaced him. Did she get notification of the old doctor's move? Was it such a total surprise or did she just not remember . . . this dramatic change of players in her story set the stage for the traumatic experience that followed.

As she shared with Cheryl, she would never forget that doctor standing at the doorway with something behind his back, and that he never told her what he was going to do to her. She was the vulnerable recipient of medical intervention without explanation or understanding. This vulnerability was consistent through her narrative, as was the feeling from me as the reader that Janice had learned over her years as a person not to question authority and the doctor was an authority figure. No one ever asked Janice how many weeks her pregnancy was, and she assumed, which I would venture to guess most pregnant women do, that the doctors would be informed and pass on the information. What is really sad in this narrative, and I say this as a nurse, is that at two times in Janice's narrative the nurses did not agree with the physician and did not say anything . . . they too were silenced by the situation and the experience. Sadly, they did not trust their expertise to question the authority, i.e. the doctors.

You read how Janice internalized the blame of the experience. Blame and shame can truly affect the way one is in the world. She assumed blame for a situation where she experienced a rupture in trust. She assumed the doctors would take care of her and do what was in her best interest.

Janice's story reinforces the need to have a voice and to remember that you are your own advocate or at least have someone with you who can advocate for you. I do not think that this is the automatic role of the husband/partner as they are usually just as anxious and trusting of the health care providers.

Mother's Reaction

The passage of 25 years has not dulled the memory of Janice's traumatic birth. It is as though she has lived with an echo. She is to be commended for how well she has done. She should not be surprised, should not beat herself up and certainly not blame herself. She is right to be angry at what happened. She also needs support in dealing with that, so that she can go forward with a lighter load in her heart and mind, and work through the ever so vivid recall that she has. She should be kind to herself during her therapy period, as it will be tough, but can yet know that she is strong, as she has survived. The depression and anxiety that she has suffered will lift, and the trauma of the events will not be ever present in the future. Her caregivers need to reflect on how they would feel if they were treated in the way that treated Janice.

Pain (Nicole's Story)

Nicole was single and 31 when she became pregnant with her first child. She went into labor 2 weeks early. After 9 hours of back pain she arrived at the hospital and was 1 centimeter dilated. She settled into her birthing room. Four hours later, when she was 4 centimeters dilated, her membranes ruptured. Contractions were really strong and long and close together. Finally after more hours of labor she was fully dilated. The doctor came in and looked at the monitor and said, "The baby is distressed." The following is some of the narrative of her story.

> The nurse pulled my left knee down and kept her eye on the monitor while the doctor peered between my legs and told me to push. I pushed and I pushed and I pushed and I felt I would burst. I squatted forwards and rocked and cried and pushed and broke the ruby beads around my neck. Then I lay back down again and then somehow rolled over and squatted with my back to the doctor. Still crying, still saying I couldn't do this anymore. No-one seemed to get it: I had NO more energy. The baby was NOT moving. I couldn't get it out. It was STUCK in there. The nurse protested that she couldn't monitor the baby that way. I had to get on my back. They put my legs in stirrups and hoisted them up, and the nurse pushed me up into a sitting position. I screamed at them. This was NOT a comfortable position. It was not even a practical one. It certainly wasn't a natural one. I was lost in this unending world of pain and they kept telling me to push and not push (still in stirrups with my legs in the air and me sitting up). I had no out. I was panicking. It was not coming out. It

would not come out. It would NEVER come out. There was simply no way. No way to get this thing out of me. It would be like this forever. I lay back. The nurse had let me go. She was at the monitor. She said to the doctor, "We've lost the baby. Can we save the mother"—The doctor said: "PUSH!"; I yelled: "I can't! I can't!" The nurse said: "Shut up your yelling and put your energy into pushing." Someone came to the door and said: "You're waking up all the mothers and distressing them" and then she came in the door and saw between my legs and said: "Oh my God." The doctor kept saying "Push!" and "Stop pushing!" and "Don't push now!" I yelled "Knock me out!" The doctor said she had nothing to knock me out with. I yelled.

The attending was saying: "We've lost the baby." I felt that I was drowning in an endless, bottomless, thick sea of pain. I had thought I'd known pain before. I had *never* known pain before. I had never imagined it. I could never have imagined it. I had expected childbirth pain to be 10/10. This was 75/10. The voices became thick and far away. Then I was back and there was more to the pain and it was sheer and sharp and unmerciful. My sister was crying and begging the doctor to give me something. She said to me: "I can't give you anything for the pain because I really need you to push." Then I was off again, drowning in the pain. There was a roaring sound and the noise and the pushing and the pain went on and on and on.

Now there was a man down between my legs with the doctor. I hadn't seen him come in. He didn't speak to me. He and my doctor both had bloodied hands and he was talking to her—"If you can get hold of the shoulder, I'll turn the head around," then: "This baby's stuck." Somebody said they'd try the vacuum extractor. They had my baby's head on the vacuum extractor for an hour and then just as he said: "Here's the head—DAMN—it's gone back in." And they started all over. Both doctors. Both sets of hands up me, trying to push the shoulder and get the head turned again to get the extractor back on. The obstetrician (presumably) muttered to the doctor: "Why didn't you call me before?" The nurse was saying *she'd* wanted to, and telling me to shut up and push. They spent another hour with the vacuum extractor. The obstetrician said no, it was too late for an emergency cesarean, this baby is truly stuck.

Now they're acting like I'm not there. Incredible, unbelievable, unimaginable PAIN. I am the pain, and the pain is me. That's all there is. There's no way out. Then the obstetrician says something about having to take the head. I don't know what they're talking about. I'm lost in pain. The nurse sits me up again—pushes me up. My legs are still in stirrups. This can't be happening. This is unbelievable. This is worse than my worst imaginings of anything. They wheel in a stretcher. There are now about four people—fiddling with instruments, picking things up, each one gasping over the mess between my legs, each one being told by the first that the baby's gone—what baby? All I know is there's something HUGE stuck up me and NO ONE CAN GET IT OUT! IT'S IMPOSSIBLE TO

GET IT OUT! There's a saw-looking thing—are they going to cut through my pelvic bone? Thank God, they're going to have to knock me out. I scream: "Please knock me out!" They've got me sitting up and my legs are up in the air strapped up in those stirrups and I've got to push. But I can't push because my body isn't there, it's mashed up from the waist down and there are no muscles and there's this huge, huge, huge thing inside of the mashed me and it can never come out of me. I'm inside my head and my head floats away. The noise is loud, deafening me, but a long way off and I'm in a cave and it's pitch black and the walls are rough. I know there's an entrance somewhere here—who's blocked it off? I've got to get to the tunnel on the other side. I know there's a light there that I've got to get to, but they won't let me through. I'm aware there's someone in here with me—someone very small and to my right—but I have no idea who. Let me through! I know someone's on the other side of the entrance—it's got to be here—but they won't let me find it and they won't let me through. I'm back on the table. I open my eyes and I see this ENORMOUS set of garden shears—the man has them. I scream "NO!!!" and I push with every fiber of my being. It's OUT. OH, IT'S OUT. "It's a GIRL!" What's a girl? What the hell are you talking about? And I'm looking at her. The doctor's holding her up, she's staring at me—staring into my soul—and she sighs—this one, big sigh. She has a look on her face that says, "Well, that took you long enough." The doctor puts her on my chest and says: "Here's your daughter" and she's all bloody and she's got this extra purple head—one huge purple dome rising up and out of the left-hand side of her head and I think she's the most beautiful two-purple-headed baby I've ever seen. It's daylight and I feel like I've literally entered a new life. It's raining lightly. It's cold for summer. I go to take a shower. I see my face in the mirror and I look like a stranger, a stranger who's been to hell and back. It's all so surreal and I realize that I am in shock.

Clinician's Reaction

Nicole's story in many ways shows how what can start out as a low stress experience can change at the flick of a switch. Having a baby is a life-altering experience and in Nicole's case, she dissociated from her body and describes a "near death experience" but could not find the entrance to the tunnel. Something happened to her that gave her super-human strength to push her daughter through the birth canal. She does not describe any interpersonal connection with any of the providers; they are taking from her but not giving anything back to her, especially in the form of empathic connection. The nurse was defensive and did not speak out very loudly to the physicians. Nicole's dissociation, where she left her body, is the mind's protective ability to remove her from a life-threatening experience. Events were happening but it felt like she was outside of her body. When her daughter was born, she is elated as well as in shock; as she looks into the mirror, she sees that she has changed and at that moment she has no idea how true those words were. She had seen the other side and would need, in my opinion, mental health care to process the events and be able to integrate the experience in a way that is congruent with her strength and sense of self.

Mother's Reaction

Pure horror, is all that can be said. In this instance, such a birth would be automatic professional referral for help for Nicole. Yet at her pace and at her wellness quotient. Yes, these kinds of births do happen, and in this day and age cannot be assigned to the "Here is your baby, now be grateful and move on" category. Nicole, via good support, care and therapy, will be able to recover and love her beautiful baby. In talking to Nicole, I would gently suggest that she begin to write her story down by hand, rather than on a computer. There is power and healing in the act of writing. As this can be done in a measured way. At the pace of the writer. At home. So safe, so private. Then "post" these papers into a beautiful storage box. And then return to the writings or simply post more, as the need arises. Writing means that the invasive thoughts are anchored down. And the writing can be events related, "letters" to those involved, and even assigning different colored paper to help. Nowadays there would be an expectation that reviewing the birth would happen. My thought here too goes to the health professionals involved, how is their self-care too?

Helplessness (Sherri's Story)

Sherri was a primipara, married, and in her twenties. She labored at home for 16 hours before she headed to the hospital with her husband. A vaginal exam revealed she was barely dilated. Sherri eventually agreed to some demerol and that helped her to doze and rest and she then dilated to 4 cm in the process. Her labor was becoming very intense. In Sherri's words:

> We tried all sorts of "comfort options." The bath was very nice, but coming out felt terrible. The cold air on my wet body made the contractions come on so strong and fast, I couldn't stand it. My doula kept saying: "These are good contractions because they're bringing the baby," and I swear I wanted to hit her. We tried a birthing ball and laughing gas, but I found neither to be especially helpful. I remember thinking that labor was total hell just about then. I lost all my reserve and was crying out. I was thinking that this must sound so very alarming but I couldn't stop myself. By then my husband had gone to take a nap and my doula was back on duty. She had this trick of placing her fingers in a circle around my head and pressing. This was supposed to be some kind of relaxation or acupressure device, but the truth is I found it to be annoying. But the nurse on duty then was just wonderful. Her name was Denise, and while I remember all the different nurses who were there that night, hers is the only name I remember.

During each contraction, she would rub my back at just the right place, at the right moment, and with the right pressure.

But finally—despite the help of this kind nurse—I couldn't take it anymore. I gave up and asked for an epidural. Everyone tried to dissuade me, and I insisted.

It feels like things began to go wrong after I'd given in and asked for that epidural. It was a relief to be free of pain for a while. I was still feeling positive that I would finish dilating by early morning and then be well rested for the pushing stage.

But when my doctor came to visit early in the morning, I was given another vaginal exam, and this one showed that I'd stop dilating at 9 centimeters. A lip had formed on the cervix. Now I was starting to get anxious. I was ordered not to move about anymore, lest I make the swelling lip even worse.

From that moment onward, I felt like I was somebody's science experiment. Nothing was in my control anymore. All I could do was to lie there and accept whatever course of action was offered. (This feeling of helplessness was significant. It is as if this was a turning point and once my spirits fell, so too did my labor stop proceeding.) The doctor first decided that maybe breaking my water would help. I had a lot of fluid to lose and the nurse that was supposed to be looking after me complained that I was making too big a mess. I was so humiliated. Time passed by. There was another shift change. A new nurse came in and I had yet another vaginal exam. No progress. Now my doctor tried adding pitocin to my IV. It didn't help. The baby began trying to move upward and dilation began to regress.

I was getting very frustrated by now. My doula tried to comfort me and said, "At least you don't have to have internal fetal monitoring." A few minutes later, the doctor ordered internal fetal monitoring. I felt like there were too many wires and tubes attached to me, I just couldn't stand it. Clearly the baby didn't like it either. He moved around a lot, and the wires kept slipping off. Of course, this showed up as an irregular heartbeat. The doctor then gave up on the internal monitoring, but had the nurse look closely at the external fetal monitor. More time passed. The nurse looked very concerned each time she looked at the tape, and she would leave the room and come back and repeat the process, but she wouldn't tell me anything.

At that time, I knew that something was going very wrong, but it was still a complete shock when a complete stranger walked in and told me she had to perform a cesarean section on me right away. I asked if there was no other choice and she said there was no choice. (I don't even remember the name of this surgeon and I don't want to. Imagine not wanting to know the name of the person who delivered your child.)

I mentally gave up. I signed the forms they shoved under my nose and I just figured nothing mattered anymore. I let them shave me and attach a catheter, and it was humiliating, but I just didn't have the strength to deal with anything anymore. The tears started falling and I just didn't care.

I could feel my emotional self retracting inward into my shell. Suddenly it was as if there was a clear glass wall between the world and me. It was like watching it all happening on television. I remember my doctor rushing in to be there and as I was being pushed into the operating room, she asked if I was okay. I said I wasn't okay, and she said that once I saw the baby, I wouldn't care how he'd gotten there.

I'd seen an episode of M★A★S★H once where they showed the experience through the eyes of a soldier being wheeled in on a stretcher to an army hospital. What I experienced seemed very similar, like I was watching television, and none of this was really happening to me. The operating room nurses came close to my face and introduced themselves, and it looked like a camera was zooming in and out. But it had no impact on me, because it didn't seem real anymore. The anesthetist was giving us a play-by-play of what was happening (the way he talked seemed like he was telling me about a football game). If he said anything encouraging, I don't really remember it. I know my husband was holding my hand and encouraging me and I can still remember some of the exact words he'd used, but at the time, they had no impact at all, because I was so far gone, I may as well not have been there. I can even remember hearing the words, and thinking that they seemed to be coming from very far away. No one on the other side of the curtain bothered to talk to me (or maybe they did, but I can't remember). The surgeon and her assistants were joking among themselves. They were trying to guess if it would be a boy or girl, and the surgeon said it must be a boy because he was causing so much trouble. I felt like I didn't matter anymore. My presence wasn't needed there. I'd failed at laboring, my body was impeding the whole process.

Again, in hindsight I believe that there is significance to this feeling and that the operating staff could have acted with more sensitivity. When a woman gives birth vaginally, she is usually encouraged and still treated as if she is the one doing the birthing. When a baby is extracted via cesarean, the mother is completely disconnected from her body and treated like an object. I've heard it said that because the cesarean is an emergency procedure, emotions have to take second seat to making sure that the job is done safely. But if my surgeon had enough energy to yammer her mouth off and joke away to her cohorts, then how difficult would it have been for her to say a few encouraging words to me instead? How difficult would it have been just to say "You're doing great, mom, your baby is almost here"? It was my body that they were cutting open, and they should have treated me, the owner, with more respect.

When my son was extracted, the surgeon called out that it was a boy. I can still remember my exact thoughts at this moment. If I could put them into words they might sound something like: "Oh no! This is too overwhelming and I can't handle it." And I started crying afresh. There was no euphoria. There was none of that motherly bliss that I'd seen in the pictures. There was just exhaustion and shock. All I could catch was a quick glimpse of him before they carried him off to be examined. I heard the "baby crew" call out "All clear here." I knew then that my baby was okay, but I'd barely even seen him. Someone (my husband?) held him close to my head, but all I could see was the side of his head and his ear, and that was through my peripheral vision. I tried to reach up to touch him, but the blood pressure monitor restricted my motion. I think I complained about it, but I don't remember if anybody answered.

Then suddenly I was left alone in the recovery room. I had a fleeting view of my doctor leaving and pulling off her operating room mask and headgear. My husband was gone. The baby was gone. Someone told me they'd be taking my son somewhere to get warmed and undergo more tests. I don't remember exactly what the reason was. I do remember feeling a certain sense of surprise at the words "your son." I remember various people congratulated me, and I honestly thought "What for?" I was shivering uncontrollably, and eventually someone had the sense to cover me with a warm blanket.

I later learned that apparently, my husband had been told he had to fill out some forms, and that it was my doula that was holding MY baby in the corridor. To this day, I feel resentment about being left alone like that. Why was my doula—a complete stranger—given the privilege of holding my son before me? Would it have been too much to at least have granted me that? And why couldn't my husband stay with me in the recovery room. What paperwork was so pressing that it couldn't wait a few more minutes?

Clinician's Reaction

It is so hard to listen to the stories of women who are experiencing PTSD secondary to birth trauma and in so many ways you are missing the whole other reality of the other participants at the birth. What is often missing is, as Sherri described, that she felt as though she, as a person, was not even given any consideration. She shares how she felt it would have helped her if the surgeon had just acknowledged her and given her some encouragement rather than talking with the surgical nurses and assistants. She is going through a life-altering experience and she had disconnected from her body and the room, basic human survival skills. What happens during these episodes in the birth process when things do not go as expected? I would imagine that each participant is processing based on their own reality and the stress levels are maximum . . . how do we protect and care for the woman who is experiencing the trauma? How do we help all the members of the team, including the mother, feel connected and empathically held? As we know, everyone in that delivery room was in some sort of panic, traumatic state. As Cheryl described and named in some future research, which we will discuss in a later chapter, it is truly a "failure to rescue" that occurs, and the trust that is often automatically given to health care providers by women who are pregnant and birthing is ruptured and the reality of that woman altered.

Mother's Reaction

"Boy, oh Boy!" This story strikes at the heart of the "It's a day at the office" attitudes of health professionals! Surely, some acts of kindness towards Sherri would have made all the difference. The newborn should never ever be given to anyone else to hold, if at all possible—to have placed this baby on Sherri's chest would have made all the difference. While it is an emergency, the woman is seeing it all in slow motion, hence the ability to "see it all so very, very clearly." A woman in labor is in a timeless zone and is acutely aware of everything going on around her, picking up the stress, the concern and the actions of everyone. It is the working environment for the medical staff, HOWEVER, for many it is a first time in the setting. NOTHING should be assumed. Gentle communication is paramount. Sherri was prepared for birth, clung to the goodness happening around her: Denise, the duty nurse, and her husband. Sherri can be assured that she is not alone, she will get better—it is for her to be strong, communicate to those who she wishes to, work through her anger and love her son!

Postpartum Hemorrhage (Michelle's Story)

Michelle is a pediatrician with three young children. There were no contractions with these births. Now full term carrying her fourth child, Michelle started to have contractions every 5 minutes. She and her husband went to the hospital and she was 4 cm dilated. The OB hospitalist checked with her private OB and she was discharged in "false labor." That same day her membranes ruptured and she started having contractions every minute. After a frantic drive to the hospital, she was rushed in a stretcher to the delivery room as the baby was crowning in the hallway en route and the daughter was born there. Michelle's story continues in her own words:

> I was left lying in the delivery room, torn open with the placenta still inside until my obstetrician finally arrived. When he finally sauntered in, I asked: "Where were you?" and he answered: "Oh, I'm not allowed to come until they call me." He yanked the placenta out of my body so hard I bit my lip to keep from crying out. When he was sewing up the tear and at one point I exclaimed, "Ouch, that hurts! I can feel that!" He replied: "Aww, that's just the deepest one" and kept right on going. He disappeared as soon as he was done.
>
> My baby and I were finally taken upstairs. I had no idea then that my nightmare had only just begun. Around 5am I hemorrhaged. One minute, I felt weak, dizzy, and unable to verbalize anything other than "Somebody help me, I just don't feel well." The next thing I know, there was blood everywhere, spurting out of my body, blood clots the size of frying pans shooting out. I thought I was going to die. Panicky nurses and doctors rushed into the room, the crash cart was wheeled in, my baby was wheeled out. My husband was shouting: "Please, somebody, get our doctor!" We

were desperate to see a familiar face in the midst of the most frightening moment of our lives. I was being stuck everywhere for an IV, but I had no strength to flinch or even move. Another hospitalist OB came in. I was told that there would be a "procedure," and then my legs were forced open and she shoved her entire arm into my uterus and pulled out clots three times and I screamed and screamed and screamed. The pain was unbearable, and I felt like I was being raped and murdered.

Afterwards, I was cleaned up and hooked up to IV fluids and pitocin. No one ever came in afterwards to debrief, counsel, or even explain to me why, how, or what happened. When my husband walked down the hall to get coffee, he was met by other new mothers at the doorways of their rooms, asking if his wife was okay after what they had heard. They were the only ones who would ever ask if I was all right. We saw the doctor on his rounds the next morning. The first words out of his mouth were: "Well, you doctors make the worst patients." The second words out of his mouth were to ask if I was up for an early discharge. At that point, I couldn't even sit up. He was defensive and completely insensitive, and made more eye contact with the chart than with me. I never saw or heard from him again.

Subsequent to such a horrific birth experience, I developed PTSD. My family and I have suffered and continue to suffer on a daily basis and struggle to recover emotionally. The careless, uncompassionate, and utterly callous attitude of the staff and physicians was so atrocious. Women such as myself entrusted our lives and that of our newborn infants to your care, and you betrayed it.

Two years later after her traumatic birth Michelle still is not practicing pediatrics because as she said: "Too many moms and babies, entails rounding on the maternity ward where I delivered—collateral damage from the PTSD."

Clinician's Reaction

"Well, you doctors make the worst patients." How many of us have heard that comment, also usually including nurses too? Is this a projection onto the victim of the provider's anxiety? Although, it is in my mind based on assumptions, expectation, and fears. What makes health care providers, which is a role they assume after education and clinical practice, different than any other pregnant and/or birthing woman? Why would one believe that your professional role could influence your physiology and reproductive function? What an easy way of passing on blame. These comments cause emotional distress over and above the experience that Michelle already had and, as she shared with Cheryl, changed her career trajectory. This is another example of how the trauma experience impacts the life of the birthing woman/new mother. As we read these stories and narratives, what comes into your mind? Why and how do you think these scenarios could have been changed? What comes through loud and clear is what appears to be a lack of an advocate, an emotional support person for the woman, one who does not leave her side (and that of her husband, partner, lover) so that she is connected to the reality experience at a moment-to-moment level. Are you considering ways that these situations could have been handled differently? We also know that it is the "eye of the beholder." Some women have a vulnerability that is not clearly identified nor described in the initial OB assessment, nor are the psychosocial aspects of care often considered as a major part of the care plan. It is the individual who is experiencing the birth, and, as an individual, there is no clear trajectory for the experience. Each birth is unique and special and, in my mind, needs to be cared for that way. The woman has never had a baby before or if she has, this experience will be different as this baby is different; no two experiences are ever the same. We enter each experience with conscious and unconscious issues based on our current reality and so often, the issues are not clear or easy to describe. This is the basis of the essential nursing skill of establishing a relationship with our patients and respecting the trust that we are so willingly given by our patients.

Mother's Reaction

Michelle approached birth as a mother, not as a doctor. Her treatment was shameful. Again, in her traumatic birth is clear evidence of the lack of empathy, and the many assumptions made. Michelle is strong, articulate, and will recover. By practicing self-care, doing activities in which she finds great reward, and within the safety of counseling, she will come back stronger for this. While this trauma was quite unnecessary, it is part of her life story. But she will recover.

Preeclampsia/HELLP (Anne's Story)

Anne was married, in her thirties, and after IVF was lucky enough to conceive her first child. Here is her story of her traumatic experience of preeclampsia and HELLP (life-threatening pregnancy syndrome of Hemolysis, Elevated Liver enzymes, and Low Platelet count) in her own words.

> This first pregnancy was wonderful, healthy, and a true blessing. I was fortunate enough to experience the onset of labor, and was allowed to attempt to deliver naturally without medications. I greatly appreciated the flexibility that my midwives and doctor showed in allowing me to experience labor; I had already been told that my pelvis was unlikely to pass a 9 pound baby. Unfortunately, after 22 hours of trying, the baby was brow presenting and I developed a fever that was suspected to indicate a uterine infection. An emergency C-section was performed, which I was able to partake in (although barely, since I nearly passed out on the table from exhaustion and fever).
>
> A day after my delivery, my feet started to swell to the point of distortion. I repeatedly mentioned my concerns to the midwives, doctors, and hospital nurses and was given the canned response: "Some women hold water and

swell after a C-section." Two days after my feet started swelling, I began to have difficulty breathing. No one had any explanation, except for possible trapped gas. By that evening, I was definitely having pain in my chest/diaphragm area and once again mentioned my problem to yet another nurse. She decided to take a blood test, and half an hour later, six doctors rushed in and strapped me to a seizure padded cart. Apparently I had developed postpartum HELLP syndrome and my liver was swelling into my diaphragm. I was given such a large bolus of magnesium sulfate I lost my vision, sense of balance, and most fine motor limb movement. The high blood pressure followed. I was kept in the hospital for eight days, and I did not develop milk until I returned home. The blood pressure resolved fairly quickly. I went on to enjoy my first foray into motherhood, and was able to leave most of my life-threatening experience behind me. Or so it seemed.

Two years after this life-threatening experience, we conceived again via IVF. A nurse at the IVF clinic had concerns about my previous experience with HELLP syndrome. At the first appointment for the 6-week ultrasound, we learned that there were two implanted embryos. My blood pressure had risen from my normal $^{116}/_{65}$ to $^{145}/_{90}$, and my anxieties about a repeat performance with preeclampsia were heightened. At 8 weeks, a second ultrasound showed that the second fetus was failing. Ultimately, we lost the twin, after which my blood pressure dropped down to normal. Looking back, I can see that the underlying anxiety about my first experience pervaded my entire pregnancy. I did not feel the joy I had with the first, or the connection to the child in-utero. I had dreams where the beautifully decorated birthing rooms at the hospital were dark and sinister. Recalling the hospital brought up feelings of sadness, injustice, and fear.

By 5 months, my blood pressure started to creep up. By 7 months, I was diagnosed with preeclampsia and placed on permanent left-side prone bed rest and was monitored frequently for blood pressure, platelet counts, and protein in the urine, all indicators of the onset of HELLP. I appreciated the attentiveness to my health this time around, but it did not provide peace of mind for me. I developed HELLP in the blink of an eye after the first pregnancy, without most of these early warning signs. No one could reassure me that it would not happen again. Bed rest had its pros and cons: I got more rest and a reprieve from working, but I also was not available to my first child. My husband was under enormous pressure to be everything both for my toddler and the household. I counted down these last days that I would have alone with my beloved first born, and was unable to enjoy any of them with him. I was sad but resigned.

By 34 weeks gestation, I was in and out of the hospital and doctors' offices every other day and my blood pressure and weight gain (water retention) were out of control. My blood pressure had gone from $^{116}/_{65}$ to nearly $^{200}/_{100}$, and the readings were like a yo-yo . . . dangerously labile. Even worse, the swelling had triggered severe rhinitis and I could not breathe well through my nose. I was not allowed to take any medications to assist with the rhinitis, due to the blood pressure issue. At 35 weeks and 6 days, my routine trip to the hospital for overnight monitoring became my delivery date. I was glad to be getting this hellish pregnancy over with, but the elation disappeared when I learned I would once again have to be dosed with magnesium sulfate. In addition, I was forced to wear electrical compression stockings up to my thighs due to concern over clotting (I had experienced a superficial clot in my arm prior to conception). During the surgery my nose was swollen shut due to the rhinitis and my lungs felt numb from the anesthesia drugs. This feeling of suffocation was increasing my anxiety to the level of panic, and the anesthesiologist was kind enough to give me cold oxygen flow and some additional drug cocktails to increase my comfort level. They delivered my preterm baby girl, and allowed me to see her, and then went to work on finishing up the C-section. I heard the doctors and nurses discussing how much I was bleeding due to the mag, and they were laughing at how difficult it was to sew me up with all of the seeping. I also heard them say how calcified my placenta was. I tried to tune out their disturbing analysis by singing country music songs, which they also found quite amusing.

Things went downhill from there, in regards to my mental state. My baby was in the NICU and I could not interact with her. There were too many wires between the two of us, and we were tangled up in IVs. I began to detach from her, knowing my husband would be there for her, and focused on my own predicament. My blood pressure continued to hover at $^{200}/_{100}$ and we waited anxiously for the HELLP to manifest again. I did not sleep for nearly three days in a row, because of my difficulty breathing, my discomfort with feeling drugged, and because of the ever-moving compression leggings. Those stockings in combination with the feeling of suffocation due to the nose/throat swelling made me feel as if I was being tortured. My legs would move up and down, up and down, up and down. I was supposed to "rest" under these conditions? I was molested by nursing staff and doctors every hour, as I swelled and developed odd reflex behavior in my ankles. My oxygen levels dropped due to the difficulty in breathing. I developed body tremors, and my panic was such that I was afraid to close my eyes. I fought sleep at all cost, begging my mother to stay with me to help me reduce my panic to a reasonable level of mere anxiety. I did not want my husband with me, as I knew he could not help me through the crisis I was facing. My primal instinct was to turn to my mother, like a child who wants to crawl back into the womb where it is safe. At the same time, I tried to maintain my identity as a mother myself. But, the one time I was able to hold my own baby, my blood pressure shot up and the nurses ripped her out of my arms due to fear that I would drop her. I was shown little compassion. This was the only time I cried during the whole miserable affair—I felt I had earned the right to at least hold my baby and to try to bond with her. I was in a complete state of despair, but there was a silver lining: at least I did not develop HELLP syndrome again, just preeclampsia and went on to be diagnosed with PTSD.

Clinician's Reaction

The "silver lining" was PTSD versus HELLP? Again, we are hearing the story from the woman's perspective but again the health care providers are the enemy. They were not emotionally responsive, in this woman's mind and in fact she felt judged by them as she sang country songs during the closing of the cesarean incision as they discussed the bleeding situation secondary to the magnesium sulfate. Again I am struck with the individuality of experiences and how we each see things through our own eyes, perceptions, and embedded realities. We know that health care professionals suffer from compassion fatigue, burnout, as well as vicarious traumatization (see Chapter 17), but what do we do for them? Perhaps if more attention was paid to the mental health of the care providers, we would find less of this rupture in the caring relationship. I don't know but as the trends of increased diagnosis of PTSD secondary to birth trauma increase, we need to look at strategies to change the dynamic.

Mother's Reaction

Simple acts of compassion and listening to her would have made all the difference to this complication in Anne's pregnancy and birth. Careful compassionate listening and acceptance of what she says would help her. Childbirth often takes turns that obstetric staff do not expect, but they must still pay attention to what mothers tell them. Mothers know themselves, even in the midst of trauma. Any effort to preserve the mothering relationship between Anne and her newborn would have turned this situation around. Proceed gently with counseling; you are strong.

Perinatal Loss/Uncaring Labor and Delivery Staff (Marie's Story)

Thirteen years ago Marie became the mother of triplets named Michael, Paul, and Ellen. Here is Marie's heart-wrenching story in her own words of her devastating multiple losses of her beloved children.

> At 21 plus weeks I had premature labor, and Michael was born and died. Only hours later, my CBC came back. I had gone into labor because I had maternal sepsis with a white count of 28, high bands and a bad shift to the left. I was told by the doctor that they would be delivering the remaining triplets and a hysterectomy was planned for me in the morning. I remember every detail in excruciating, agonizing, and astonishing clarity. I desperately needed a nurse. I was terrified, in shock, in severe emotional distress, had some physical pain and felt tremendous guilt. In that moment, I did not believe I would survive the deaths of all my babies. The grief of it would surely kill me and if the grief didn't, I would surely finish the job. I was oozing ache. The profound depth of my despair, I could never have

imagined. Not one nurse spoke to me, not one. They abandoned me to labor alone and left me without care of any kind, only coming in and tweaking up the pitocin and then literally running from the room. Twice, alone except for my husband, I delivered something or someone in the bed. I was terrified and screamed to my husband, "Is it a baby?" "It's red and bloody," my husband said. "Is it moving? Any arms or legs?" I asked. "I don't know," my husband said with panic, "I'll get the nurse." The nurse seemed irritated at having to come in the room at all. "It's only the placenta from the first abortion," she carelessly said. "I didn't have an abortion. I had a baby, his name was Michael." I told her. Michael had lived for over an hour gasping and blue but was alive all the same. She removed his placenta and literally ran from the room. Many things about this hospitalization were horrendous and traumatizing and a case study in how not to do things and I could have healed from everything else that happened and gone on and even the deaths of my beloved, wanted children. But what happened when I delivered my precious beloved Ellen has impacted my life in as profound a way I could not have imagined. I have re-run the trauma of it many thousands of times in astonishing detail and the memory of it is burned on my brain and it will stay with me forever.

When it was time to deliver Ellen, I had the tap water at the bedside to baptize her as no chaplain was available, after all, premature babies this age don't last long and I wanted to be prepared. Right after she was born, I calmly requested, "Please, give me my baby." There were three people with "RN" engraved on their nametag in the room but they did not move or speak or acknowledge my request. There was deafening silence in the room. I repeated it several more times in a calm, polite, controlled and rational manner. No one moved, no one spoke, no one even looked in my direction. Instead, the "nurse" put my sweet baby girl, Ellen, on a cold metal counter next to the sink to die like she was discarding a piece of garbage. Then, over the course of the next 11 minutes I repeatedly and with increased escalation screamed for her at the top of my lungs over and over and over again and no one handed Ellen to me. I sobbed and begged and reached out yet no one responded. They stood like deer in the headlights, immobile, like statues, doing nothing but standing there when they could be handing my baby to me. "She'll die!" I screamed, "Give her to me!!!" I could see her. I raised up on my elbows and rough, uncaring hands pushed me down into the bed saying "You're busy!" "I'm not too busy to hold my baby! She'll die! Ellen, Ellen, Ellen!!!!" My baby was dying unbaptized, gasping and blue and cold on a hard metal surface and I only had moments or minutes to be her mother to comfort and to hold her and to love her and talk to her while she died and the "nurses" absolutely refused to hand her to me. Was she in pain? Did it hurt to die? She needed her mother! I could not get up because I was delivering another baby, Paul, or I surely would have bolted from the bed. I was beyond desperate for her. There was nothing in this world I had ever wanted more or will ever want more. I was spiraling into a hopeless, cold black hole so deep, I knew I would never climb out and I knew it was something that I would never be able to recover from. If I could have dissociated and jumped out of my body to go to her, I would have. After 11 agonizing minutes, the doctor said, "Give her the baby!" But it was already too late, Ellen was dead, cold and alone. She died on a cold hard metal counter top, in pain, and without the warmth and love of her mother. The other babies lived for over an hour but Ellen's death was expedited by the "nurses." Also, she was unbaptized, maybe regulated to limbo or hell according to my parents' religious beliefs. The doctor then handed Paul, who was still alive and kicking to me and I did baptize him in time. Michael and Paul, two babies in heaven, poor Ellen in hell/limbo.

Decent human behavior? Not on the "nurses" radar. How would I explain to my own parents the gross lack of parenting I displayed when I was unable to baptize my own baby in time? Maybe the truth was that I had not fought hard enough, screamed loud enough, although I could not imagine what else I could have done. I had only 11 minutes to be a mother while Ellen was alive and those "nurses" cruelly and intentionally denied me that. I've forgiven them, but cannot forget and they continue to remain monsters to me.

Clinician's Reaction

Oh, how I hope that this story is never repeated. What a sad commentary on death and dying in the obstetrical arena. True, most of the time the experience of birthing is warm, happy, and exhausting but there are untoward events that occur during the "normal process" and as health care providers we need to be prepared and ready for those events when they do occur. Marie so clearly describes what the experience felt like for her, she can forgive but cannot forget. There is a basic reality, and it is the golden rule, "do unto others." What happened during Marie's experience? Where were the human care and concern from the staff as she was birthing her babies and watching them die, her hopes and dreams shattered? All the plans she had imagined during her pregnancy, her role as a mother, watching her children grow, all ended that day and she did not feel as though anyone helped her.

In so many ways we are a death-denying culture; we tend to isolate and ignore issues pertaining to unhappy endings. Is it because "there but for the grace of God go I"? What is wrong with speaking from the heart and caring for Marie and women like her as we would want someone to care for us? Again, much needs to be done to support the staff in the obstetrical divisions when it comes to untoward endings. How does the system provide emotional support to them? The purpose of this book is to increase awareness on the part of health care providers and health systems. These women's stories are real and powerful, take this opportunity to meditate upon what you as a health professional need to do for yourself to help you integrate the sad experiences that you encounter in your clinical life and vow to take care of yourself: emotionally, physically, and spiritually. That self-care will allow you to be there for your patients in their hours of need.

Mother's Reaction

Marie's story is familiar in many ways, and she is not alone. Good support would be empathic, and let Marie lead the way. Support would not lead to judgment of or challenge to Marie's reaction. If she has not already done so, she would find a listening ear with one of the many baby loss support groups. She and her husband need to keep talking and to use every ounce of strength, resolve, and determination to regain their former selves, and perhaps "feed back" to the institution where this occurred. They must be strong.

Preterm Birth/NICU (Christine's Story)

The following is one mother's story of her traumatic experience of her preterm infant's birth and stay in the NICU. This mom had participated in Beck's (2004a; 2004b) earlier studies on birth trauma and its resulting PTSD.

Christine started her story with the telling fact that it had been eight years since her traumatic birth experience. It took her that length of time to be able to manage writing her story about her preterm birth. In Christine's own words:

> I was pregnant with my first baby and I planned to have a home birth. When I was seven months pregnant, I started to bleed and I was rushed to the hospital at around 7am. The first doctor said I would be having a cesarean that morning. Forms were given to me to sign. Drips and monitoring devices were set up. I insisted that they at least try to find out what was going on and as long as there was no fetal distress, we would wait and see. A thorough ultrasound showed nothing amiss. The blood loss had slowed but hospital staff insisted that I was in labor so I reluctantly signed forms which basically said they could do whatever they thought was necessary to my premature baby. If I didn't sign, they said they would not be able to care for him.
>
> When they were putting on a fetal scalp monitor clip, I passed a massive blood clot. I had three blood transfusions and I possibly had a near-death experience. I felt like I was floating above my body and I saw everyone running around me. Throughout the day there were staff changes, different people coming in to check on me and on the baby, etc. Luckily for me, other women came to the hospital who needed emergency cesareans so I just waited. The original doctor went off and I had a new doctor that evening who decided my baby should be born now. I was taken to a delivery room. I had an epidural and syntocinon (a variation of pitocin). I was fully dilated and the doctor said I had 20 minutes to deliver the baby myself then

he left. I had two great midwives helping me delivery. One of them said to me: "Push this baby out or he will come back" and she made a scissors sign with her fingers. My baby was delivered by the midwives. Then the doctor came back in and said, "Oh, it's out." I held my baby for about 2 seconds then he was taken away and my trauma began.

My trauma is not so much about the birth as it is about the next 25 days when my baby was in the neonatal intensive care unit. I cried for 25 days. The staff couldn't work out why I was so upset all the time. I had a tiny baby, stuck in an incubator. I couldn't hold him. I couldn't breastfeed him. And they wondered why I was so upset! I stayed in the maternity ward for two nights then I was sent home—with no baby.

At home, I felt so far away from my baby. I had lots of support. My husband was fantastic. My mother came to stay and do all the housework, meals, and everyday stuff. I saw a lactation consultant. The midwives were great and kept coming to see me. But I was so devastated that I couldn't have my baby. I felt so robbed and so useless and so helpless. I couldn't stop crying. The NICU staff sent me to see a chaplain who asked me—was my marriage OK? Did I have financial problems? How did I think all the other mothers of premature babies were coping? They weren't crying all the time. What was wrong with me? Did I believe in God? This barrage of questions was unhelpful and, in my opinion, unnecessary and even irrelevant. I was sent off for a blood test. They decided I must have been anemic. I wasn't. Even the person who did the blood test asked me a question and when I said "I don't know," she replied: "We don't know much, do we?" I was severely traumatized and medical staff were being rude to me.

All this time I was expressing breast milk to feed my baby by nasogastric tube. I bought my own breast pump attachments so I had them to use whenever I wanted to. The hospital ones were not always available. One day someone stole my attachments which was devastating to me. Little things like that, I just couldn't handle. Finally after 25 agonizing days, after several overnight stints, and after rooming in for the last few nights, I was able to take my baby home. At that time I didn't realize the effect that this experience had had on me. I thought I was OK. I thought once I got home, everything would be perfect. Looking back now I realize a lot of my coping mechanisms were shattered and my perspective was radically altered. This led to an extremely tumultuous year. I finally got referred to a mental health specialist and was diagnosed with PTSD. I cannot emphasize enough how important it is to have support from helpful people after a traumatic experience. I found out the hard way that not getting that support can have devastating consequences.

Clinician's Reaction

Christine's story is very common in that mothers who birth premature babies often experience postpartum depression in addition to some having PTSD. The striking thing with Christine's story is again, how clear her memory was of an event that had occurred more than eight years before she wrote her narrative for Cheryl's study. The memories are clear and the feelings are like it had happened yesterday. What an impact the NICU experience had on Christine! Her crying was a symptom that had meaning but rather than try to find the meaning, her behavior was judged and devalued. She was told that none of the other NICU moms were crying all the time. I wonder how many of those mothers were crying but no one was really asking them how they felt either. Christine had just delivered a premature baby. She began her journey of becoming a mother in a NICU where she felt criticized, judged and was clearly not seen as a unique individual with an experience that had only happened to her. She was not like everyone else, nor should she be. Each person has their own way of dealing with stress, loss, and grief. She had to learn to parent in a sort of fish bowl, the NICU, where she probably felt she was being watched by others all the time. An additional event that caused even more grief was the loss of her pumping equipment in the NICU, a personal assault added to the loss of the experience of birthing and mothering that she had hoped and dreamed of. Again, this is her story but one hears the continual theme that is present in these women's narratives of feeling uncared for, of feeling judged, devalued, and in many ways "not seen." We need to consider how the system and the professions can take these stories and change policy and procedure. The sad part is that we cannot make people learn how to feel!

Mother's Reaction

The NICU experience can be turned to good or increase the trauma. Sadly, for Christine, it was the latter, with the focus being on the well-being of the baby, and the prolonged shock of 25 days of waiting, waiting to be that mother. Her tears were eloquent. Their message was missed. However, you say both your mother and husband were fantastic, what a close unit you are! As with many mothers, she keenly felt her trauma, but the staff did not appreciate it. The dynamics of NICU have changed, and the voices of parents need to be heeded. Good support will help resolve Christine's trauma, and help her continue as a mother.

Childhood Sexual Abuse (Kerry's Story)

One mother, who had participated in Beck and Watson's (2010) study of subsequent childbirth after a previous birth trauma, courageously shared her story of her childhood sexual abuse. In her own words:

> I suppose I need to begin by saying that as a victim of childhood sexual abuse (a constant thing perpetuated by my father), I came into motherhood already plagued, unbeknownst to me, by PTSD. Pregnancy and labor and delivery exacerbated an already present issue. My subsequent experiences

were as much a symptom of where I was in my healing journey as they were symptomatic of treatment by hospital staff. Telling my birthing stories always begins with the abuse and is told from that standpoint. I guess when I think about my third birth, the one that stands out in my mind is the dread and the panic. It wasn't like the pregnancy wasn't planned, it was planned. I was in the shower when the panic hit. I had been thinking about the new baby, due in the summer, when it hit me. In seven short months I was going to have to endure labor and delivery again. I literally bent over in fear. I couldn't breathe. I felt sick to my stomach. I panicked. I contacted a friend of mine and in an email told her my struggles learning I would have to give birth again. My friend cut and pasted what I had written and prefaced it with, "How unspeakable the crime that robs you of the joy of childbirth." Here is what she sent me:

> I am so sorry. Inhuman, diabolical, filthy sin. If you ever, ever wonder in your weak moments if there is enough evidence to "prove" what you know is true really happening—just read the following as you wrote it.

>> But what about the pain and the out of control and the mistreatment?
>> I feel like it is an intrusion by other people.
>> It feels, well, it reminds me of the abuse.
>> My body but not MY body.
>> Other people's hands and opinions and wills where only mine should be.
>> I must suck it up and endure it until it is over.
>> They weren't 'horrible' but they were the stuff of nightmares
>> Some man pushing his will and not even discussing it with me.
>> And the pain, I lost it from the pain this last time, that was embarrassing to me.
>> I won't feel like a piece of meat.
>> Not knowing who to trust (and not trusting anyone).
>> Clean up after it's over, yuck.

I replied to my friend, there it was in black and white on my computer screen, my words, and I couldn't ignore them. The abuse. Labor and delivery mirrored the sexual abuse. I was overwhelmed at this realization but I didn't really know what to do with it. What could I do? I was pregnant. There was no way out other than labor and delivery. When I caught myself thinking first about demanding a c-section, no, that won't work—it's more invasive than vaginal delivery, and then about having an abortion I decided to take my despair seriously. I wasn't concerned that I'd actually have an abortion. I am morally opposed to most reasons for abortion and, more than anything, I WANTED this baby. He was a part of me, a part of my family and we wouldn't be complete without him. But if my brain was so tormented by the possibility of another labor and delivery that it was desperately looking for options to get out of it, then I needed to take this seriously.

I think that if my births were absolutely perfect, I would still have problems due to the other people—doctors and nurses—that must touch me to help. Honestly, I get those same feelings just from a routine pap smear or if a guy stares at me too long at the supermarket. I feel vulnerable (vulnerable, that's it in a nutshell), out of control, and unable to protect myself. In a very real way, that is what labor and delivery are. The thing that makes this so hard for someone like me is that those feelings of vulnerability were exploited, through the abuse, for so long in my life that I automatically associate vulnerability with abuse.

For my third birth, I was checked in and pronounced "in labor" and given the option of having my water broken. I remember that my midwife came into my room and that as soon as I saw her, I was overwhelmed with relief that we'd done it. I'd managed to get to the hospital on time with my doula in tow and my midwife was there and available. Already, this birth was looking far more positive than my first two. My midwife offered me a choice to have my water broken or not. I felt panicked and an overwhelming amount of pressure to answer correctly but, now, I knew that panic was my biggest enemy and that I had to fight my way clear. I realized that everything that I let "slide" would come back to haunt me afterwards. So, instead of shutting down, I ask her to leave and to give me time to "discuss it" with my husband. I already knew that I didn't want her to break my water but I needed the support of my doula and my husband before I could verbalize it. So, after she left the room, I was more able to calm myself down and focus on what I wanted. I said to my doula: "If she breaks my water, that could make my contractions harder, right?" The doula said: "Yes, that is a possibility." I said: "Well, I don't want that, so we won't do it." I honestly believed that if this labor and delivery were anything like the last, we wouldn't need to do it. Everybody seemed to be in agreement with me and that let me feel as though someone had "my back," like I was really going to be able to make this decision.

I chose to labor in the tub. It was great. The warm water helped me to relax, which I had never been able to do in labor and delivery before. But, more than anything, the water felt like a giant cover, like it was hiding me from everybody else. I would be able to labor with the comfortable feeling of security and isolation without actually being isolated. The tub afforded me the opportunity to move around. I could respond to the pain. I didn't have to lie there like an animal on a slab and try not to move.

I could feel that the baby was getting closer and closer, with every push, to crowning. I was totally terrified. My pain was horrible but THAT I knew would make my present pain feel like menstrual cramps. I've tried to think of a way to describe this to my husband and the only thing that I can think of is fire. It's like you have already put your hand so close to the fire that it is burning your skin and you don't think you can stand that level of pain for any longer. You feel desperate to stop but you also know that you have to somehow find the will power to force yourself to actually put your hand into the flame and hold it there. It is pain beyond belief with the knowledge that it has to get much, much worse. And you have to do it to yourself. I'm not sure he gets it and, really, how could he?

My babies don't seem to crown once. They crown several times and each time is more horrible than the last and there is no relief in between. It is the most excruciating time of the delivery and this time was no different. I began to feel like I was losing control. I felt overwhelmed by panic. I felt like I was clutching my fists, hanging desperately onto life but coming to the end of my last breath underneath that dark sea, and where was my life jacket? Where were my rescuers? My doula had disappeared. She was at the foot of the tub taking pictures. Each flash from her camera made me feel exposed. When I'd asked her earlier what her job was as doula, she said that it was to support me and then she added that she also would take a few pictures. I figured this meant that she'd take a FEW pictures, maybe right after he was born, maybe of him, his dad and me. Not that she'd document the whole thing like it was some independent film for PBS. Right when I needed her the most, she was gone. This is the part that I am the most angry about. I was struggling, struggling, struggling. I needed a constant and steady, "I am here, you are safe" voice to help ground me, someone to help me know that I was in a safe place and that I'd be okay. Someone to give me enough encouragement to get past this final hurdle and what I got are pictures that, honestly, I don't want. And can't throw away! They're pictures of my baby's birth but also of "angry vaginas" and stuff I don't want to remember. On the one hand, sacred, on the other, humiliating. And when I look at them I can't help but remember that she wasn't with me when she took them. I feel trapped in ambivalence about these photos. I'd hired that doula so that someone would be all about ME during my labor and delivery because everybody else would be so focused on the baby and I needed someone focused on me. The doula made it about the baby but she also made it about herself. It was as if *she* was present at the birth of my child and that was what was most important. I wanted her to be present at *my* labor and delivery. I wanted that to be what was most important to her as doula. That is what I hired her for. In her defense, I am sure that I appeared calm and together and in control but, and here is where she needed her sexual abuse survivor training, abuse survivors shut down. They become quiet and non-combative. It's not that they're in control. It's that they've gone deep into survival mode like a deer before you hit it with your car. That "deer in the headlights" thing is real and I had it big time. What I wanted her to know was that I needed her more, not less, at that time. I remember that I kept thinking to myself, *Get back up here! I need you!* But I couldn't say it out loud. I was having to concentrate too hard on dealing with the pain.

About this time, the midwife said: "He has dark hair, keep pushing. You'll see him soon!" which I'm sure was meant to encourage me. Here again, you have to know your patient. My dad has dark hair so what flew through my mind was, "*Oh no! He's going to be just like my dad.*" A feeling of grief and desperation threatened to overtake me. I had to forcibly shake myself out of it, "*No, he's not! Kerry! And if you think like that, you'll never get through this. Push Kerry! He is NOT your dad!*" The midwife had just told me that, in essence, I was giving birth to a monster. How was she supposed to know that every abuse survivor worries that the abuse is genetic, that she herself will turn out to be abusive or that she'll give birth to an abuser? That those fears strike at the very heart of who she is as a person and as a mother? That such a seemingly positive statement could have such negative connotations? The midwife didn't know because she didn't ask. She didn't ask because, honestly, she probably wasn't trained to deal with that information or to know that I would take special dealings. Maybe, she had her own undealt with trauma. Clinicians need to be taught about survivors of childhood sexual abuse. We are "special needs." There are so many of us and we're being hurt by the very systems that are trying to help us.

One of the neatest things that happened afterwards while everybody else was occupied with doing the "baby stuff" was that the midwife showed me the placenta. First off, delivering the placenta was an open part of the procedure. I could easily see what the midwife was doing, how she took hold of it and waited for my body to expel it. In the past I had laid blind and dumb and mind reeling after delivery and a nurse had walked over and pressed on my abdomen hard and when I'd call out in pain she said, "Sorry, it has to be done." It was days before I realized that the doctor was removing the placenta then. This time the midwife waited for my body to let it go, no pain. Then still immersed in the bloody water, I asked to see the placenta and she showed it to me. She showed me how it worked, where the baby had been connected. I could see the blood vessels and for the first time the whole process felt like it was a normal, healthy, miraculous function of my body. Always before, labor and delivery had seemed like something that was being done TO me, like a hellish roller-coaster ride. I was strapped in and headed over the drop-off, the whole car might come completely off the tracks but there was nothing I could do but hold on and scream.

Today, 16 months after this happened, I am still amazed at that thought process. Of course, I was going "to do this." Who else was going to do it? And I'd had two babies already. But I do think that it points to the depths of my insecurity about childbirth. One thing that I'd noticed when I was a child was that when my parents got together with other adults, the talk eventually turned to two things: for my father (a war veteran) and the other men, the talk turned to the war and interestingly, to me as a small child, for my mother and the other women, the talk always turned to childbirth. It was as if, from a young age, for me the connections between the two were drawn. A man is tested through war; a woman is tested through childbirth. My dad, as abusive as he was, was considered a "good man" because he'd been a soldier and so I reasoned forward with a child's intelligence, that all that really mattered for a woman was to be strong and capable in childbirth. And I failed. In the past, with the previous two births (particularly with the one that resulted in PTSD) that is what it felt like. I failed at being a woman. I don't think I am alone in my feeling. I have a sneaking suspicion that this is pretty universal. Just as a man who "talks" under torture in a POW situations feels as though he's failed, a woman who can't "handle" tortuous situations during childbirth feels like she's failed. It is not true. But it feels true. My dad received two Purple Hearts and a Bronze Star during the war. He, by most standards, would be considered a hero. Where are my Purple Hearts? My Bronze Star? I've fought a war no less terrifying, no less destroying but there are no accolades. At least that is what it feels like. I am viewed as flawed if not downright strange that I find labor and delivery so terrifying. The medical establishment thinks that I am "mental" and I have no common ground on which to discuss my childbirth experiences with "normal" women. I know. I've tried. And that makes me feel isolated and inferior.

Clinician's Reaction

Kerry writes poignantly of her experiences of labor and delivery through the eyes of a survivor of sexual abuse. She clearly puts into words her thoughts and feelings regarding similarities and the need for health care providers to pay attention, especially in that for many survivors of abuse, childbirth can be a trigger. Simpkin and Klaus (2004), in their book *When Survivors Give Birth*, provide guidelines for professionals into understanding and healing the effects of sexual abuse and the impact on childbearing women. It is so important for obstetrical staff to be aware and cognizant that any women who comes in to their system to have a baby can have a history of physical, emotional, and/or sexual abuse, but not aware of the potential impact of pregnancy, labor, and delivery as triggers to the memories of those experiences.

Kerry clearly shares with us how she was thinking as a survivor and how the behavior of her midwife triggered her emotional responses even though she was empathic to the needs and behavior of the doula, especially with regard to taking the pictures. As she states: "You have to know your patient." It was not intentional that the doula lost the connection, but in many ways she was not focusing on what her role was during the birth, to be with the patient (Kerry), not taking pictures.

Remember to keep that focus as you care for women, "you have to know your patient," each patient is unique and special in her own way. All behavior has meaning, we just have to take the time to find out what that meaning is rather than judge, devalue, personalize, and react to it.

Mother's Reaction: The Desire to Hug

Kerry tells her story simply and beautifully. As a survivor, her trauma responses are absolutely reasonable in view of her abuse. This is NOT her fault. She can go forward in strength and courage. Thankfully, health professionals are increasingly mindful about what pre-existing trauma can mean for birthing mothers. By way of a path forward, she can tell these caregivers how it was for her, so that this does not happen again for others. For survivors, both self-awareness and articulating their needs are important.

Reflections from TABS

Upon reading these stories and also the wonderful clinician's comments, again, we are reminded why we first embarked on our journey of supporting families troubled by this devastating condition of PTSD. The stories have many threads entwining them. Allow me to name a few.

A Day at the Office

The staff here would be well advised to reframe their thinking. What is their 'office' setting will be absolutely new, overwhelming, or even frightening. What they may have seen a thousand times before also falls under this framework. Every birth situation needs to be approached with the focus on the couple, following their lead perhaps. Casualness or being blasé may cause distress, disempowerment, or even fear. For women who come to birth, it might be their first ever time to be in a hospital. Yes, even if they look like they might know better, or appear as seasoned regulars.

Where Is the Compassion?

This relates to above. Staff who display kindness, care, understanding, honesty, telling the truth, "take time"—are remembered just as clearly as the "other" in traumatic births. We were always keen to listen for these elements that did come when stories were being told. The "gems" were held dearly and gave equilibrium. Sadly, it was the lack of compassion that featured all too well. Therefore, the style of the staff members had a great influence in swinging the pendulum.

Be Wary of Silence

Looking into the eyes would be good. Therefore embarking on forms of non-verbal communication is imperative, even flash cards with words as simple, "Yes," "No," "Wait," and "I have a question," would be so empowering. Check in with the support people present.

Acts of Kindness, Display Your Own Humanity

These are worth a mention in their own right. They speak volumes. Be real, be vulnerable, it's OK.

Conclusion

The mothers' narratives of their risk factors, which were so courageously shared with Cheryl in her research studies on birth trauma (Beck, 2004a), and PTSD following traumatic childbirth (Beck, 2004b), powerfully bring these risk factors to life for clinicians and researchers.

In Chapter 6, first, the neurobiology of the brain is described. The assessment and diagnosis of PTSD related to birth trauma are then presented. Use of the Earthquake Assessment Model is highlighted as this model is based on a stress model of neurobiology and can highlight potential vulnerabilities. Some women may be living with a pre-existing history that may lead to a diagnosis of PTSD related to traumatic childbirth.

References

Beck, C. T. (2004a). Birth trauma: In the eye of the beholder. *Nursing Research, 53,* 28–35.

——— (2004b). PTSD due to childbirth: The aftermath. *Nursing Research, 53,* 216–224.

Beck, C. T., & Watson, S. (2010). Subsequent childbirth after a previous traumatic birth. *Nursing Research, 59,* 241–249.

Simpkin, P., & Klaus, P. (2004). *When survivors give birth: Understanding and healing the effects of early sexual abuse on childbearing women.* Seattle, WA: Classic Day Publishing.

6   Assessment and Diagnosis

In this chapter we will discuss the assessment and diagnosis of PTSD related to birth trauma. Use of the Earthquake Assessment Model is highlighted as this model is based on a stress model of neurobiology and can highlight potential vulnerabilities that some women may be living with as a warning of pre-existing history that may lead to a diagnosis of PTSD related to birth trauma.

Introduction

Why do some women experience a birth as a trauma resulting in a posttraumatic episode while for other women the experience leads to a posttraumatic disorder? As witness to women's narratives regarding their birth experiences, Jeanne has wondered why there are times when she is flinching inside, while the women sharing their stories seem to move from the onset to the finale and they are euthymic and accepting. She ponders as to what it could be about their biochemical foundations that allows them to cope at that level. On the other hand, she has described sitting with other women who share the stories of their birth experiences and it appears that a crisis in that experience can trigger physiological and psychological responses that become a full-blown traumatic disorder.

This again reminds us of that expression that "beauty is in the eye of the beholder." It is this metaphor that describes the concept of perceptive reality. How we each see the world through our own personal lenses and the experiences that we have in the past affect how we interpret the world today. We are each unique in our way of viewing the world as well as in our responses to that view at a basic neurological/psychological level. As we learn more about the workings of the brain, through non-invasive neurological imaging, we can begin to understand more of the underpinnings of the symptom presentations and perhaps treatment methodologies for posttraumatic stress disorder related to birth trauma.

Pregnancy, labor, and delivery are stressful times for women biologically, psychologically, culturally, and spiritually. As many women have shared with me, "The experience changed my life." Pregnancy, in many ways, is like a biochemical storm or assault. Reproductive hormonal levels surge to their highest levels which would then have to have an impact on the other aspects of her biology. There is an exquisite interaction between reproductive bio-chemistry and neurochemistry. We know so much more today about the concept of stress and how we are biochemically affected by the response system and how it presents itself. It is this information that is changing the treatment models of PTSD and emotional disorders.

When we think about emotional symptoms, we need to remember that it is the way our brain tells us that something is going on and we need to pay attention to it. Over the past decade there has been a focus on the aspects of neurobiology and that changing how we see the world can change the physical structure of the brain. Neuroscience has been informing us that we can change the circuitry of the brain and how critical attachment and relationships are to the development of these neural circuits (Siegel, 1999, 2004, 2007). The term to describe this capacity of the brain to create and grow neurons and neural connections in response to experiences is called neuroplasticity. It is this healing process in the brain that is the basis for the treatment methods that have developed and continue to be discovered for the treatment of trauma reactions and PTSD. These treatments will be discussed throughout the rest of the book.

In order to understand the concepts of stress and trauma, one has to have a sense of how the brain has evolved and how it functions. Knowledge is power and the more a woman can learn about her biology and physiology, the more she can be an active partner in her treatment and her healing trajectory. The following discussion is very limited and simplified in that none of this book's authors are neuroscientists. There are references in the bibliography that the reader can access to further their personal understanding of the brain structure and function.

The following discussion is information that Jeanne provides to her patients as a way to help them understand what has happened to them at a physiological level. She feels that it gives patients a better understanding about what happens biochemically and neurochemically in response to stress and/or trauma. This information regarding brain structure and function also provides the foundation for elements of the Earthquake Assessment Model (Sichel & Driscoll, 1999).

Structure and Function of the Brain

Over the years, research into brain biology and neuroscience has been rampant and exciting. The brain is an amazing, sensitive, complex organ. It is indeed the "master computer" that controls and regulates your physiological functions, coordination, balance, and emotional reactions, to name a few specific things. The brain is continuously responding to your world both internally and externally, organizing behaviors in response to stressors through your decision-making, moods, actions, etc.

MacLean had described the structure of the brain as a "a brain with a brain within a brain" (1990, p. 8): brain stem, limbic brain, and cortical brain. The structure and function of specific aspects of the brain will be described (see

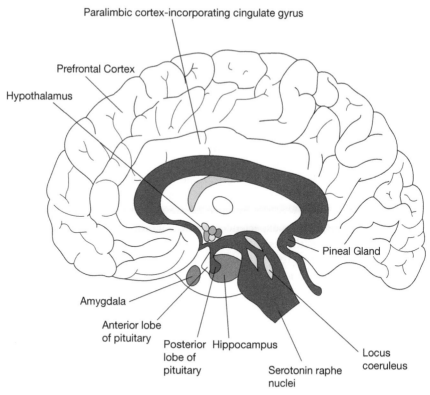

Figure 6.1 The structure of the brain

Source: From *Women's Moods* by Deborah Sichel and Jeanne Watson Driscoll © 1999 by Deborah Sichel and Jeanne Watson Driscoll. Courtesy of HarperCollins Publishers, p. 40.

Figure 6.1). The brain stem governs arousal, contains nerve cells that are responsible for the automatic, physiological functions of breathing, heartbeat, states of alertness and sleepiness, aspects of the primitive "fight or flight" mechanism, and digestion. This part of the brain connects to the spinal cord and is located at the base of the brain. It is well developed at birth and is the oldest area of the brain.

Around this brain stem is the limbic brain. This area of the brain evolved when reptiles developed into mammals and has many critical functions. The hypothalamus gland is located in the limbic brain and is critical in orchestrating menstrual cycle, thyroid function, physiological stress, body, and temperature, sleep–wake cycle, appetite, growth and milk production in lactation, aggressive impulses, attachment, memory (processing events into factual and autobiographical forms), the appraisal of meaning and the creation of affect, and our inner sensations of emotion. The limbic area of the brain regulates the functions that sustain and protect life and is the area that is crucial in how we form relationships and attachments.

Also located in the limbic brain are two other critical structures: the amygdala and the hippocampus. The amygdala regulates emotion and fear responses, and participates in the establishment of memory. It is thought to modulate the production of the neurotransmitters serotonin and norepinephrine which are implicated in mood and anxiety symptoms. The hippocampus is the structure that plays an active role in how memories are made, stored, and retrieved. Additionally, the hippocampus has a role in the modulation of stress responses and emotions (McEwen, 1995, 2005, 2006; Sichel & Driscoll, 1999; Siegel, 2011).

The hypothalamus gland, the master endocrine control center, is also located in the limbic brain and plays a critical role in our physiological response to stress. The hypothalamus gland connects with the pituitary gland and in turn the adrenal gland (located on the kidney). This interconnection, known as the HPA Axis (hypothalamic-pituitary-adrenal axis) is the main stress response system in the body. The stress response triggers the "fight or flight" mechanism and works fine in "normal" life situations. If, however, there is overload or continual stress for a significant time, the body will move into becoming in many ways exhausted and be unable to respond and reset when the stress is over. This chronic dysregulation may lead to changes in the cardiac system and the immune system to name a few. It has been called allostatic loading (McEwen, 1993, 1995, 1998; McEwen & Stellar, 1993) (see Figure 6.2).

The hippocampus is a seahorse-shaped structure, located in the limbic brain. It develops gradually through the early years and continues to grow new connections and new neurons throughout the life span. It integrates basic forms of emotional and perceptual memory into factual and autobiographical recollections (Siegel, 2011, p. 19).

The cortex is the outer part of the brain. The cortex "creates more intricate firing patterns that represent the three-dimensional world beyond bodily functions and survival reactions mediated by the lower subcortical regions" (Siegel, 2011, p. 19). The posterior cortex is the area of the brain that is the "master mapmaker of our physical experience, generating our perceptions of the outer world" (Siegel, 2011, p. 20). The prefrontal cortex is the area behind your forehead and has evolved only in human beings. It is in this prefrontal cortex that we create representations of concepts such as time, sense of self, and moral judgments. It is the middle prefrontal cortex that connects everything. The prefrontal cortex makes complex representations that permit concepts in the present, think of experiences from the past and plan and make images of the future (Siegel, 2011, p. 9). It is responsible for the neural representations that enable us to make images of the mind itself. Siegel calls these representations "Mindsight maps" (2011, p. 8) and he has a wonderful "hand model of the brain" that he has developed to help educate patients regarding where the structures of the brain are located. He instructs the readers to "take your hand and put your thumb in the middle and curl your fingers over the top, you'll have a readily accessible and fairly accurate mode of the brain." I recommend his book *Mindsight* (2011) to my patients as part of bibliotherapy for

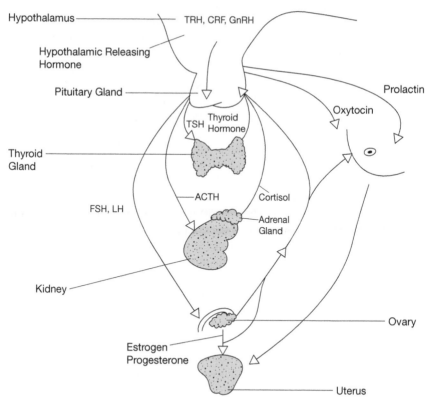

Figure 6.2 Hormonal relationships in the woman

Source: From *Women's Moods* by Deborah Sichel and Jeanne Watson Driscoll © 1999 by Deborah Sichel and Jeanne Watson Driscoll. Courtesy of HarperCollins Publishers, p. 98.

further explanations and descriptions of brain structure and function. The book also provides treatment strategies to help to quiet the biological responses of the brain to stress.

There are three levels of information processing—cognitive, emotional, and sensorimotor—which can be thought of as correlating with the three levels of brain architecture—brain stem, limbic, and cortical—together (Ogden, Minton, & Pain, 2006, p. 5). These three levels may not, however, always work together. It has been stated by van der Kolk that the dysregulated arousal caused by trauma may drive the person's emotional and cognitive processing adrift, causing emotions to escalate, and thoughts to spin, and to misinterpret the present environmental cues as those of the past trauma (van der Kolk, 1996, 2006; van der Kolk, McFarlane, & Weisaeth, 2007). This is perhaps why, for women experiencing PTSD after birth, they are often not sure why their emotions are responding to present life situations that on an intellectual level do not seem that bad. It is perhaps how the present reality triggers the past emotional response and why mindfulness, sensorimotor psychotherapy, eye movement desensitization and reprocessing (EMDR), cognitive behavioral therapy (CBT), and dialectical behavioral therapy (DBT) are treatment methods that help patients become empowered with the body awareness and be able to respond in a more self-aware way. These treatment methods will be discussed throughout the book in regard to specific case studies as well as in Chapter 13.

There are many models that are being investigated to uncover the basis of the PTSD at a biochemical level and psychological level but there is no one model that captures all the aspects of this disorder (Committee on the Assessment of Ongoing Effects in the Treatment of Posttraumatic Stress Disorder, 2012). Some of the models that are being researched are: animal models of fear conditioning and extinction; homologous brain structures in animals that are similar in humans; human studies using positron emission tomography (PET scans) and functional MRI studies, as well as structural MRI studies (Committee on the Assessment of Ongoing Effects in the Treatment of Posttraumatic Stress Disorder, 2012). Research continues and at present there is no one specific agreed upon theory for the basis of the symptoms of PTSD.

The Earthquake Assessment Model (© Sichel & Driscoll, 1999)

In 1999, the Earthquake Assessment Model was published in the book *Women's Moods* by Jeanne and Deborah Sichel, MD. The model is based on the ecological model of earthquakes and tremors and uses the life span approach for data collection. This model has its underpinnings based on the concepts of allostasis and allostatic loading (Post, 1992; McEwen, 1993, 1995). The premise of this foundation is that with the accumulation of stress responses biochemically on the brain, the physiological aspects of the neurological system are sensitized in the brain, loading, and straining the mood pathways. Traumatic events stimulate the stress response, resulting in the complex cascade of cortisol and other hormones in the brain and body. This physiological action can alter the brain's self-regulatory capacity (McEwen, 1998).

McEwen and Lasley state that a major paradox of stress is that it "protects under acute conditions but when activated chronically it can cause damage and accelerate disease" (2002, p. 4). Allostasis (McEwen, 1998) is produced by a swift communication system in the brain: the brain perceives an event, and then the endocrine system (HPA axis) responds by mobilizing the body and the immune system to activate to protect the inner body. The goal is to get the maximum energy to the parts of the body that need it: the fight or flight response. The purpose of allostasis is to help the body remain stable in the face of any change and provide the body with the energy it needs to cope with any challenge. Allostatic load, however, is the damage that the allostatic response causes when it is not functioning properly. The allostatic response may not shut off over time and may move to a state of continual dysregulation. Genetics and sex seem to play a significant role in what becomes allostatic load to some people as opposed to others, similar to how some women will perceive birth as a traumatic event while others may not (McEwen, 1998; McEwen & Lasley, 2002). Interestingly, there is beginning to be research data suggesting that sex hormones, i.e. estrogen and progesterone, may be involved in modulating memory formation in women in ways that impact their control of fear (Protopopescu et al., 2005; Goldstein et al., 2010; Zeidan et al., 2011). Pregnancy is a time of extremely high sex hormones. Future research will be very informative regarding sex-specific differences in stress responses and PTSD.

As previously stated, McEwen (1995) describes allostatic loading as the process where the brain, over time, becomes overloaded with stress and loses its ability to cope. Sichel and Driscoll (1999) refer to this process as "brain strain." Brain strain manifests itself in feelings of being overwhelmed and difficulty concentrating. Additionally the physical symptom of headaches, anxiety, fatigue, etc. can represent brain strain. Brain strain symptoms are, in essence, the way the body tells you to pay attention; something is out of order and needs to be addressed. These symptoms are often described as psychiatric symptoms: sleep dysregulation, appetite changes, bowel and bladder changes, feelings of anxiety, anger, rage, irritability, fatigue, and/or hypomania or manic-like symptoms. The body cannot continue to function at a homeostatic level if it is constantly being challenged and stressed. Something has to give and it is usually demonstrated by how we feel. In essence, behavior has meaning; we are just not always clear as to the cause, psychologically or physiologically.

The Earthquake Model of assessment uses the ecological model of earthquakes and tremors (alterations in the fault lines of the earth). Earthquakes occur when the internal pressure of the earth's fault lines become overwhelmed or to use the vernacular "stressed to the max." To relieve the internal pressure, the fault lines shift and move, causing a tremor or tremors. If the pressures get too high, an earthquake occurs. When the event has quieted and the earth has resettled, the fault line has shifted into a new position and is now in a state of altered quiescence, waiting for the pressure cycle to build again. Generally there are tremors that are experienced prior to "the big one," reminding us that there is instability below. We can equate basic brain biochemistry to these fault lines under the earth. With tremors, there are felt shakes, however; there are no breaks in the earth's foundation although they are a reminder of the pressures underneath. Metaphorically these fault lines and their reactions to the subterranean pressure can be compared to the presentation of symptoms of mood and anxiety disorders. PTSD is a type of anxiety disorder.

Life brings with it stress, conflict, interpersonal issues, feelings, and emotions. The response of each person to these experiences is based on their genetic foundations and learned coping strategies as well as relationships and support. So when the fault lines are homeostatic and responsive to life as it is lived, the subterranean pressure may lead to slight or even moderate tremors. These tremors may present as mild symptoms of anxiety, sadness, depression, or a various myriad of feelings. The feelings are felt and coping strategies are utilized and the event and the response to the event pass. Often these experiences can be positive learning experiences for a person to increase their repertoire of coping skills. However, if the events are life-altering, persistent, repetitive, and overwhelming, the coping that used to work does not and the person enters into a crisis and/or experiences an earthquake. They cannot achieve home-ostasis or balance and they have moved into the physiological and psychological process of allostatic loading (McEwen, 1995) and dysregulated neurobiology. The fault line erupts and the earthquake occurs. This earthquake represents metaphorically a psychiatric disorder. The symptoms increase in frequency, duration, and intensity. The woman does not feel that she can take control of how she feels and her daily life is now being altered or compromised. So it is with birth trauma. A woman can have an earthquake response to her birth experience. This response is to how she perceives the events, not the observer. If she comes into the birth experience with a history of minor and major tremors (life experiences) or earthquakes, she has an increased vulnerability or propensity to experience a traumatic response to a birth experience. Again, this is an individually perceptive experience. It is uncertain what it is that triggers this major response in some women and not in others.

Let's discuss the key elements of the Earthquake Assessment Model (© Sichel and Driscoll, 1999). There are three domains that are critical in the assessment. These are: family history; life events/stressors and responses; and reproductive history. The three domains are assessed and the information is used to obtain a base of how the woman's brain has responded to those elements in her life both

External
appearance: _____

Biochemical
fault line: --

Emotional/social
stressors: --

Hormonal State:
(normal
reproductive
events): --

Age _____
         10 12 14 15 16 17 18 19 20 21 22 23 24 25 26 27 28 29 30 31 32 33 34 35 36 37 38 39 40 41 42

Figure 6.3 The Earthquake Assessment

Source: From *Women's Moods* by Deborah Sichel and Jeanne Watson Driscoll © 1999 by Deborah Sichel and Jeanne Watson Driscoll. Courtesy of HarperCollins Publishers, p. 100.

physiologically and psychologically, her allostasis and allostatic loading. This information is then charted on the assessment chart (Figure 6.3).

Key information that is needed under each domain includes some of the following:

1   Genetic family history: This domain provides us with information pertaining to the biochemical propensity and/or genetic loading of the woman's brain. The questions include: family history of mental illness and/or emotional problems, propensity to a biological/organic/mental/emotional event or response. Any family history of drug and/or alcohol abuse? If a woman has a positive family history of mood swing or bipolar disorders, this is a critical piece of information that will be important in the treatment plan, especially if psychopharmacological therapy is to be considered. If the woman has a positive family history, this gives her an altered baseline (or biochemical fault line), so that she has a genetic propensity toward vulnerability to mood and or anxiety disorders.

2   Life events/stressor history: With this domain the assessment focuses on the events of a woman's life and her responses to them, her coping strategies. The woman is asked to describe any positive or negative events in her early life, grade school life, high school, etc. History of physical/sexual/emotional abuse? Were there events that triggered emotional responses in her: bullying at school, death of a sibling, traumatic event(s) in her family of origin, relationship conflicts, issues, living with a parent with emotional/mental/ physical illness, alcohol/substance use/abuse? This information gives some clues as to how her brain has responded in the past and her psychological responses to specific events. This information will allow you to fill in the information on the external presentation line as a shift in baseline to an elevation: Did she experience mood and/or anxiety symptoms in response to life stressors? Eating disorder, cutting, depression, suicidal thoughts, attempts, phobias, compulsive thoughts, behaviors, etc.? These presentations will cause an alteration in her basic fault line of external appearances: the symptoms were present and felt.

3   Reproductive history: When did she get her first period? Were there any physiological issues that presented around that time? Did she have headaches, stomach aches, feelings of sadness, anxiety, depression? Did she proceed to have regular menstrual cycles? Were there any issues with cramps, school/work absence, feeling incapacitated? Had she ever taken oral contraceptive agents and was there any physical and/or emotional response to them? Any experience with depot contraceptives; any physical and/or emotional response to those agents? Any history of pregnancy, reproductive assisted technology, miscarriage, elective termination? What were her responses to these events? It is necessary to go through each pregnancy, trimester by trimester, to ascertain any mood/anxiety issues and have her describe if there were any. Asking her to describe her birth experience: onset and duration of labor, description of pushing, if a vaginal

birth; if a cesarean birth, what does she remember of that experience? Also important is information about her first postpartum day, her emotional state, e.g. euthymic, hypomanic. The data collected in this domain will potentially move her baseline up depending on her experiences.

By completing this assessment, both you and the woman get a sense of what has happened in her life and her brain's response. The Earthquake Assessment Chart can show her, via a graphic representation, her current fault line or mental health status. It is through the use of these metaphors of tremors and earthquakes that we can understand the concepts of allostasis, allostatic loading, and her risk factors and vulnerabilities. This helps the clinician in formulating a diagnosis. The graphic representation can be very comforting to the woman as you discuss her risk factors and how we can strategize the care plan based on who she is and what her life experience has been. It also takes away the issue of judgment and blame. Brain biochemistry is not static but rather constantly changing . . . the earthquake model helps women to understand what may have brought them to their today reality as well as a way to remember that "the brain you were born with is not the same brain you have today" (Sichel & Driscoll, 1999, p. 104). Remember that knowledge is power and women want to make sense of what they are feeling so that they can integrate, heal, and move on.

After the assessment is complete, the clinician will go through their formulation process to arrive at the diagnosis. The diagnosis of posttraumatic stress disorder secondary to birth trauma is based on the diagnostic category in the DSM-IV (APA, 2000). The diagnostic criteria of PTSD are as follows:

The person has been exposed to a traumatic event in which both of the following were present:

(1) The person experienced, witnessed, or was confronted with an event or events that involved actual or threatened death or serious injury, or a threat to the physical integrity of self or others.
(2) The person's response involved intense fear, helplessness, or horror.

B. The traumatic event is persistently re-experienced in one (or more) of the following ways:

(1) Recurrent and intrusive distressing recollections of the event, including images, thoughts, or perceptions.
(2) Recurrent distressing dreams of the event.
(3) Acting or feeling as if the traumatic event were recurring (includes a sense of reliving the experience, illusions, hallucinations and dissociative flashback episodes, including those that occur on awakening or when intoxicated).
(4) Intense psychological distress at exposure to internal or external cues that symbolize or resemble an aspect of the traumatic event.
(5) Physiological reactivity on exposure to internal or external cues that symbolize or resemble an aspect of the traumatic event.

C. Persistent avoidance of stimuli associated with the trauma and numbing of general responsiveness (not present before the trauma), as indicated by three (or more) of the following:

(1) Efforts to avoid thoughts, feelings, or conversations associated with the trauma.
(2) Efforts to avoid activities, places, or people that arouse recollections of the trauma.
(3) Inability to recall an important aspect of the trauma.
(4) Markedly diminished interest or participation in significant activities.
(5) Feeling of detachment or estrangement from others.
(6) Restricted range of affect.
(7) Sense of a foreshortened future.

D. Persistent symptoms of increased arousal (not present before the trauma), as indicated by two (or more) of the following:

(1) Difficulty falling or staying asleep.
(2) Irritability or outbursts of anger.
(3) Difficulty concentrating.
(4) Hypervigilance.
(5) Exaggerated startle response.

E. Duration of the disturbance (symptoms in Criteria B, C, and D) is more than 1 month.
F. The disturbance causes clinically significant distress or impairment in social, occupational, or other important areas of functioning.

(Reprinted with permission from the American Psychiatric Association, 2000, pp. 467–468.)

To make the diagnosis, based on the DSM-IV, women need to present with symptoms of re-experiencing the event, avoidance, and arousal. These symptoms are interfering with her everyday living and causing significant issues in her interpersonal relationships and way of being in the world. Much of the information can be obtained from the assessment interview but there are also instruments that can be used to augment the diagnostic process. These instruments are available to clinicians for use in routine screening of new mothers and can provide the clinician with quantitative evaluation data that are useful in assessing the efficacy of the treatment modalities in the reduction of symptoms. Chapter 8 will provide the reader with a review of some of the current instruments used to screen for PTSD.

Diagnostic Parsimony

There is substantial evidence for the co-morbidity between depression and PTSD in the general population. Recent evidence is now accruing to also support this co-morbidity in the postpartum period. Significant correlations between elevated symptoms of posttraumatic stress symptoms and postpartum depressive symptoms have been reported in numerous countries such as the USA (Beck, Gable, Sakala, & Declercq, 2011; Sorenson & Tschetter, 2010), Australia (White, Matthey, Boyd, & Barnett, 2006), Italy (Maggioni, Margola, & Filipp, 2006), Sweden (Soderquist, Wijma, & Wijma, 2006), Switzerland (Zaers, Waschke, & Ehlert, 2008), and Israel (Lev-Wiesel, Daphna-Tekoah, & Hallak, 2009). In the national U.S. Listening to Mothers II Postpartum Survey of 903 women, postpartum depressive symptoms accounted for 51% of the variance in women's scores on the Posttraumatic Stress Symptom Scale-Self Report (PSS-SR) (Beck et al., 2011).

Why are women suffering from PTSD due to childbirth not given this diagnosis? Why does a diagnosis of postpartum depression tend to trump a diagnosis of PTSD following a traumatic birth? One possible answer is the principle of diagnostic parsimony. Goldberg (1984) coined this phrase to describe how physicians are taught to choose the single most likely cause for a specific symptom. So in psychiatry even though it is well documented there is co-morbidity of depression and anxiety, a person who experiences depression and anxiety will often be given the diagnosis of depression. The anxiety may not be addressed or maybe underscored as not of primary concern. Diagnostic parsimony may be one reason for the failure to detect women suffering from PTSD due to birth trauma.

Below are two stories that illustrate the lengthy time it took for mothers to be given the correct diagnosis of PTSD due to their traumatic childbirth experiences. Both mothers had participated in Beck's (2004) study on PTSD following birth trauma.

Rachel's Story

Rachel had postpartum depression after the birth of her first baby. Her physician had prescribed antidepressants. After a couple of months of medication and counseling, she was starting to feel right again. So good in fact that she suggested to her husband that they should have another baby. At this stage their son was 10 months old. Here is Rachel's story in her own words of her second childbirth, recurrence of postpartum depression, and co-morbidity with PTSD.

> At 41 weeks I went into the hospital. I had been having mild contractions on and off for a couple of days but my waters hadn't broken. My waters were broken not long after we got there. But as the day wore on, there seemed to be one complication after another. Labor was very slow to progress. Contractions were strong and regular but 20 minutes apart. There was meconium in my waters which seemed to gush out all day. I vomited up my food. After lots of internal exams during the day, the decision was made to give me syntocinon via a drip late in the afternoon. It didn't seem to do anything at first so after an hour or two, the hospital midwives pumped a bit more into me. By 7 p.m. my own midwife had arrived and I was pushing uncontrollably. At 7.30 p.m. I knew something was wrong. I

had been through childbirth before and this just didn't feel right and I said so to my midwife. At 8 p.m. she knew I should have had the baby out by then. It was then she discovered that my baby was stuck, jammed. He wasn't going anywhere. Unfortunately because of the amount of syntocinon I had been given to get the labor going, I now couldn't stop pushing. It was uncontrollable. It was the most horrible feeling knowing that he was stuck but I wouldn't stop pushing him. With every contraction I had, his heart beat dropped. By now I had several drips in one arm (syntocinon, antibiotics, pethadine, etc.) and blood was being taken out of the other arm as there was protein in my urine and my blood pressure was high. I felt incredibly out of control of my body. It was a new feeling for me. I had felt completely in control of my body when giving birth to my first baby. Between the hours of 8 and 11 p.m. I had numerous internal exams by two specialists and my midwife. They couldn't agree on what position the baby was in and what action to take. So for that whole three hours I was pushing, knowing he was stuck! I was so tired. It had been a long day. My midwife and I talked about a cesarean. I felt so relieved. It was what I wanted by then so I signed the forms. The doctor decided she wanted to do one more exam to see if the baby had changed positions. She did that and said she thought using a ventouse would be a better option than a cesarean so I countersigned the cesarean forms. I was prepped for the delivery room (in case a cesarean needed to happen) and taken there. I remember screaming my way through the hospital corridors and in the elevator. We got to the delivery room and now not only had I lost control of my body but my dignity too. My feet were put up in stirrups and half the table was collapsed under me. I was exposed—not just to my midwife and the doctor, but to 13 various hospital staff (pediatrics, obstetrics, anesthetists, etc.). Everything around me shocked me. All these people looking at me, the lights above me. The ventouse was not the little rubber suction cup I had imagined or read about but a large metal thing with a chain on it. It was all very surreal. The actual ventouse delivery went well. It was sheer hell for me while the doctor was getting it in place on my baby's head but once it was on, my baby was out with only a few pushes/pulls and no rips or tears. But the drama wasn't over. My son was taken to the other side of the room away from me to be checked out. His collarbone had been broken during delivery. While that was happening, I had trouble delivering the placenta. I was given an injection of something to help it along but it didn't work. After about 25 minutes the doctor said I needed to push it out or she was going to have to put her hand inside me to pull it out. That was enough for me to summon up the strength to give one last almighty push. The placenta came out. It was huge. The doctor didn't quite catch it in time and it fell to the ground splattering everyone around the table with my blood. It was quite humiliating.

I experienced postpartum depression after having my first baby. With the help of my counselor and knowledge from reading, I had put in place things to help prevent me from having postpartum depression again and support that I might need if I did get it again. I was sure I wouldn't get it the second time around. My family (in particular my mom) was around to help this time. My mother even started helping out when I was pregnant and sick with the gestational diabetes. I had two good friends who knew me very well and were there to help if I needed them, or even just to talk. My husband took time off work and was there every day and some nights while we were in the hospital. But when I was in the hospital, I just couldn't stop crying. I couldn't get over what I had just been through. I didn't feel a bond at all with my baby. I knew I had it again. I decided to wait to see if things improved when I got home, but they didn't. My son was 5 weeks old when I asked my doctor for help and got in touch with my therapist again. The reason being the postpartum depression was different this time. It wasn't lack of support and loneliness like the last time. It was the traumatic birth my son and I had been through. He put me on antidepressant medication and said I had postpartum depression again.

During one of the home visits by the nurse I mentioned to her the flashbacks and emotional outbursts I had been having since my son's birth, the unwilling reliving of his birth over and over in my mind. It wouldn't go away and neither would the negative feelings I had about the whole experience. I felt that there were some things quite different happening to me in comparison to when I had postpartum depression after my first baby was born. It was quite apparent I had postpartum depression again, but something else was happening too. The nurse gave me some information on PTSD and the TABS website. I had a look on the Internet and it all made sense to me. I read about other women who were feeling the same as me. It was during a visit from my counselor that we talked about PTSD. Within the mental health team that my therapist works in, there was a psychiatrist who administers my medication and a psychologist whom I see on a regular basis. My appointments with the psychologist started when my son was about 4 months old I think and they have been absolutely invaluable to me. She diagnosed me with also having PTSD. She has helped me to reflect on his birth and accept that that is what happened. She has even helped me to come to terms with some of the finer details, like why wasn't I given a cesarean I wanted, and why did I have to have so many internal exams. I now have no flashbacks or emotional outbursts relating to my son's birth. We have both recovered physically with no long-term effects. I have accepted his birth, nothing was his fault. I have now bonded beautifully with him and I am pleased to say that I am proud to have been able to breastfeed my son for 3 months, especially under the circumstances of a traumatic birth.

Clinician's Reaction

It is not uncommon for the diagnosis of PTSD to be misinterpreted as postpartum depression (PPD), especially in a case where a woman has had a history of PPD with treatment. Oftentimes the assumption is made that there is a recurrence as that happens in a large percentage of women. The clinician needs to take a new assessment of the woman's symptoms and events that precipitated the onset of symptoms. Having spent over 30 years caring for women with mood and anxiety disorders that occur during the childbearing years, I am exquisitely aware of the unique aspects of each birth and its lived experience. Each pregnancy, labor, delivery, and postpartum experience is distinctive and unique. The woman enters the childbearing experience with familiarity but quickly becomes aware that each experience is a once in a lifetime. Often I have shared with women that when you begin your personal childbearing trajectory, you become quickly aware that you control only your perception of the experience but not the events as they unfold in the process. It is this sense of personal perception and resiliency that seems to have an impact on the experiential process of integrating childbearing experiences. We know from research that women live with risk factors of perinatal mood and/or anxiety disorders; history of mood and/or anxiety prior to any pregnancies, childhood sexual abuse, experiencing fetal loss, miscarriage, elective termination, premature labor/delivery, babies in the NICU, and a history of physical/emotional/sexual abuse are some of the high risk factors that can lead to vulnerability to the potential for PTSD secondary to birth trauma.

Rachel's experience reminds clinicians to pay attention to the circumstances of the birth experience and assess the lived experience as it is in the now, not just the history.

Mother's Reaction

It could be that this mother came to us after she had begun her journey of recovery. Yes, whilst in the midst of this challenging, but worthwhile process, it is necessary to regain one's emotional well-being and to even to start to feel normal during the day. Thank goodness that Rachel was not put in the "too hard basket" and not heard, when relaying the very clear "non-" mood troubles happening for her. She did very well to be articulate and state her symptoms and her very strong self-awareness of "something is quite different happening to me, in comparison to when I had postpartum depression." PTSD sufferers are very clear in their mind about their "reactive" living, rather than the low mood state. For Rachel, I would have affirmed her, encouraged her to be strong, to always find something healthy and comforting for herself, and to know the therapy is worth it in the long term. Your voice will be your friend. Continue with this skillful counselor. The pain will ease and not be so acute for you, and you will see that the sky is in fact blue. Well done!

Jennie's Story

It took 23 years for Jennie to finally be diagnosed with PTSD due to her traumatic birth that she described in her own words:

I went into labor three days after my due date at around 10 p.m. When I arrived in the labor area I was handed over to a nurse. I needed to use the bathroom and went to the bathroom and closed the door. The nurse immediately opened it (there were no locks) and yelled at me for closing it. She stood by and watched while I vomited some more, had a bowel movement, and cleaned myself up. I was put back in bed and given a vaginal exam by this nurse. Then three more people showed up and did the same thing. I protested this lack of privacy but was ignored. I tried to catch their eyes with mine so I would be harder to ignore but they wouldn't look at me. A discussion ensured about how far everyone thought I was dilated. No one could agree but the final general consensus was either 2 or 3 cm. It was still early on but I already felt violated and humiliated.

I was hooked up to a monitoring system right after this. They were done routinely in the hospital I delivered in. My husband and four other people (three of them students) were present during this procedure. I didn't want this and said so but I was dismissed and ignored again. One of the students accused me of being a bad mother because I wasn't considering my baby. By the time the external and internal monitoring devices were attached to my abdomen and inside my uterus and on my baby's scalp, my contractions were coming so fast that one wasn't finished before the next one started. The machine wasn't registering this. The nurse called me a drama queen and was explaining to my husband what was "really" happening. I was trying to explain to my husband that they were wrong but I could see he believed them. This went on for about 10 minutes before they realized that the monitoring device wasn't working properly. I received no apology for the treatment I received. They called for a machine technician to repair the equipment.

I had genuinely expected the hospital and my husband to support and care for me. The sense of betrayal when neither of those things happened was profound. I kept asking where my obstetrician was because I hoped she would care for me in a humane way. I was told she hadn't been called and she wouldn't be for a while. The first time I remember seeing her was in the delivery room. I had discussed labor and delivery with her during a prenatal visit and I was assured that pain relief would be available. The machine technician showed up. I was not covered in his presence. When I tried to cover myself, the nurse slapped me. The machine technician wasn't able to get the equipment working and they unhooked me and took everything out of the room.

The next 2 to 3 hours are etched in my mind as well. Things were really just more of the same except there wasn't monitoring equipment. The pain was excruciating and I was denied pain relief. If I asked for it, I was told that it may cause fetal distress and "Didn't I care about my baby?" Of course, I did. This was a constant fear. I was afraid that we would both die. I longed for the times when I was left alone by hospital staff. I was treated with disrespect and a complete lack of privacy. Exams were done without my permission or consent. Several people were there while they were done. I had no control over who was there or what was done to me. They talked amongst themselves but never to me. I wasn't prepared for the complete disregard of my human rights. I couldn't even protest anymore because I couldn't speak. The pain was too severe.

I have no memory of the next 2 or 3 hours except for two clear exceptions. The first was while I was still in the labor room. I remember being alone with a kind nurse who was holding my hand and telling me she would protect me. I remember crying at this unexpected kindness. The second was while I was being pushed down the hallway to the delivery room. I knew without being told that I was going to have a cesarean and I didn't consider this a failure. I was relieved that my ordeal was ending. I had an oxygen mask on my face that I tried to take off because I felt I couldn't breathe. The nurse kept pushing it back on and holding it on my face. I was trying to ask if my baby was OK. She ignored me. I was handed off to the surgical team waiting for me. They stripped me from the waist down and the anesthesiologist began ridiculing me and making rude gestures. My obstetrician made a slashing movement across her throat to stop him when she realized I was aware of my surroundings. The oxygen mask was removed while they draped me in blue sheets and it was replaced with the mask for general anesthesia. I remember nothing more until recovery.

I was hovering between unconscious and barely conscious when my husband came in holding my daughter. I don't know how long that was after she was born. I remember two things about this. One, I was so happy that my daughter had survived and since I was aware of this, it must mean I survived as well. I was also aware I was the last one to see my baby. What I wanted was to have time alone with my baby but I was so drugged I couldn't hold her. She lay beside me on the bed and I couldn't focus or lift my arms.

My nightmares started about 3 weeks after I gave birth and they have continued episodically throughout my life for the past 23 years. There are triggers and one of them is anything related to childbirth. When episodes are triggered, I have reoccurring intrusive thoughts, memories, and nightmares. I feel anger. My body experiences symptoms of stress. I have shortness of breath and chest constriction. My pulse races. I am afraid to go to sleep because the nightmares will come. Insomnia and the resulting fatigue are big problems. These episodes can last for a few days or several weeks. I have no control over when they start and how long they last. I am very adept at avoiding situations that trigger these episodes but it is often very difficult to avoid them. I listen empathetically to other women's birth experiences because I want to be supportive and I understand how much they need to decompress and find validation but these horror stories always trigger episodes. If I can avoid these stories, I do and I feel guilty for doing that. I can't watch movies that aren't light comedies. I am always on guard for situations that may be harmful to me. Social injustice reduces me to tears. My teeth are cracked from grinding them at night. I need to wear a mouth guard to sleep when the nightmares are a problem. I use avoidance, distraction, and stress management techniques to cope with PTSD. I'm very adept at tuning things out. If I told people I had PTSD, they wouldn't believe it. People who know me may comment that I'm quieter than usual or that I seem preoccupied during the episodes. Sometimes they point out that I look tired. Outwardly I am a quiet, calm, efficient person just as I was before having my child.

I tried to get help when my nightmares first started but the stigma attached to women who suffered during their postpartum was evident. I was told to move on and to be thankful I had a healthy baby. I never mentioned the problem again to anyone. I also tried to get my medical records so I could fill in the time where I have no memory but I was told I had no right to them. I didn't find out that what I was experiencing all these years was called PTSD until two years ago! I googled my symptoms and sat stunned when I recognized myself in the description. Finally I had some validation and I learned that many other women suffered the same way. I wasn't alone. I learned many other women used the same language of sexual assault to describe childbirth as I did. I wasn't the only one to feel brutalized and violated. I sought help with a psychiatrist and was diagnosed with PTSD. It took 23 years to be diagnosed with PTSD due to my traumatic birth.

Clinician's Reaction

Jennie describes in her narrative an experience that happened over 23 years ago. Her clear, concise memory of the events of her daughter's birth give validation to the embedded impact of the experience on the individual woman and the fact that she was not heard by clinicians when she tried to get help demonstrates again the need to listen to the perceptive reality of the woman and her story, not your belief in what you, the clinician, imagined to have happened, even if you were there.

Early in Jennie's hospital experience she described feeling disrespected and invisible to the health care team. She described how eye contact was avoided and this is a way to not be in connection or to disconnect from the relationship. Perhaps these providers were dealing with their own traumatic responses to their jobs in that they were using defensive, protective strategies to disconnect from the relationship? The woman felt ignored, not acknowledged as a human much less as a laboring woman. Jennie describes feeling betrayed by her husband. I often wonder what we expect of the partner, husband, lover in these critical life situations. They are often just as scared, isolated, and disconnected but are not always acknowledged for their feelings. Sadly, their behavior is interpreted as betrayal by their partner. Perhaps we need to do more education regarding the "coaches," partners, husbands, lovers in their role in the birth experience. Here is, in my professional mind, part of the nursing care of the couple. We need to remember that they are both novices in this experience. We as the care providers have experience and it is not our personal experience, it is not our body nor our wife, partner, lover. This allows for some objective participation but does not provide us with a rationale to provide less than quality, interpersonal, empathic, connected care.

We must continually remember that our patients are our priority and we need to do our own emotional and psychological work to help us provide our patients with the care they deserve, especially during this close to death experience of childbirth.

Mother's Reaction

If I had had the pleasure of chatting with Jennie, I would have said, "Well done, you strong and wonderful woman, and, yes, now is the time to press forward in your recovery." I would ask, "What is most important for you right now?" and just listen and listen, and respond encouragingly to her content. I would say, "Your story we have heard before and your sharing as you have, will 'turn the light on for others'." Her counseling might be quite tough, and there could be many ways for her to be helped. We are firm believers in the power of the pen and paper. Write down what pours out of you and then file it away in a treasured place or even rip it up! Do what is best of you. Recovery is here.

Conclusion

Once the diagnosis is made, the discussion will take place regarding the appropriate treatment plan for the patient. Treatment methods are discussed in Chapter 13. The treatment needs to be individualized for each woman, as one size does not fit all. Chapter 7 will present a case study from Jeanne's practice which will utilize the Earthquake Assessment (© Sichel & Driscoll, 1999) as well as describe the care plan development and treatment experience.

References

American Psychiatric Association (2000). *Diagnostic and statistical manual of mental disorders*. Washington, DC: American Psychiatric Association.

Beck, C. T. (2004). Posttraumatic stress disorder due to childbirth: The aftermath. *Nursing Research, 53,* 216–224.

Beck, C. T., Gable, R. K., Sakala, C., & Declercq, E. R. (2011). Posttraumatic stress disorders in new mothers: Results from a two-stage U.S. National Survey. *Birth, 38,* 216–227.

Committee on the Assessment of Ongoing Effects in the Treatment of Posttraumatic Stress Disorder (2012). *Treatment of Posttraumatic Stress Disorder in military and veteran populations: Initial assessment.* Washington, DC: National Academy of Sciences.

Goldberg, D. (1984). The recognition of psychiatric illness by non-psychiatrists. *Australian and New Zealand Journal of Psychiatry, 18,* 128–133.

Goldstein, J. M., Jerram, M., Apps, B., Whitfield-Gavrieli, S., & Makris, N. (2010). Sex differences in stress response circuitry activation dependent on female hormonal cycle. *Journal of Neuroscience, 30*(2), 431–438.

Lev-Wiesel, R., Daphna-Tekoah, S., & Hallak, M. (2009). Childhood sexual abuse as a predictor of birth-related posttraumatic stress and postpartum posttraumatic stress. *Child Abuse and Neglect, 33,* 877–887.

MacLean, P. D. (1990). *The triune brain in evolution.* New York: Plenum Press.

Maggioni, C., Margola, D., & Filipp, F. (2006). PTSD, risk factors, and expectations among women having a baby: A two-wave longitudinal study. *Journal of Psychosomatic Obstetrics and Gynecology, 27,* 81–90.

McEwen, B. S. (1993). Stress and the individual: Mechanisms leading to disease. *Archives of Internal Medicine, 153,* 2093–2101.

—— (1995). Stressful experience, brain, and emotions: Developmental, genetic, and hormonal influences. In M. S. Gazzaniga (Ed.). *The cognitive neurosciences.* Cambridge, MA: The MIT Press.

—— (1998). Protective and damaging effects of stress mediators. *The New England Journal of Medicine, 338,* 171–179.

—— (2005). Glucocorticoids, depression and mood disorders: Structural remodeling of the brain. *Metabolism Clinical and Experimentation, 54*(Suppl. 1), 20–23.

—— (2006). Protective and damaging effects of stress mediators: central role of the brain. *Dialogues in Clinical Neuroscience, 8*(4), 367–381.

McEwen, B. S., & Lasley, E. N. (2002). *The end of stress as we know it.* Washington, DC: Joseph Henry Press.

McEwen, B. S., & Stellar, E. (1993). Stress and the individual: Mechanisms leading to disease. *Archives of Internal Medicine, 152,* 2093–2101.

Ogden, P., Minton, K., & Pain, C. (2006). *Trauma and the body: A sensorimotor approach to psychotherapy.* New York: W. W. Norton & Company.

Post, R. M. (1992). Transduction of psychosocial stress into neurobiology of recurrent affective disorder. *American Journal of Psychiatry, 149,* 999–1010.

Protopopescu, X., Pan, H., Altemus, M., Tuescher, O., Polanecsky, M., McEwen, B. S., Silbersweig, D., & Stern, E. (2005). Orbitofrontal cortex activity related to emotional processing changes across the menstrual cycle. *Proceedings of the National Academy of Sciences in the United States of America, 102*(44), 16060–16065.

Sichel, D., & Driscoll, J. W. (1999). *Women's moods: What every woman must know about hormones, the brain, and emotional health.* New York: William Morrow and Company, Inc.

Siegel, D. J. (1999). *The developing mind: How relationships and the brain interact to shape who we are.* New York: Guilford Press.

—— (2004). *The present moment in psychotherapy and everyday life.* New York: W. W. Norton & Company.

—— (2007). *The mindful brain: Reflection and Attunement in the cultivation of well-being.* New York: W.W. Norton & Company.

—— (2011). *Mindsight: The new science of personal transformation.* New York: Bantam Books Trade Paperbacks.

Soderquist, J., Wijma, B., & Wijma, K. (2006). The longitudinal course of post-traumatic stress after childbirth. *Journal of Psychosomatic Obstetrics and Gynecology, 27,* 113–119.

Sorenson, D. S., & Tschetter, L. (2010). Prevalence of negative birth perception, disaffirmation, perinatal trauma symptoms, and depression among postpartum women. *Perspectives in Psychiatric Care, 46,* 14–25.

van der Kolk, B. A. (1996). The complexity of adaptation to trauma: Self-regulation, stimulus discrimination, and characterological development. In B.A. van der Kolk, A. C. McFarlane, & L. Weisaeth (Eds.). *Traumatic stress: The effects of overwhelming experience on mind, body and society* (pp. 182–213). New York: Guilford Press.

—— (2006). Foreword. In P. Ogden, K. Minton, & C. Pain (Eds.). *Trauma and the body: a sensorimotor approach to psychotherapy*. New York: W.W. Norton & Company.

van der Kolk, B. A., McFarlane, A. C., & Weisaeth, L. (Eds.). (2007). *Traumatic stress: The effects of overwhelming experience on mind, body and society*. New York: Guilford Press.

White, T., Matthey, S., Boyd, K., & Barnett, B. (2006). Postnatal depression and post-traumatic stress after childbirth: Prevalence, course and co-occurrence. *Journal of Reproductive and Infant Psychology, 24*, 107–120.

Zaers, S., Waschke, M., & Ehlert, U. (2008). Depressive symptoms and symptoms of posttraumatic stress disorder in women after childbirth. *Journal of Psychosomatic Obstetrics and Gynecology, 29*, 61–71.

Zeidan, M. A., Igoe, S. A., Linnman, C., Vitalol, A., Levine, J. B., Klibanski, A., Goldstein, J. M., & Milad, M. R. (2011). Estradiol modulates medial prefrontal cortex and amygdala activity during fear extinction in women and female rats. *Biological Psychiatry, 70*(10), 920–927.

7   Case Study 1: Carol

I received a call from Carol. She had heard about me from her colleagues where she worked as a nurse. She had had a baby about 6 months earlier and was currently, "not feeling very well." She described that she felt her "heart pounding" and her hands were "shaky all the time." "I just feel lost." She went on to describe that she only felt safe at home and that was not acceptable as she had to go out into the world and could not just stay home. She had a 6-month-old daughter and felt that the birth experience was "horrific" but felt she should be able "to get through it." We agreed to meet the next day for an evaluation and I informed her that she could indeed bring her baby to the appointment as it is my practice to include children. I include babies whenever possible as it is a perfect way to assess the maternal–infant attachment/relationship which can be affected by a mood and/or anxiety disorder that occurs during the childbearing years. Carol was relieved to hear that she could bring her baby in that she did not have child care and her husband could not take the day off from work.

The next day I met Carol and her daughter, Madeleine. Carol sat on the couch in my office, and picked up her daughter and held her close. I felt that Carol was very anxious and not sure of me at all. My priority was to help to decrease her anxiety so that she could interact with calmness and ease. I shared with her how scary it must be for her to be experiencing the feelings she had described to me on the phone yesterday, and to meet a complete stranger who is a psychiatric mental health provider. She nodded and said that she had never felt that she would ever need a "shrink" and that she was terrified that she was "losing my mind." I encouraged her to take some deep breaths and that we would be collecting a bit of information as to what had been happening to her so that I could come up with a formulation and a care plan that we could agree upon. I explained how I would be collecting information pertaining to her family history, her response to life events as well as her menstrual history. I told her that my basic philosophy is that all that information would help us to understand how she perceives the world and the impact on her biology of the lived experience of her life. I believe that the brain gives off symptoms that are what we call psychiatric in response to the biochemical changes the brain experiences. I encouraged her to get comfortable, nurse and/or feed her baby as needed as well as let me know if she needed a break, etc.

We were going to start with the family history to ascertain if there were any genetic high risk factors that we needed to take into consideration. I have also found that family history is a bit more objective and does not cause as much stress as discussing a woman's life events and responses.

Based on my model of the Earthquake (Sichel & Driscoll, 1999) I would be assessing her "fault lines" and ascertaining if there had been any previous tremors or earthquakes prior to this episode (see Figure 7.1 for Carol's assessment). Carol was 31 years old and a nurse by profession. She worked in a small community hospital as a staff nurse in obstetrics. When she told me that piece of information, red lights were going off in my brain. I was wondering about expectations, what she had seen prior to her birth experience, etc. All these experiences would affect how Carol perceived the world based on her personal and professional encounters. So this information was tucked into the assessment side of my brain as I began to ask Carol to describe her family history for me.

Carol was the older of two children; she had a brother who was three years younger. She described her mother as a quiet, passive woman who deferred to her father all the time. She verbalized that her mother's philosophy was "don't rock the boat" and "just put things behind you . . . move on." Carol described that her mother's parents had died when her mother was a teenager so that Carol never knew them. She did know, however, that her mother's mom did not think there was any problem with hitting her children since her own mother regularly spanked her. Carol believed that her mother gave over the

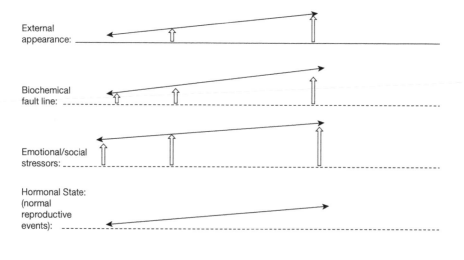

Figure 7.1 Carol's Earthquake Assessment

Source: From *Women's Moods* by Deborah Sichel and Jeanne Watson Driscoll © 1999 by Deborah Sichel and Jeanne Watson Driscoll. Courtesy of HarperCollins Publishers.

responsibility of disciplining the children to her father, "He would punish us and she would just stand back . . . then she would come up to my room later and tell me that he did not mean to be so mean . . . it was crazy making . . . and I just never felt totally safe."

Carol felt that her mom was the "queen of pretending." "My mom wants to believe that my childhood was wonderful. She does not want to talk about how I experienced my childhood, and she just wants everything to be fine." Carol's mother considers that Carol is her friend yet Carol is not too sure about how she feels.

> I can remember when I was getting on the plane to go off to college for my freshman year, imagine I was going off to college all by myself . . . my mom just watched. She didn't even fight with my father to at least go with me to see the campus, get me settled, I was all alone and so scared . . . she just watched.

As I listened I was wondering what it must be like for Carol to grow up not feeling safe, nor feel protected, in essence, by either of her parents.

Carol described that her father's father had committed suicide when he was 17 and that that was a big family secret.

> I was terrified of my father until I became 17, then I got a job after school and I just worked all the time so I didn't have much to do with him. I would come home from work and go to my room to study. I stayed away from him.

Carol went on to describe many incidents of verbal and physical abuse at the hands of her father. She described that he would drink and have "temper tantrums" and that she would feel "numb" whenever he talked to her about anything. Carol described that she felt most of her life that you were only as valuable as others thought you were, so she worked hard to be the best she could be, school-wise and life-wise. "I am a bit obsessive and try to take care of everything." Carol's father died last year and she is still trying to figure out what to do with the feelings of rage and hatred that she has for him.

"In my family, you do not talk about how you feel to anyone. This is so hard to be sitting here answering your questions and talking about my family." I shared with Carol how I agreed that this must be very hard for her and asked if she needed a break. She said, no that she could continue but that "this was hard." I reassured her that it was indeed hard to share family stories when that was so counter to what she had been raised to do. I also encouraged her to take a break whenever she felt she needed one. She then looked at me and said, "It hurts but it feels good to finally tell someone." I felt we were establishing a rapport and that she was feeling safe in the relationship. She seemed encouraged by this process.

I asked her to describe her relationship with her father. "He was strict, verbally abusive; hit me when I was growing up. I even had a black eye once and told everyone at school that I had fallen down." "I would always try to please him. I tried to do everything perfectly so he would not get disappointed or angry. He was scary and yet he was my father." Carol's ambivalence was palpable. She needed some time to process this relationship and knew this work would be happening down the road in our work together.

Carol did not know of any other family history of mood and/or anxiety problems as "no one ever talked about family issues . . . remember, it was just the way it was and move on."

As stated earlier, Carol's brother was three years younger. "He was the prince . . . he could do no wrong . . . I was supposed to take care of him. He never got into any trouble with my father . . . he was the son . . . yet in my mind he was lazy and selfish." She described that they were not close even now as adult siblings and that he lived a few towns over but she never sees him. She believes that he has some depression or "something" because he is not able to hold down a job and just "doesn't seem happy."

Up to this point, I had learned that Carol grew up in a strict environment, had experienced both physical and emotional abuse and that there were problems with emotional regulation on both sides of her family of origin. So there would be an increased genetic propensity to mood and anxiety disorders for Carol, as well as traumatic life experiences. Carol shared with me how she turned her anxiety into perfectionism and obsessive behaviors doing all she could to be "the best and the nicest." Carol came from a family of aggression, anger, alcoholism, depression, avoidance, denial, and numbness. She had what sounded like a rigid upbringing with many rules and regulations for performance in her family of origin. In my nurse therapist mind I was wondering where her anger was directed. It seemed to be definitely redirected into herself as she describes that she is "never good enough" and "just has to work so darn hard to get through one day at a time." There was not a lot of room for play in Carol's life. She lived with very high levels of performance criteria.

We moved our assessment process to the area of her responses to her life stressors: good and bad. I learned early on that most of her childhood was filled with severe anxiety and fear related to her father and stifled anger at her own mother for not protecting her. She studied hard, got good grades, and was very involved with extra-curricular activities. She remembers feeling her best when she got a job at 17 and "now I had my own money . . . I would work as much as I could." She had good friends in grammar and high school and no one knew what went on in her home with her father's rage as she never brought anyone home. She does remember that when she went off to college, she did it all herself and really felt that she needed to go away. Her father was not at all supportive of her getting a college degree but she knew she had to do that. She flew off to college and describes that she had a big adjustment being so far away from home but that once she made friends, it was "great . . . I loved my teachers, enjoyed living in the dorm and I only had to take care of me and my patients . . . I loved nursing school." She had a number of nurturing faculty members and really felt that it was a good move for her to find herself. After college, she moved back to the area and started work on a medical surgical unit in the local, community hospital. "I really wanted to work in obstetrics so it took some time and then I transferred to that specialty . . . I am a good nurse."

Carol met her husband, Harry, at a party.

> It was love at first sight in my book. He is two years older than me and he became, really, my best friend, I can tell him anything and he makes me laugh. He knows all about my crazy family and what it was like for me growing up. He is very supportive to me although, I have to say he didn't step up to the plate with this birth.

This was an area we would definitely return to later in our assessment process.

When we moved the assessment into Carol's reproductive life, I was going to learn all about what had happened to her with her baby's birth. She had experienced menarche at 13 years old. "My mother gave me a book and some sanitary napkins . . . it is not her comfort zone to talk about periods." She described that she had been on oral contraceptives for about a year after she and Harry were married with no problems.

So tell me about the pregnancy, was my lead-in question and Carol began to sob. She was holding Madeleine who was sleeping so she just kept hugging her, sobbing, and rocking back and forth. I sat quietly in my chair and just sat, providing an accepting environment so that she could feel what she was feeling at that moment in time. Slowly she regulated her breathing and she looked at me and began to share her story. I knew that she had a lot to tell me and I wanted this to happen gently and with some control. I didn't want her being re-traumatized just telling me the story. I responded to Carol by telling her that I had a feeling that this story was going to be very hard for her to talk about and she could start wherever she wanted and we could fill the missing puzzle pieces over time, she could proceed in whatever direction she wanted and I was listening.

Slowly, Carol's breathing recaptured a rhythm and I felt like she was present in the room. For a while I felt she had dissociated a bit in that she had a glazed look in her eyes while she had been sobbing and rocking.

> I don't know where to start . . . I don't know what happened . . . I had seen so many births in my career . . . some where women screamed and cried, I did not want to be one of those women . . . a screaming banshee, but that is what I became . . . it was the birth from hell *and I cannot forget it and move on!*

The last part of this phrase was yelled at me. I felt she was responding to someone that was not me, and I remembered that she described that her mother's way of being was to move on and basically pretend that nothing had happened. There was a definite trigger.

Carol described that the pregnancy was planned and they were very excited when they learned she was pregnant. They had been trying for about 6 months before she conceived. She described the first trimester as relatively uneventful.

"I was tired. My stomach was queasy but I didn't really have to throw up, just low grade nausea all the time." She had an obstetrician associated with the hospital where she worked. "I was very comfortable in my early pregnancy, planning on birthing my baby at the hospital where I worked. I knew my friends would take good care of me."

The second trimester continued to be relatively calm with no problems. As she moved into her third trimester, she describes beginning to get a "bit anxious" and began to have a small increase in her blood pressure, "but I watched my salt intake, continued to work and rested when I wasn't working."

When I asked her to begin to describe her labor experience, she looked at me like a deer in the headlights. "Oh, my God, I really don't want to talk about this . . . I think I am going to throw up . . ." I encouraged Carol to just sit up and breathe in and out; we would proceed at whatever pace worked well for her. It took her some time to regulate her breathing and to be a bit more focused on her story.

"I thought I would be safe delivering at the hospital that I worked in but that did not work out at all." She went on to describe how she was always terrified at the idea of screaming in labor, or acting "out of control." She went into the hospital at about 4 centimeters. "I had been in labor all night, but I could walk and talk so we did not rush to call the doctor." When she was admitted, her friend admitted her and she felt that things were going to be alright. She felt safe and cared for. "Boy, did that change quickly." She went on to describe how she felt like she was "abandoned." She had expected that her friend would stay with her but the unit was very busy on that day and Carol and Harry were left alone. She went on to describe,

> In the beginning that was fine, I thought, but as the contractions were getting harder, Harry was not as helpful as I had hoped. We did go to childbirth classes but he just sat back and kept telling me to breathe. I wanted to throw something at him and when I called for my nurse, they did not rush to check on me. In fact, I was told how busy they were.

I was just sitting in my chair feeling so sad for Carol in that it was sounding like this birth experience would be a repetition of how she felt growing up: being alone and not having anyone to protect you and stay with you.

When she was 6 centimeters, she asked for an epidural.

> I did not have any strong feelings prior to going into labor about an epidural or not. I had always figured I would just play it by ear, but this was painful and I was really feeling so anxious. I don't think anyone knew how anxious and scared I really was.

In many ways, Carol was right, remember she had learned early on to look good and be well behaved; she was not going to change that even now. She shared with me that when the anesthesiologist came in,

> She had an attitude, until she learned that I worked there . . . she was nice
> for a while and then when she inserted the epidural, I felt this shooting
> pain down my leg. I started to scream. Then it felt like I had a gun shot to
> my head. She told me to breathe and then gave me some Demerol and left
> the room.

Carol continues as she describes that when she rolled over there was spinal fluid
all over the bed.

> I guess she made a mistake. Now I would have a spinal headache, and I
> knew I didn't move when she was putting it in. I was screaming but I kept
> still. No wonder she left. I kept screaming, Take it out!

She went on to describe how she felt like such a mess in front of her colleagues
and knew that she was going to have a spinal headache.
  When a new anesthesiologist came into her room,

> He fixed the epidural but in many ways the damage was already done. I
> couldn't pick up my head. It was killing me . . . then it just started to go
> crazy. I was so scared and now I was shaking, turned out I had a fever of
> 102. Where did that come from? I did not think that I had ruptured
> membranes, yet what was happening . . . next thing I know they are giving
> me antibiotics and I just felt crazy.

She went on to describe that when the obstetrician came in to do a vaginal
exam, she felt the gloved hand enter her vagina and, "it felt like his hand was
going to come out my mouth . . . I wanted to throw up. I wanted to scream for
someone to help me. I thought that we were both going to die." She went on
to describe how she remembered

> Staring at the knob on the baby warmer. I tried breathing, tried to get my
> mind focused, moved to fantasy land, pictured my cat . . . I fixated on that
> knob and I had no idea, I was holding my mouth shut because I didn't
> want to scream and be one of *those* women in labor. I felt that I had no
> connection with reality. My friend who was now at my side kept asking
> me what I wanted. I didn't know. My head was killing me and the
> contractions were on top of each other. I had pressure in my butt. I wanted
> to move my bowels. I was embarrassing myself to death yet, what was
> happening?

She remembered that she was thinking

> dead baby . . . I was trying to push, but I couldn't hold my head up. There
> were so many people in the room and they were all telling me what to do.
> Where the hell was Harry? I couldn't find him at all . . . I felt I was going

to die. Then I heard the doctor say that he was going to use the mighty vac to pull out the baby . . . I heard him whisper that to someone. Then I feel this incredible pressure in my butt and felt my body being yanked off the table . . . they were yanking this kid out of me. I felt this burn; felt I was going to die. My legs fell off the stirrups. Everyone ran over with the baby . . . I did not hear any crying . . . I must have a dead baby. I did remember it was a girl and I was screaming at them to tell me what she looked like and then someone moved and I saw this black face. I thought I just had a dead baby and I just remember shutting down. The doctor sewed up the episiotomy and the third degree tear and he left. At that time I remember just thinking that I wanted to die if my baby was dead.

I was told that I was lucky I didn't have to have a cesarean by my dear friends . . . no, I didn't have to have a cesarean but I gave birth to a dead baby with a ripped face in a room of a 100 people and no one spoke . . . Harry just moved around like he had seen a ghost.

She was crying and intermittently gasping for breath while she was telling me her story.

Madeleine did indeed begin to breathe and had a laceration on her cheek as well as looked "black" when Carol saw her from across the room. Eventually the baby cried very loudly and the room began to get noisy again . . . relief was felt by all was what I imagined, except perhaps Carol. She was at that time, not really even in the room anymore. "I had just checked out."

When they transferred her to the postpartum room with her baby, she again began to describe feeling disappointment and in many ways abandoned by her friends and colleagues. She remembered an episode of being helped into the shower then no one ever came back to help her. She had lost a significant amount of blood and did indeed feel light-headed but "there was no one there . . . even Harry was gone . . . I don't even remember where he went. . . . oh wait, yes, he went home to change his clothes!"

She described getting herself from the shower to the bed and pulling the curtain around her bed. "I was afraid if I made a peep everyone would hear me, I just sobbed into my pillow and I didn't know where Harry was and none of my 'so-called friends' were around." She went on to describe that it was the evening nurse who informed her that "I needed to request a blood patch for my spinal headache and to try to lay flat until the next day . . . I couldn't even hold my new baby girl. It was a horrific experience."

Carol went on to describe the days in the hospital. She did have the "blood patch" procedure to treat the spinal headache and that was a relief in that she could then sit up and tend to her baby, Madeleine. "She just looked so traumatized. She had a cut on her cheek and her head was so bruised. She looked like she had gone through a war, and in many ways she had." Carol showed me some of the pictures of those first few days and indeed Madeleine did look bruised and what was more telling were the expressions on Carol's face in the pictures. She just looked empty and just "not there."

"It took about a week for Madeleine's bruising to heal and fortunately her behaviors were fine. She nursed well, and was just an even-tempered baby. Thank goodness because I was a mess," said Carol. When she went home from the hospital, Harry stayed home for a week and the three of them connected and became a family.

> My mother did drop-off meals but I had asked her to just leave us alone and she did, as did everyone else. It was a nice week as Harry and I were able to talk about what had happened. I cried a lot. He cried and told me how helpless he had felt. I tried to just let the experience go. It was over and there was nothing I could do about it.

She went on to tell me that in many ways she had fooled herself into believing it was over until the past few months.

She described how she noticed she was having lots of anxiety as it came closer to going for her 6-week obstetrical checkup.

> I noticed that I was having a difficult time catching my breath. I felt like I had constant shortness of breath. I didn't want to see the doctor. I was angry at him for the whole birth experience, for him letting me push so long and then pulling my baby out with the damn vacuum extractor and for not even talking to me about any of it. It was, like, in his mind, it was over and that was it. I had a baby and the birth was over.

Carol was shaking again on the couch as she started to share this part of her story. She went on to describe that prior to the doctor's visit, not only did she have respiratory changes but she was having nightmares regularly and kept remembering the sounds of the delivery room or rather lack of sounds in the room when her baby was born. She had been trying to figure out ways not to go for the checkup but she knew she had to and she would just "suck it up."

The checkup visit was uneventful, according to Carol. "As I thought, he did not bring up any of the birth experience, just acted like everything was fine." She described that that was when she began to think that something was very wrong with her but she would just keep moving forward, as she had done most of her life, not touch the feelings, and not talk about them and just move forward. She did tell me that secondary to the episiotomy and the vaginal tear that she was having a very difficult time with sexual intercourse and "I couldn't care less if we ever do that again."

So Carol was trying to live her life, dedicated to her daughter and her husband as she said "moving forward" until it was time to consider going back to work every other weekend at the hospital of the birth and where she had worked for years prior. She then began to experience what she called "panic attacks," and she cannot understand, why now? She feels that since she had been at work she just "numbs up and wants to be invisible. I don't really want to talk about anything with my nurse colleagues. Why me, am I crazy?" she asks. She describes that many nights she can't get to sleep, has nightmares, and is restless all night. Sometimes "I feel like I want to jump out of my skin and I think it would be easier to be dead but what about Harry and Madeleine?" She does go to work, "I am the great pretender" as she describes acting like nothing is wrong when she goes to work and all the other times in between but she is "a mess."

I sat back and took a deep breath and shared with Carol that I felt she had posttraumatic stress disorder secondary to the birth trauma that she experienced. I also felt that even prior to the birth she had grown up in a somewhat unpredictable house and survived her father's abuse and her mother's disconnection and had a pervasive underlying anxiety disorder already with her perfectionistic behaviors having been developed as a coping strategy that was both a gift and a curse. It helped her with focus, organization and feeling in control while at the same time causing anxiety, obsessions, worries and performance criteria that were hard to meet regularly. She was very hard on herself and her being. We looked at Carol's Earthquake Assessment (see Figure 7.1). I shared with her that based on her genetic history, she had a propensity toward mood and anxiety symptoms and indeed during her childhood and college years she described anxiety, sadness, fear, depression and other feelings that she experienced in response to life events and family dynamics. This genetic vulnerability and her responses to life events had set the stage for a major earthquake that came as a result of the birth trauma. She had had many "tremors" prior to Madeleine's birth. She could see them represented on the earthquake chart. We discussed the need to formulate a care plan that would take all her history into consideration and develop treatment strategies that would help to quiet her neurobiology which was leading to symptoms of anxiety, fear, nightmares, sleep dysregulation, sadness, and depression, her "just not feeling good."

I asked Carol if she felt she could work with me, was she comfortable in the relationship? She said she felt safe and that she wanted to work with me so she could feel better for herself and her family. We then went on to develop the care plan, i.e. The NURSE Program (© Sichel & Driscoll, 1999). We took each element and created strategies of intervention that we would reassess at each meeting.

- *Nourishment and needs*: I felt that some medication would be helpful especially to help quiet down the biology that led to the anxiety, sleep problems and shortness of breath. Carol shared with me that she was really against medication. "I am not crazy and I don't want to be addicted to anything." I let her tell me all the reasons why she did not want medication and we decided that we would wait on that aspect of the care plan. I didn't want to add any more stress to Carol's already stressed self-system at this time, so we would continue that conversation at our next session.

  We talked about her nutrition: water intake, protein intake, daily multivitamin, calcium supplements and vitamin D. We went over her caffeine intake; she drank about five cups of coffee and/or tea a day, so she was going to work on decreasing those numbers and gradually modifying her caffeine intake.

- *Understanding*: I suggested that Carol come to see me for weekly sessions so that she could have a safe place to feel her feelings and share her experiences and her emotions so that she could begin to feel empowered and authentic in what she felt, rather than shamed, and judged.
- *Rest and relaxation*: We went over some meditation strategies that she could implement prior to going to bed as she needed to be able to have some full nights sleep without restlessness and hopefully no more nightmares. She did not want any medication at this time so we were going to use a body relaxation method she had learned in childbirth classes. Also meditation strategies have been found to be helpful in quieting some of the parasympathetic responses to anxiety and fear with trauma situations (Siegel, 2011).
- *Spirituality*: Carol described a strong belief in God and that she did have faith that she would get better. She prayed a lot and was very active in her church although she had not shared her experiences with any of the church community at this time.
- *Exercise*: Currently, she had no formal exercise program in place. "I take Madeleine for walks almost every day." In our discussion, I learned that she had a treadmill in her basement and I suggested that she set it up so she could watch one half-hour television show in the evening when Harry was home and he could watch Madeleine. That would give her about 30 minutes a day of aerobic exercise which helps anxiety and mood. She agreed to try to do that this week.

I felt we had made a good connection and that my goals were to continue to establish a strong rapport with Carol in this relationship and help her be able to feel her emotions without judgment and criticism, to learn to be kinder to herself. I would continue to assess her biochemical responses to the emotions/ feelings and educate her regarding medication as I felt that medication would help her feel a bit better sooner, especially a small amount of a benzodiazepine to quiet her anxiety. I had learned to trust the process and with our relational development over time, we could address the medication issue in the future. We agreed to meet next week and she knew she could call me with any concerns or questions.

Carol came back the next week. She described that she was glad that we had met the week before and hoped that coming to see me would help her. She had a "tough" week as she had worked over the weekend and felt "triggered" a lot during the weekend.

There were two births over the weekend that were horrible and I watched the women and all I could do was feel panic and anxiety. I took care of them in the postpartum unit and I just worked very hard to have them tell me what they were feeling and what I could do to help them. Then when I went home at night, I just sobbed.

We talked about how these experiences re-triggered her own memory of her experiences and that that was not uncommon after a traumatic episode. I explained some of the biochemistry of the "fight and flight" reaction and how the brain/body responds to the events and experiences. We had to hold and honor her emotions and strategize ways for her to feel the feelings, honor them and then let them go. She was not the feeling, but it was what she was feeling. "I feel so helpless and at the same time so angry, why did this happen to me? I am a nice person who works very hard to help others, why me?"

As we developed our relationship over time, Carol agreed to try some low dose clonazepam to help treat her anxiety/panic. She had a positive response to this medication and felt that it helped her to feel more connected and less disconnected when she had the anxious feelings. She also responded well to a low dose of serotonergic reuptake inhibitor, sertraline. We spent many sessions working on understanding how the medication may help in essence "turn down the heat" of the biochemical responses to the trauma while we were cognitively processing the experiences and her new strategies of being in the world with emotional regulation and self-loving care. She came to therapy weekly for about a year. Over that time she was able to integrate her birth experience. She wrote a letter to her obstetrician describing her experience and making suggestions to him about what he needed to do for women in the future, and began to plan for her next child. Although she did not receive a response to her letter from the physician, she felt proud of herself that she had done it as it was a positive thing for her to do to help with some resolution of her experience.

Our relationship continued and after about two years, Carol began to talk about having another baby. She was able to verbalize her level of fear re: birth experience and wanting to be more in control if that was at all possible with the second birth experience. The second birth event would need to be a corrective experience for Carol and we spent many sessions discussing what the key elements she needed to help her feel supported and encouraged through the birth. Carol did a lot of work in finding a new obstetrical care provider and wanted to have an elective cesarean birth so that she did not have to go through labor again and panic with the repeat of that previous experience. She was also going to birth her baby at a different hospital and had asked me to attend the birth as a support person. I was honored to be asked to attend this birth as I had attended many in my old career as a childbirth educator/lactation consultant, so it felt very comfortable for me to say yes to this request. We also spoke about ways to protect our relationship as I am a very public nurse person, and my client didn't want anyone to know I was her patient as she was still not that comfortable with being a "therapy patient." So we processed the issues and when she went into labor, I showed up at the hospital as a labor support person in addition to Harry. The elective cesarean birth was a positive experience for Carol. She felt listened to, honored, and cared for by the anesthesiologist and the obstetrician as she had done a lot of pre-op interviewing and shared with her providers why she wanted this birth to be as "controlled" as it could be. She was awake and aware.

She heard her son cry as soon as he came out of her uterus and then Harry brought the baby to her head and the three of them sat there during the closure of the operative site. It was an amazing experience for me to see her smile, to see the tears of joy stream down from her eyes as her baby made his first cry . . . a healing experience, to say the least.

Carol's postpartum experience was uneventful. Breastfeeding went well. She felt listened to by the nurses and it was on the whole a wonderful corrective experience. When she came back to therapy a few weeks later she was able to talk about how in many ways she felt so sad that Madeleine's birth was so horrific and that David's birth was so different. So some of our work was based on integration of both experiences and how the experience was just that, "an experience," it was not about who she was. She did the best she could do with each and she was working on honoring who she was and who she had become.

Conclusion

Caring for women living with PTSD after the birth is a positive experience for me as I see them make sense of an experience that in so many ways does not make any sense. Paying attention to the unique perceptive realities of each women and her experience is essential. Also, we bring ourselves into all our experience, consciously and unconsciously. The past does affect the present but it does not have to control the future. So often it is the expectations that get blown away, so adjusting expectations, working with a sense of being present in the moment makes it sometimes easier to adapt and adjust. I am, however, constantly amazed and saddened when I realize how critical interpersonal relationships are in the world. How would the situations have been different for these women, including Carol, if someone had really focused and prioritized them as the primary patient in the room?

In Chapter 8, instruments available to clinicians for use in routine screening of posttraumatic stress symptoms in new mothers are presented. The instruments that will be described include: the Posttraumatic Stress Disorder Symptom Scale-Self Report (PSS-SR), the Posttraumatic Diagnostic Scale (PTDS), the Traumatic Event Scale (TES), the Impact of Event Scale (IES), and the Perinatal Posttraumatic Stress Disorder Questionnaire (PPQ).

References

Sichel, D. & Driscoll, J. W. (1999). *Women's moods: What every woman must know about hormones, the brain, and emotional health.* New York: HarperCollins.

Siegel, D. J. (2011). *Mindsight: The new science of personal transformation.* New York: Bantam Books Trade Paperbacks.

8   Instruments to Screen for Posttraumatic Stress Disorder

In this chapter instruments that assess the level of posttraumatic stress symptoms in new mothers will be described. The instruments that will be described include: the Posttraumatic Stress Disorder Symptom Scale-Self Report (PSS-SR), the Posttraumatic Diagnostic Scale (PTDS), the Traumatic Event Scale (TES), the Impact of Event Scale (IES), and the Perinatal Posttraumatic Stress Disorder Questionnaire (PPQ) (Table 8.1). These instruments are available to clinicians for use in routine screening of new mothers and can provide the clinician with quantitative evaluation data that is useful in assessing the efficacy of the treatment modalities in the reduction of symptoms.

Posttraumatic Stress Disorder Symptom Scale-Self Report (PSS-SR)

Foa, Riggs, Dancu, and Rothbaum (1993) developed the PSS-SR which consists of 17 items that correspond to the symptoms of PTSD, according to the DSM-IV diagnostic criteria. These 17 items are categorized into three symptom clusters: 4 items (intrusion subscale), 7 items (avoidance subscale), and 6 items (arousal subscale). Subjects are asked to rate the severity of each symptom over the last two weeks on a 4-point Likert scale (0 = not at all, 1 = a little bit, 2 = somewhat, and 3 = very much). Total scores can range from 0 to 51. A total PSS-SR score of 12 or higher is indicative that a woman is experiencing elevated posttraumatic stress symptoms. A positive screen for meeting the DSM-IV criteria for diagnosis of PTSD can be made when a person endorses at least one item from the intrusion symptom cluster, three items from avoidance, and two items from the arousal symptom cluster. Severity scores can be calculated for each of these three symptom clusters.

Foa et al. (1993) assessed the psychometric properties of the PSS-SR with 118 recent rape and nonsexual assaulted victims. Cronbach's alpha was 0.91 for the total scale and 0.78, 0.80, and 0.82 for intrusion, avoidance, and arousal symptom clusters, respectively. Zaers et al. (2008) reported a reliability of 0.80 at 6 weeks postpartum and 0.85 at 6 months postpartum in 47 new mothers using the PSS-SR. This type of reliability assesses the degree of consistency with which the scale measures posttraumatic stress symptoms.

Table 8.1 Instruments to measure posttraumatic stress symptoms

Instrument	Author/year	Format	Sample	Reliability
Traumatic Event Scale (TES)	Wijma et al. (1997)	17 PTSD symptoms, 10 of these are specific to childbirth	1640 mothers	r = .84
Impact of Event Scale (IES)	Horowitz et al. (1979)	15 items of PTSD symptoms, 7 items (intrusion), 8 items (avoidance), no arousal items	66 adults with serious life events	r = .79 intrusion r = .82 avoidance
Impact of Event Scale–Revised (IES–R)	Weiss & Marmam (1979)	6 items (arousal) added to IES	429 adults emergency personnel	r = .87 intrusion r = .85 avoidance
Perinatal PTSD Questionnaire (PPQ)	Hynan (1998)/ De Mier et al. (1996)	14 yes/no items of PTSD symptoms specific to childbirth, 3 items intrusion, 6 items avoidance, 5 items arousal	92 mothers of high risk infants & 50 mothers of full-term infants	r = .85
	Callahan et al. (1996)	Modified PPQ to 5-point Likert format	47 mothers of preterm infants, 11 mothers of fragile infants & 86 mothers of healthy infants	r = .86
Post Traumatic Stress Symptom Scale (PSS–SR)	Foa et al. (1993)	17 items based on DSM-III-R	46 female rape victims and 72 female non-sexual assault victims	r = .91 total scale r = .78 intrusion r = .80 avoidance r = .82 arousal
Posttraumatic Diagnostic Scale (PTDS)	Foa et al. (1997)	Part I: Checklist of 12 trauma events; Part II, 9 items of impairment in family relationships and work	264 adults with various traumas	r = .92 total scale r = .78 intrusion r = .84 avoidance r = .84 arousal

When the PSS-SR was used as a diagnostic scale, the sensitivity was 0.62 and the specificity was 1.0 using the Structured Clinical Interview for DSM-IV Axis 1 Disorders (SCID). Sensitivity refers to the ability of a screening scale to correctly diagnose a condition. The PSS-SR correctly identified 86% of the sample. Using the PSS-SR in the Netherlands, Olde et al. (2006) reported a reliability = 0.81 with 140 women in the first 3 months postpartum. Also in the Netherlands, in a study of 428 mothers 2–6 months after delivery, the PSS-SR achieved an internal consistency reliability = 0.82 (Stramrood et al., 2010).

Ayers and Pickering (2001) adapted the PSS-SR to make it event-specific with its items referring to childbirth. Examples of some items include the following: "In the past few weeks have you had upsetting thoughts or images about childbirth that come into your head when you do not want them to?" "In the past few weeks have you been making efforts to avoid activities, situations, or places which remind you of childbirth?" Alpha coefficients for this childbirth-specific version of the PSS-SR have been reported to be 0.90 for the total PSS-SR scale and 0.91 (intrusion subscale), 0.81 (avoidance subscale), and 0.84 (arousal subscale).

Posttraumatic Diagnostic Scale (PTDS)

The PSS-SR (Foa et al., 1993) provides information about the symptoms of PTSD like similar scales, however, it does not assess whether the aversive event meets the criteria for trauma as defined by the DSM-IV, nor does it assess the degree of impairment in persons. Foa, Cashman, Jaycox, and Perry (1997) revised the PSS-SR to include these additional criteria for PTSD and named the instrument the Posttraumatic Diagnostic Scale (PTDS). The first part of the PTDS consists of a checklist of 12 traumatic events (one of which is "other" category) in which persons indicate which of these traumas they have either experienced or witnessed. Then individuals are asked to pick the traumatic event that has disturbed them the most in the past four weeks. The person is then instructed to refer to this event when completing the remainder of the items in the scale. The second part of the PTDS consists of the 17 items of PTSD symptoms. The final (third) section of the PTDS consists of 9 items that assess impairment in areas such as family relationships and work.

Foa et al. (1997) assessed the PTDS' psychometrics with 264 individuals who had experienced a variety of traumas such as sexual assault, accident or fire, and combat. Internal consistency reliability for this sample was 0.92 for the total symptom severity and 0.78 (intrusions), 0.84 (avoidance), and 0.84 (arousal). Test–retest reliability over a 2–3 week period was reported as 0.83 (total symptom severity), 0.77 (intrusions), 0.81 (avoidance), and 0.85 (arousal). The psychometrics of this scale need to be assessed with samples of women with PTSD secondary to traumatic childbirth.

Traumatic Event Scale (TES)

The TES was developed to correspond with the DSM-IV criteria for PTSD (Wijma, Soderquist, & Wijma, 1997). Four statements specifically assess childbirth as the stressor criterion:

- The childbirth was a trying experience.
- The childbirth was a threat to my physical integrity.
- During the childbirth I was afraid that I was going to die.
- During the childbirth I felt anxious/helpless/horrified.

(Wijma, Soderquist, & Wijma, 1997, p. 590)

After these stressor statements, the TES consists of 17 DSM-IV PTSD symptoms. Ten of these 17 items are specific to the childbirth experience. Women first rate the frequency of these symptoms and then the severity on a Likert scale. Wijma and colleagues reported a Cronbach's alpha = 0.84 for the TES. Stramrood et al. (2010), for example, reported the internal consistency reliability for the TES was r = .87 for their sample of 428 women 2–6 months postpartum in the Netherlands.

Impact of Event Scale (IES)

The IES is a 15-item scale that measures PTSD symptoms of intrusions (7 items) and avoidance (8 items) but not arousal (Horowitz, Wilner, & Alvarez, 1979). The internal consistency reliabilities of r = 0.79 for the intrusion subscale and r = 0.82 for the avoidance subscale were reported by Horowitz and colleagues. Each subscale is totaled separately. The intrusion subscale score ranges from 0–35 and the avoidance subscale score ranges from 0–40.

Impact of Event Scale Revised (IES–R)

In 1997, Weiss and Marmar revised the IES to include items to assess the third symptom cluster of PTSD, that being arousal. The original IES only assessed intrusion and avoidance. Weiss and Marmar added six symptoms to measure arousal such as anger/irritability, exaggerated startle response, and difficulty concentrating. Olde, Kleber, van der Hart, and Pop (2006) assessed the psychometrics of the IES-R in a sample of 435 Dutch women 3 months after birth. Cronbach's alpha for the total TES-R was 0.89 and internal consistency reliabilities for the subscales were: intrusion (r = 0.84), avoidance (r = 0.79), and arousal (r = 0.68).

The IES-R has also been used to assess posttraumatic stress due to childbirth in Germany (Kersting et al., 2004) and in Switzerland (Lemola, Stadlmayr, & Grob, 2007). The psychometrics of the scale were not reported in these studies.

Perinatal Posttraumatic Stress Disorder Questionnaire (PPQ)

Hynan (1998) developed the PPQ which is a 14-item, yes/no survey to measure symptoms of PTSD specifically related to childbirth. The first three items on the PPQ measure intrusion symptoms such as having bad dreams of childbirth or of the infant's hospital stay. Symptoms of avoidance or numbing of responsiveness are the focus of the next 6 items. Examples of these items include avoidance of things that remind the mother about her childbirth or infant's hospital stay and difficulty remembering parts of her childbirth. The remaining 5 items measure arousal symptoms such as feeling jumpy or irritable.

DeMier, Hynan, Harris, and Maniello (1996) reported the reliability to be 0.85 for the PPQ and test–retest reliability of 0.92 for an interval of 2–4 weeks. Reliability was assessed in a sample of 92 mothers of high-risk infants and 50 mothers of full-term, healthy infants. Quinnell and Hynan (1999) reported substantial support for convergent and divergent validity of the PPQ in a sample of 83 mothers of preterm infants, 51 mothers of full-term, healthy infants, and 8 women whose full-term infants were in the NICU. Convergent validity measures the degree to which two methods of measuring a concept are similar. Divergent validity assesses the degree to which two methods of measuring a concept are different. The mean length of time since birth for this sample was 7 years. Women completed the PPQ, the IES (Horowitz et al., 1979), and the Need for Cognition Scale (NCS; Cacaioppo & Petty, 1982). Correlation of the PPQ with the convergent measure of the IES was 0.78 and with the NCS, the divergent measure was $-.025$.

Callahan and Hynan (2002) further assessed the construct validity of the PPQ with 111 mothers of preterm infants, 10 mothers of fragile infants in NICU, and 52 mothers of full-term, healthy infants. Construct validity assessed the extent to which a scale measures the concept it is supposed to be measuring. The mean length of time since birth for this sample was 3 years. Women were asked to answer yes to the items only if they had experienced the symptom for longer than 1 month during the time frame of 4–18 months postpartum. The PPQ had a significant positive correlation with the IES ($r = 0.61$) and the Beck Depression Inventory-II (BDI-II; Beck, Steer, & Brown, 1996) ($r = 0.58$). The correlation with the divergent measure of the Openness Scale (Costa & McCrae, 1992) was nonsignificant.

The PPQ was modified to change the item response options from a dichotomous yes/no choice to a 5-point Likert scale format where mothers respond to the frequency of each of the 14 symptoms (Callahan, Borja, & Hynan, 2006). Response scale and scoring weight for each items are as follows: 0 = not at all, 1 = once or twice, 2 = sometimes, 3 = often, but less than 1 month, and 4 = often, for more than a month. The total possible range of scores on the modified PPQ is $0 - 56$. A Likert scale consists of a set of items that participants rate their degree of agreement or disagreement with. In their study conducted via the Internet, 179 women completed the modified PPQ.

In this sample 47 mothers had preterm infants, 11 fragile infants, and 86 full-term, healthy infants. Internal consistency reliability was 0.86 for the total scale. Internal consistency refers to the degree to which items on an instrument are all measuring the same attribute or concept. Convergent and divergent validity were supported by a significant positive correlation of the modified PPQ and IES ($r = 0.74$) and the BDI-II ($r = .52$). The modified PPQ was not significantly correlated with the Openness Scale, thus supporting divergent validity.

Conclusion

In this chapter five instruments were reviewed that are available to clinicians for use in screening women for posttraumatic stress symptoms. In Chapter 9, the focus is on the impact of traumatic childbirth on mothers' experiences of breastfeeding.

References

Ayers, S., & Pickering, A. D. (2001). Do women get posttraumatic stress disorder as a result of childbirth? A prospective study of incidence. *Birth, 28,* 111–118.

Beck, A. T., Steer, R. A., & Brown, G. K. (1996). *Beck Depression Inventory* (2nd ed.). San Antonio, TX: Psychological Corporation.

Cacaioppo, J. T., & Petty, R. E. (1982). The need for cognition. *Journal of Personality and Social Psychology, 42,* 116–131.

Callahan, J. L., & Hynan, M. T. (2002). Identifying mothers at risk for postnatal emotional distress: Further evidence for the validity of the Perinatal Posttraumatic Stress Disorder Questionnaire. *Journal of Perinatology, 22,* 448–454.

Callahan, J. L., Borja, S. E., & Hynan, M. T. (2006). Modification of the Perinatal PTSD Questionnaire to enhance clinical utility. *Journal of Perinatology, 26,* 533–539.

Costa, P. T., & McCrae, R. R. (1992). *Revised NEO Personality Inventory (NEO-PI-R) and NEO Five Factor Inventory (NEO-FFI).* Odessa, FL: Psychological Assessment Resources.

DeMier, R. L., Hynan, M. T., Harris, H. B., & Maniello, R. L. (1996). Perinatal stressors as predictors of symptoms of posttraumatic stress in mothers of high-risk infants. *Journal of Perinatology, 16,* 276–280.

Foa, E. B., Cashman, L., Jaycox, L., & Perry, K. (1997). The validation of a self-report measure of posttraumatic stress disorder: The Posttraumatic Diagnostic Scale. *Psychological Assessment, 9,* 445–451.

Foa, E. B., Riggs, D. S., Dancu, C. V., & Rothbaum, B. O. (1993). Reliability and validity of a brief instrument for assessing posttraumatic stress disorder (PSS-SR). *Journal of Traumatic Stress, 6,* 459–473.

Horowitz, M., Wilner, N., & Alvarez, W. (1979). Impact of Event Scale: A measure of subjective stress. *Psychosomatic Medicine, 41,* 209–218.

Hynan, M. T. (1998). The Perinatal Posttraumatic Stress Disorder (PTSD) Questionnaire (PPQ). In R. Wood, & C. P. Zalaquette (Eds.). *Evaluating stress: A handbook of resources* (Vol. 2; pp. 199–220). Lanham, MD: Scarecrow Press.

Kersting, A., Dorsch, M., Wesselmann, U., Ludorff, K., Witthaut, J., Ohrmann, P., Hornig-Franz, I., Klockenbusch, W., Harms, E., & Arolt, V. (2004). Maternal posttraumatic stress response after the birth of a very low-birth-weight infant. *Journal of Psychosomatic Research, 57,* 473–476.

Lemola, S., Stadlmayr, W., & Grob, A. (2007). Maternal adjustment 5 months after birth: The impact of the subjective experience of childbirth and emotional support from the partner. *Journal of Reproductive and Infant Psychology, 25,* 190–202.

Olde, E., Kleber, R. J., van der Hart, O., & Pop, V. J. M. (2006). Childbirth and posttraumatic stress responses: A validation study of the Dutch Impact of Event Scale-Revised. *European Journal of Psychological Assessment, 22,* 259–267.

Quinnell, F. A., & Hynan, M. T. (1999). Convergent and discriminant validity of the Perinatal PTSD Questionnaire (PPQ): A preliminary study. *Journal of Traumatic Stress, 12,* 193–199.

Stramrood, C., Huis In 't Veld, E. M. J., van Pampus, M. G., Berger, L. W. A., Vingerhoets, J. J. M., Weijmar Schultz, W. C. M., van den Berg, P. P., van Sonderen, E. L. P., & Paarlberg, K. M. (2010). Measuring posttraumatic stress following childbirth: A critical evaluation of instruments. *Journal of Psychosomatic Obstetrics & Gynecology, 31,* 40–49.

Weiss, D. S., & Marmar, C. R. (1997). The Impact of Event Scale-Revised. In J. P. Wilson, & T. M. Keane (Eds.). *Assessing psychological trauma and PTSD: A handbook for practitioners* (pp. 399–411). New York: Guilford.

Wijma, K., Soderquist, M. A., & Wijma, B. (1997). Posttraumatic stress disorder after childbirth: A cross sectional study. *Journal of Anxiety Disorders, 11,* 587–597.

Zaers, S., Waschke, M., & Ehlert, U. (2008). Depressive symptoms and symptoms of posttraumatic stress disorder on women after childbirth. *Journal of Psychosomatic Obstetrics and Gynecology, 29,* 61–71.

9 Impact of Traumatic Childbirth on Breastfeeding

A question that was triggered as part of the process of Cheryl and Sue's research and the narratives that women emailed to them led to the investigation of the breastfeeding relationship. Was there an impact on this relationship positively, negatively, or not at all? In this chapter, first, is a review of the literature highlighting factors that have been reported to impact mothers' breastfeeding experiences. Next, Cheryl and Sue's qualitative study is described (Beck & Watson, 2008).

Delivery Type

Conflicting findings have been reported in the literature between type of delivery and breastfeeding. Janke (1988) did not find any difference in breast-feeding rates at 6 weeks postpartum for women who had vaginal and cesarean births. Reasons for stopping breastfeeding were similar for both groups of women. In a randomized control trial study, conducted by Hannah and colleagues (2002), no differences at 3 months postpartum in breastfeeding rates were found between women who had planned cesarean as opposed to planned vaginal delivery for breech presentation. On the other hand, in another study when compared to women who delivered vaginally, mothers who had cesarean births were more likely not to breastfeed and those who did choose to breastfeed were more likely to stop within the first 2 weeks after delivery (Samuels, Margen, & Schoen, 1985). In an earlier study, Procianoy, Fernandes-Filhio, Lazaro, and Sartori (1984) reported that mothers who had cesarean births were significantly less likely to breastfeed at 2 months postpartum compared to women who had given birth vaginally. These two groups did not differ significantly in socioeconomic, prenatal, and neonatal factors. Nissen et al. (1996) reported that compared to women who had vaginal births, mothers who had cesarean deliveries had lower pulsatile oxytocin release patterns and lower levels of prolactin. Both oxytocin and prolactin hormones are critical hormones needed for successful lactation. Oxytocin is the hormone that is connected to milk ejection or let down and prolactin is involved in milk production.

Compounding this physiological research finding about the hormonal levels is the issue that there seems to be a delay in the sucking responses in babies born via cesarean delivery. Otamiri, Berg, Leden, Leijon, and Tagercrantz (1991) reported delayed neurological adaptation in infants delivered by cesarean during the first 2 days after birth. Infants born by cesarean birth were less excitable and had a significantly decreased number of optimal responses compared to infants born vaginally. On day 5 postpartum, there were no significant neurological differences reported between these two groups of infants. On a practical level, these early days are when the lactogenesis and milk ejection reflexes are maturing; the infant's delay in early suckling can alter the maternal feelings of success with breastfeeding so the health care providers need to support and encourage the aspects of learning new behaviors and trusting the process that the baby will indeed become an active participant in the breastfeeding relationship. The mother may need to be taught pumping skills so that she can be working physiologically along with her body while her baby responds to extrauterine life and suckling.

Labor Stress and Lactogenesis

In a sample of 40 women at delivery, it was reported that the mothers who had experienced longer labors had elevated stress hormone levels in their blood, and lower breastfeeding frequency on the first day postpartum (Chen, Nommsen-Rivers, Dewey, & Lonnerdal, 1998). Also in Chen et al.'s study on day 5 postpartum, primiparas who had a long duration of labor had a lower milk volume. Dewey (2001) reported that a delay in lactogenesis (milk making) was related to prolonged duration of labor and emergency cesarean delivery. In a sample of 136 Guatemalan women Grajeda and Perez-Escamilla (2002) reported that stress during labor and delivery, as reflected by cortisol levels, was a significant risk factor for delayed onset of lactation. Primiparous women who had emergency cesarean births were more likely to have a significant delay in onset of lactation compared to the rest of the sample.

Postpartum Mood and Anxiety Disorders

The only research located on the impact of any postpartum mood and anxiety disorder on breastfeeding focused on postpartum depression. No consistent pattern has been confirmed in the literature between breastfeeding onset or duration and postpartum depressive symptomatology. No studies, quantitative or qualitative, examined the impact of PTSD due to birth trauma on breastfeeding until 2008 when Beck and Watson conducted a qualitative study on mothers' perceptions of the impact of traumatic childbirth on their breastfeeding experiences.

Beck and Watson (2008) conducted an Internet qualitative study with an international sample of 52 mothers who experienced a traumatic birth. In the study, women were asked to describe how their birth trauma impacted their breastfeeding experiences. The range of duration of breastfeeding for these mothers was from 48 hours to 27 months. Eight themes emerged from the

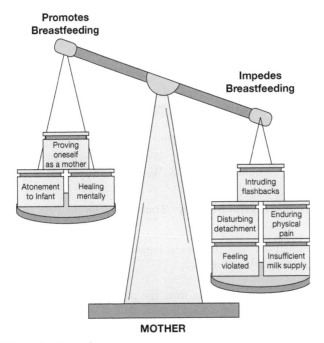

Figure 9.1 Breastfeeding scale

Source: Reprinted with permission from Beck & Watson (2008, p. 232).

analysis of the mothers' stories. These themes revealed that the impact of traumatic childbirth on mothers' breastfeeding experiences can lead women down two strikingly different paths to either impede or promote their breastfeeding attempts. The eight themes were portrayed as weights on a scale (Figure 9.1). Three of the themes helped to promote breastfeeding while five themes impeded or disrupted the women's experiences related to breastfeeding. Not every mother experienced all eight of the themes. Each woman experienced a different combination of the themes and it was the individual combinations which determined which path the women followed; which direction the breastfeeding scale tipped. The first three themes dealt with aspects of birth trauma that *facilitated* mothers' breastfeeding attempts.

Theme 1: Proving Oneself as a Mother: Sheer Determination to Succeed

Women who had a traumatic birth often felt as if they had "failed" at giving birth. In their eyes they needed to succeed at breastfeeding to "prove" to themselves and to others that they could do something right in motherhood. Women were tenacious in their desire to breastfeed. As one mother shared, "It was part of my crusade, so to speak, to prove myself as a mother and . . . being able to breastfeed successfully was the only and last chance I had to 'normalize' my horrible experience with giving birth" (Beck & Watson, 2008, p. 233).

Theme 2: Making up for an Awful Arrival: Atonement to the Baby

Women were steadfast in their resolve to make amends to their infants for the traumatic way they were brought into the world. Mothers felt strongly that they had to atone for their "sin" of the traumatic birth. As one mother in this sample, who breastfed the longest time, explained: "Breastfeeding became a form of forgiveness for me. Giving my daughter the best possible start, I breastfed her for 27 months" (Beck & Watson, 2008, p. 233).

Theme 3: Helping to Heal Mentally: Time-Out from the Pain in One's Head

For some women the time they spent breastfeeding their infants was soothing for them. As one mother shared:

> Breastfeeding was a time-out from the pain in my head. It was a "current reality"—a way to cling onto some "real life." Whereas all the trauma that continued to live on in my head belonged to the past even though I couldn't seem to keep it there.
>
> (Beck & Watson, 2008, p. 233)

Successful breastfeeding helped mothers to heal by restoring their faith in their bodies and increasing their self-esteem as illustrated by the following quote:

> My body's ability to produce milk, and so the sustenance to keep my baby alive also helped to restore my faith in my body, which at some core level, I felt had really let me down, due to a terrible pregnancy, labor and birth. It helped to build my confidence in my body and as a mother. It helped me heal and feel connected to my baby.
>
> (Beck & Watson, 2008, p. 233)

This theme was validated in the literature by a study conducted by Olza-Fernandez, Garcia-Murillo, and Palanca-Maresca in 2011. They reported in their case study that breastfeeding helped calm a mother with PTSD due to her emergency peripartum hysterectomy and helped her to feel more attached to her infant.

The remaining five themes focused on aspects of birth trauma that *hindered* women's breastfeeding attempts.

Theme 4: Just One More Thing to Be Violated: Mothers' Breasts

Frequently women admitted that their childbirth felt like they had been raped with everyone watching and no one offering to help them. They felt as if their bodies had been violated and they had been stripped of their dignity. Protecting their bodies from being further violated became paramount as they needed to regain control of their bodies. The following quote from a mother who had been traumatized giving birth illustrates this vigilance to protect especially one part of her body, namely her breasts:

> I was sick of everyone grabbing my breasts like they didn't even belong to me. My breasts were just another thing to be taken away and violated. When I breastfed my baby, I felt like it was one more invasion on my body and I couldn't handle that after the labor I had suffered. Whenever I put her to breast, I wanted to scream and vomit at the same time. After a horrible 8 weeks, I made the decision to stop breastfeeding. It was crucial to me in reclaiming some power for myself, in taking back control of my life, my body and my right to choose what kind of care was best for my child.
>
> (Beck & Watson, 2008, p. 233)

Theme 5: Enduring the Physical Pain: Seeming at Times an Insurmountable Ordeal

Not only did psychological trauma impact breastfeeding but also physical trauma as vividly explained by one woman:

> Nursing required sitting up, putting pressure on my pointless episiotomy. When the nurses would check my bottom, they would visibly wince before pulling the blanket back up. I snuck a peak at myself at one point and was appalled to see that my labia were so swollen that they looked like testicles. I hated breastfeeding because it hurt to try and sit to do it. I couldn't seem to manage lying down. I was cheated out of breastfeeding. I feel I have been cheated out of something exceptional.
>
> (Beck & Watson, 2008, p. 234)

Theme 6: Dangerous Mix: Birth Trauma and Insufficient Milk Supply

Women described that their "meager milk supply" was due to the repercussions of their birth trauma. A mother who had a severe postpartum hemorrhage followed by a uterine infection recalled: "I think the trauma definitely affected my milk supply. It wasn't an easy decision but a continuing inadequate milk supply and a desperate need to reduce the pressure, I was forced to 'call it quits'" (Beck &Watson, 2008, p. 234).

Another mother who had suffered from preeclampsia, a torn pelvic ligament, and a severe reaction to a drug given to decrease her high blood pressure admitted that: "My body was so traumatized by the delivery and days after it that it never fully recovered from it. My milk never really came in well" (Beck & Watson, 2008, p. 234).

Theme 7: Intruding Flashbacks: Stealing Anticipated Joy

Some women, who had endured a traumatic childbirth, described that when they breastfed, intrusive, distressing flashbacks to their birth trauma haunted them. One primipara who had a long, painful labor due to an ineffective epidural, followed by a high forceps delivery, shared:

> I had flashbacks to the birth every time I would feed him. When he was put on me in the hospital, he wasn't breathing and he was blue. I kept picturing this, and could still feel what it was like. Breastfeeding him was a similar position as to the way he was put on me. I would get really upset and cry when I fed him which would cause my baby to cry.
>
> (Beck & Watson, 2008, p. 234)

Theme 8: Disturbing Detachment: An Empty Affair

This theme spotlighted the insidious effects of traumatic childbirth on mother–infant bonding. Women shared that they felt detached from their infants as this quote highlights:

> Breastfeeding my son in the first few months, certainly the first 6, but possibly as much as 9 months, was an empty affair. I felt nothing at all. Breastfeeding was just one of the many things I did while remaining totally detached from my baby.
>
> (Beck & Watson, 2008, p. 234)

Implications for Clinical Practice Based on Beck and Watson's (2008) Study

This study highlighted to the researchers the need for women to have time to process their birth experiences prior to discharge from the hospital. Health care providers need to spend time with women as they describe their perception of the birth experience, so that assessment of a traumatic experience can be completed and the care plan developed for their hospitalization as well as after discharge. The care plan needs to include the referral to mental health providers so the women's experiences are validated as real to them and they know that their experience been taken seriously by the postpartum health care providers. As we have discussed in this book, it is the perception of the experience to the individual woman that is the identifying variable in the etiology of PTSD secondary to traumatic birth, not the perceived experience of the care provider. Clinicians need to provide an empathic connection with new mothers that facilitates mental health and integration of experiences. As was also reported in this study, mothers who have experienced traumatic births may need intensive one-on-one support to establish breastfeeding. Respect must always be given to a new mother in the form of asking permission to touch her breasts when assisting with breastfeeding. Clinicians must be cognizant of body boundaries and personal space.

The disturbing detachment from their infants that some women felt when breastfeeding is alarming since during the postpartum period mothers should be developing a relationship with their infants. Traumatic childbirth can impede mother–infant bonding. Nursing staff need to watch for altered attachment in mother–baby dyads and implement a care plan that facilitates the mother–baby attachment: teaching about the unique behavioral skills of newborns, asking women to describe how they see their babies, who they look like, how they feel about them, etc. This is a time when continuity of care providers is critical.

It is important to allow and encourage women to talk about how they feel about breastfeeding rather than just assuming infant feeding methods. Clinicians should be aware of their projecting onto mothers their personal beliefs about infant feeding methods. They are vulnerable and hyper-alert to other people's body language, words, and presence. It is important to help her to process her experiences and know that she has the right to choose how she feeds her baby and need not feel guilt or judgment from others, to realize that this is HER experience and she will do what is best for her and her baby. For some women who have experienced birth trauma, pressure from clinicians, family, and/or friends to continue breastfeeding, no matter what, can complicate further their feelings of failure, shame, and inadequacy. Often, health care providers are not always conscious of the nuances of women's verbalized cues for support, guidance, and/or direction. The mother may not be able to put in clear words how she feels inside as negative emotions are not often "allowed" after the birth of the baby. People lead the conversation with their feelings, i.e. "You must be so happy about breastfeeding your baby," so clinicians should try to lead with empathic concern and open-ended questions.

The following are two mothers' experiences of their struggles and triumph at breastfeeding after their traumatic births. They both had participated in Beck and Watson's (2008) Internet study.

Debra's Story

Two hours after entering the hospital, Debra had an emergency cesarean due to severe preeclampsia. She was 31 weeks gestation and her daughter weighed 2 lbs 12 ounces and was transferred to the neonatal intensive care unit (NICU). Debra's traumatic birth of her preterm daughter set the stage for breastfeeding difficulties. Her husband said, "The NICU is its own special hell." Debra voiced that:

> Nothing can prepare you for having a child in the NICU and it takes ridiculous amounts of stubbornness and willpower to stick to the goals you had before you had your life turned inside out because of a premature birth. Stubbornness, willpower, and more support than you can imagine and from anyone, anywhere, who will give it. I had lost so much because of her

premature birth that I was going to be dammed to hell before I was going to give up on nursing her, especially before it even started.

The rest of Debra's story of the impact of her traumatic childbirth on her breastfeeding experience is as follows in her own words:

I spent the first 24 hours of my daughter's life doped up on morphine and whatever else they gave me for the pain. I spent the next 24 hours trying to get out of bed so I could finally see my daughter. The first time I saw her and changed her itty bitty diaper I thought she was a he. She had no fat on her so her little girl parts looked like little boy parts. I argued with the nurse for a minute or so over the supposed gender of my child. All of this compounded the feeling of disconnect I had between me and this little creature. It took until day three before someone finally said I should start pumping, and at that point my baby had already gotten her first bit of formula, thus negating the exclusive breastfeeding goal. However, I did not feel a feeling of failure at that time, just frustration and determination.

Pumping has to be one of the most tortuous things that one can impose on themselves. You have a cold mechanical machine forcing your gift of milk out of you and it serves mostly to remind you only that there is supposed to be a baby there at your breast. Then if you only pump a little bit, there is a strong feeling of failure and you are reminded that you didn't measure up to carrying your child, so why would you measure up here? At least that was my feeling.

The first time I pumped it barely came up to 1cc of breast milk/colostrum and if the nurses had not made a huge fuss over how amazing that was, how that little bit was still "liquid gold" and how great a job I was doing by pumping, I would have quit right there and never have forgiven myself for it. My husband was right along with them telling me what a great mother I was for doing this. I personally felt I needed to do it. I mean, damn it, I had lost nearly everything, or so it felt at the time, that there was no way I was going to lose this too. Pumping milk was the only thing that reminded me I was connected to this little creature that seemed so foreign to me.

The support of my nurse, the lactation consultant, my friends, my husband, my family, and even strangers from the Internet is the main thing that kept me from throwing in the towel. In order to keep up my supply I was suppose to pump for 15–30 minutes every 3 hours, which is an insane schedule to keep, especially when you factor in the need for sleep and to visit our child in the NICU at least once a day. I never managed to keep that schedule and sometimes I would go up to 6 hours between pumping sessions. I hated that pump so much.

Eventually my supply took a hit because of a combination of not keeping the proper pumping regime and more importantly because the pump I was renting wasn't keeping proper suction. I went from pumping 2 ounces at a time to pumping 3 ccs. I was devastated. I began doing everything I could to bring my supply back up. I pumped in hour-long sessions every 3–4 hours and I made sure to keep pictures of my baby nearby, though without feeling any motherly instinct it didn't seem to make any difference. It took a long time but I was eventually able to pump half the amount I had been up to before, and occasionally a little more, but never as much as I had gotten earlier. The supply of milk ran out and my daughter was given formula for the first time since I had started pumping. I had failed her again.

The NICU is completely counterproductive to the warm natural ways of nursing. Even with the painted walls and dimmed lights that my hospital had, it was still a cold and sterile place. Babies are fed on a schedule, which is done because there are not enough people to handle on-demand feeding. You are not allowed to put the child to your breast early on when they are still rooting and it is more instinctive to latch, which leads to babies forgetting what they were born to know. Not only do you have to pump and store, but you must also deliver the milk, which must be kept frozen. After my daughter got out of the NICU, I spent another month pumping and nursing until she finally took completely to the breast. I had to fight hard with myself and occasionally with others to get there, and once there thought I was never able to get myself to pump again.

Breastfeeding after a traumatic birth, especially one that results in a NICU stay, is almost an act of defiance. Defiance against the detachment and almost loathing you feel toward the child. Defiance against the depression that rules so much of your mind and defiance against all the people who try and switch you to formula. Breastfeeding in these circumstances has to be supported even more than in healthy normal births, the more the better, or the mother will drown.

My daughter is now 1 year old and I am still nursing her. I nearly gave up around 10 months when she was waking every hour until I finally made my husband get up with her instead and the bottle helped her sleep longer, and which made me saner. She has five teeth now and occasionally bites so thoughts of weaning her are entering my mind but I'm OK with it because I made it a year. Her pediatrician says I am one of the only mothers of a preemie that she has that was able to breastfeed at all (let alone that long). It is a source of great pride for me and has helped tremendously in overcoming the guilt I have about her birth, because I know I got this part right.

Victoria's Story

Victoria described how her traumatic birth was filled with multiple medical interventions. Her membranes had ruptured spontaneously at 36 weeks gestation and after 22 hours of labor, Victoria was only 4 centimeters dilated. The rest of the story is in Victoria's own words:

So induction drip in place, monitoring in place, pethidine (an analgesic) pain pump in place (eyes spinning in two different directions), anti-nausea stuff in one of the trios. My labor was a really medicalized situation. After 9 hours of this, I was very sensitive to the nasty side effects of pethidine but it did very little to diminish the pain. I was permanently nauseous, hallucinating, etc. The induction was badly handled and I had several bouts of hyper-reactive activity in the uterus—extremely painful.

By the time I was 10 cms, ready to push, I was utterly exhausted and couldn't even lift my eyelids let alone push. After an hour of pushing and no progress, my midwife called the on-call obstetrician. After another hour of pushing, he finally arrived. I specifically wanted an episiotomy rather than to tear but I was too stoned from the pethidine to ask for this—and thought my husband and/or midwife would remember to say this—neither did. Actually at this point in time I just wanted to die (or at least to sleep) and I desperately wanted a c-section under general—just so I could sleep—but was too stoned to ask for this. So ventouse in place, and it slipped off several times. Room now full of people who kept talking to me which I found incredibly frustrating as I couldn't properly understand them or answer them. Obstetrician now told me (after 3 hours of pushing), and I quote, "It's time to *really* push now" . . . had I been able to tell him to **** off, I would have—what did he think I had been doing for the past 3 hours?

Baby finally delivered at 9 a.m. No overwhelming sense of love, just relief. I actually said "Is that it? Thank God!", much to everyone's horror. The baby taken straight away to be checked, didn't even see her for 5 minutes, just heard her crying. Third degree tear which took an hour of painful stitching (when I told the obstetrician that it really hurt, he said, and I quote, "It can't hurt, I've given you a local") while baby had been whisked off and dressed—against my wishes for skin-to-skin contact. By the time I got the baby, she had been out for at least an hour, also against usual hospital policy. Tried to breastfeed at this time, complete failure. This is second point at which things went wrong. First, I had expected that my body would know what to do in giving birth—it didn't. Second, I had expected (and had been to classes which confirmed this), that breastfeeding would just happen—it didn't. Baby didn't even recognize that a breast was there—none of the snuggling, licking, or nuzzling that second baby did. So now I felt as though there must be something fundamentally wrong with me—my body (and indeed my baby who came out of my body) just didn't know what to do. This was compounded by a sense of failure at not having the birth I expected, and guilt at feeling that it was just a horrible, painful, bloody experience (not the wonderful empowering stuff the antenatal classes had led me to believe it would be).

I didn't actually even want to hold my baby. She looked so alien and I couldn't believe she had come out of my body. I felt guilty about this on top of the exhaustion, shock, and sense of failure. I was so exhausted that all I could think about was sleeping—for days and days and days. I couldn't sleep though, not through excitement but every time I closed my eyes, I had intense and vivid thoughts of my birth and overwhelming feelings of revulsion, fear, and failure. My poor baby spent her first weeks in a crib beside me and had hardly ever been held (guilt on top of guilt).

Second attempt at breastfeeding, same failure as first. Continued attempts to breastfeed just basically hopeless which continued for three days. My body had betrayed me again. On discharge at two days, my baby had lost an utterly 20% of her birth weight and was jaundiced. I went to a specialist postnatal facility, as before I had the baby I knew I would need more help than just two days in hospital. On admission to the postnatal facility, it was all action. Pediatrician, lactation consultant, breast pump, etc. So now, not only was I exhausted, feeling like a failure, and utterly traumatized by my birth, now I was into "rescue" mode, with a VERY sick baby that I hadn't realized was sick. More guilt. Still couldn't sleep properly.

Because our first few days breastfeeding were so incredibly unsuccessful, my milk hadn't really come as such, more like dribbled in, which compounded the problem. My baby put on no weight at all for the next three days while I was in the postnatal facility, but I was determined to get home and get on with it—feeding, pumping, and formula top-ups on a 3-hourly basis, day and night.

Breastfeeding during this time was frankly awful. In the first two days when I was just a drugged, exhausted, shell-shocked zombie, it was frustrating and I felt that it was another thing that my body didn't know how to do. When it got to panic-situations in the next few days, it felt like it was critically important, still incredibly difficult, but now it felt like life or death (probably this was a really exaggerated response). So when it still wasn't going well in these few days, it was hugely alarming. Breastfeeding became my focus for overcoming the birth and proving to everyone else (nay-sayers) and mostly to myself that there was *something* I could do right.

Because my milk supply was so low, and the baby was not gaining weight, I continued with pumping and formula top-ups. Many people, including my mother, midwife, and husband, suggesting I just get her on formula exclusively—this would mean I could actually get some sleep as the whole feed/top-up/pump cycle took at least an hour and a half. Every 3 hours, day and night. I really wanted to give breastfeeding a decent chance although most people around me felt I had done so already. In my mind, I think being able to breastfeed successfully was the only and last chance I had to "normalize" my horrible experience with giving birth so I was bloody determined to do it. Lucky that I'm incredibly bloody-minded and persistent otherwise my baby would most definitely be a bottle baby. I think, had I bottle-fed, my bond with my baby would have been even more compromised.

I was utterly shocked by my birth experience. It actually wasn't until weeks later that it really hit me and I really started having trouble sleeping, feeling anxious and indecisive, and having momentary flashbacks about parts of the birth that I had sort of forgotten. I became quite obsessed with trying to work out what had happened. Later on when I felt really comfortable with breastfeeding (probably around 4–5 months), breastfeeding was just bloody hard work. But it was part of my crusade, so to speak, to prove myself as a mother. Once breastfeeding got easier, it was just a normal part of life, but never really became something I enjoyed. It was just convenient for me and good for the baby.

Victoria breastfed for one year.

Victoria went on to have another baby. This time her childbirth was not traumatic and she could then compare the difference this made in her breastfeeding of her second baby.

With baby number two breastfeeding has been and continues to be an absolute joy. I get the rush of hormones (that the books tell you about) that makes me feel calm and relaxed and I always feel particularly "madonna and child"-like when I breastfeed him. It is, and always has been, an essential part of our bond, and something I do as much out of love as for nutrition. It was never that way with my first baby. I now feel I've cheated her out of something really special and I'm just so sad about that. No one told me that the circumstances of my birth would be so tied up on my own experience that bonding with my baby would need to be worked at. Perhaps if this emotional aspect of breastfeeding had been explained to me before I gave birth, it might have been easier.

Clinician's Reaction

These narrative stories of two women who experienced traumatic births and described breastfeeding experiences trigger such sad feelings in me as a nurse and retired lactation consultant. The mental well-being of these women is critical and I believe it is the role of the nurse to provide the individual support and care that postpartum women deserve. Each of these experiences, as described by the women, presents situations where my question is, where are the nurses? Why did these women have to be in essence re-traumatized by the breastfeeding experience? And thank goodness for their personal stubbornness and resiliency. It is physiologically known that the initiation of lactogenesis occurs secondary to suckling behavior on the nipple/areola area, be that the baby or the pump, so why didn't that happen for Debra, where were the postpartum nurses to help her initiate lactation while her baby was in NICU? An individualized care plan must be developed by the nurse on the postpartum unit in collaboration with the new mother and her unique experience. So if we think of what that might be, it basically falls into three domains: maternal care, initiation of breastfeeding, and the facilitation of maternal–infant attachment. I do believe that care of the father is also necessary in the postpartum experience as he has seen his wife go through the experience and he too needs to process the events which can affect the couple's relationship and paternal development. So let's begin with maternal care.

The physiological care of the new mother includes vital signs, assessing urination, bowel function and adequate hydration. Pain management is critical as is the application of psychosocial care principles: relationship development, emotional connection, facilitation of the integration of the experience into the woman's self system. Often when providing physical care there is an opportunity to encourage and facilitate the processing of the birth experience. Open-ended questions are especially useful in that they allow the woman to share her own unique perception and take on the birth events. An example might be, "Tell me about your birth experience, how much was it what you had imagined?" Another example, "Many women have an idea of what their birth experience will be like. How was this for you?" The woman will hopefully sense the empathic connection and feel safe to speak her voice and share her experience. It is so important that HER experience be validated, and not judged or critiqued. Remember the experience is in the "eye of the beholder."

The assistance with breastfeeding is another critical opportunity to allow for the processing of events as well as a time to support the woman's boundaries and sense of self. It is important to assess the woman's motivation and skills level and it is critical to ask permission to touch her breasts if it will be needed to guide the feeding experience. Sometimes it is helpful to put your hands over hers and guide the feeding that way. Again, be cognizant that you have no idea what the woman's past history is with regard to trauma prior to the birth, so you want to lead with respect and clear boundaries. This is another critical time for assessment of preconceived ideas regarding feeding as well as time to process the labor, delivery and birth experience.

Facilitation of maternal–infant attachment is promoted at every nursing assessment and visit, encouraging the woman to identify with her baby: What are his/her unique characteristics? Does he/she resemble anyone in the family, etc.? This is also a time to teach and demonstrate all the unique aspects of the baby: rooting reflex, self-soothing, competency, etc. These "Kodak moments" of mother–baby interaction are times of connection and care for both mother and baby. The father/partner is also a main player in the development of this trio, so make sure that he/she is being asked their perceived experiences also.

It is in the utilization of every patient encounter that the integration of birth experience takes place and the internal processing of events is given priority. If the nurse has a feeling or an intuitive awareness that this woman will need additional psychosocial services, this is a good time for referral to mental health services or to give names of resources upon discharge. Documentation is important as well as shift-to-shift reports on the emotional aspects of the mother's care.

Mother's Reaction

This is a dynamic situation. Take all cues from the mother. You will see in which direction she moves. It could be the "Lioness" syndrome, where the first three themes apply. Or, sadly, the trauma will affect or even consume her, and she will go down the "impeded" path. From the research it is clear: preparedness could be a great help for mothers and their precious babies—not to walk away from breastfeeding, but to persevere, thus giving the best start for mother and baby. The beautiful hormonal bodily gift associated with breastfeeding will help lift the mood of the mother and make it more likely that the impact of the trauma will not be so great. Yet moving into breastfeeding is still a journey in itself.

Take time to observe and then support, support, support. This would be the essence of the way forward. Affirm what the mother is saying, listen, hear, and do not judge. Be mindful of how you communicate, of what messages your body language is giving, and so on. It is a fine balance for the mother. She already knows it is best to breastfeed, so do not let this be an additional trauma. Provide whatever she is asking for by way of support.

If the trauma is ongoing, for example, preeclampsia, then there is time to set breastfeeding support in place. Start talking early. Do this, too, for a birth that follows a previous traumatic birth. Good support can come from many quarters. Think outside the square. Consider the family, the partner, the mother, and the usual health professionals in the couple's lives. Be practical. Be prepared.

For those who show the "Lioness" syndrome, success in breastfeeding is wonderful. Work with them to make it happen. But be aware that the trauma is still there, and treatment will still be necessary. As the words of the mother clearly state, this is their way to heal themselves. Affirm her actions, yet still keep the need for counseling in view.

To those who are impeded by their birth trauma, offer practical relevant support. Ask open-ended questions. Try to distinguish the psychological from the physical. Try NOT to increase the burden of failure for those who do not continue in breastfeeding. Their traumatic birth may be the most appropriate focus for them. Therefore, affirm the mothering skills you see. Celebrate what is going on, rather than censuring for what is not. Being shell-shocked and just coping is using all their available energy. Nurture the mother. Acknowledge the good that she is doing. Involve appropriate professionals, for example, chaplains, social workers, and family members too. The first phase is important. Keep the channels of communication open. Permit birth reviewing at a time that is right. Encourage the mother's delight in the relationship with baby. It is, again, her birth, and it is her equilibrium that is at stake.

Conclusion

Cheryl and Sue's qualitative research on the impact of traumatic childbirth on women's breastfeeding experiences provides clinicians with a glimpse into the world of these mothers as they struggle to breastfeed. Further research, both qualitative and quantitative, is needed to investigate the effect of birth trauma on breastfeeding. In Chapter 10, another long-term effect of traumatic childbirth on women is the focus. This time it is the anniversary of mothers' birth trauma which is always the child's birthday.

References

Beck, C. T., & Watson, S. (2008). Impact of birth trauma on breast-feeding: A tale of two pathways. *Nursing Research, 57,* 228–236.

Chen, D. C., Nommsen-Rivers, L., Dewey, K., & Lonnerdal, B. (1998). Stress during labor and delivery and early lactation performance. *American Journal of Clinical Nutrition, 68,* 335–344.

Dewey, K. G. (2001). Maternal and fetal stress are associated with impaired lactogenesis. *Journal of Nutrition, 131,* 30125–30155.

Grajeda, R., & Perez-Escamilla, R. (2002). Stress during labor and delivery is associated with delayed onset of lactation among urban Guatemalan women. *Journal of Nutrition, 132,* 3055–3060.

Hannah, M. E., Hannah, W. J., Hodnett, E. D., Chalmers, B., Kong, R., William, A., et al. (2002). Outcomes at 3 months after planned cesarean vs. planned vaginal delivery for breech presentation at term: The international randomized term breech trial. *JAMA, 287,* 1822–1831.

Janke, J. R. (1988). Breastfeeding duration following cesarean and vaginal births. *Journal of Nurse Midwifery, 33,*159–164.

Nissen, E., Uvnas-Moberg, K., Svensson, K., Stock, S., Widstrom, A. M., & Winberg, J. (1996). Different patterns of oxytocin, prolactin and cortisol release during breastfeeding in women delivered by caesarean section or by the vaginal route. *Early Human Development, 45*(1–2),103–118.

Otamiri, G., Berg, G., Leden, T., Leijon, I., & Tagercrantz, H. (1991). Delayed neurological adaptation in infants delivered by elective cesarean section and the relation to catecholamine levels. *Early Human Development, 26,* 51–60.

Procianoy, R. S., Fernandes-Filho, P. H., Lazaro, L., & Sartori, N. C. (1984). Factors affecting breastfeeding: The influence of cesarean section. *Journal of Tropical Pediatrics, 30,* 39–42.

Samuels, S. E., Margen, S., & Schoen, E. J. (1985). Incidence and duration of breastfeeding in a health maintenance organization population. *American Journal of Clinical Nutrition, 42,* 504–510.

10 Anniversary of Birth Trauma

According to the DSM-IV: "Intense psychological distress or physiological reactivity often occurs when the person is exposed to triggering events that resemble or symbolize an aspect of the traumatic event (e.g. anniversaries of the traumatic event)" (APA, 2000, p. 464).

Researchers have studied anniversary reactions to different traumatic events such as in mental health disaster relief workers following traumatic exposure at the site of the World Trade Center terrorist attacks (Daly et al., 2008). Only one study, to date, has been conducted looking at the issues pertaining to the anniversary of traumatic childbirth (Beck, 2006). This chapter focuses on describing mothers' narratives they shared in that study which allows readers a privileged insider's view of the yearly struggles these women endure.

The purpose of Cheryl's qualitative study (Beck, 2006) was to describe the essence of mothers' experiences surrounding the anniversary of their traumatic childbirth. Thirty-seven women participated in this study via the Internet. The sample was international and included mothers from the USA, New Zealand, Australia, the UK, and Canada. Women were recruited through a notice placed on the Trauma and Birth Stress (TABS) website. Women sent their anniversary stories to the researcher via attachment. What was revealed loud and clear from the mothers' stories was that the anniversary of birth trauma has a complicating element that other trauma anniversaries do not have. The anniversary of a traumatic childbirth is also the day of another event, but this event is cause for celebration. It is the birthday of the child whose birth was the original traumatic event for the mother.

As the celebration of the child's birthday took center stage, mothers struggled to survive their anniversary. Beck (2006) entitled this study, "The anniversary of birth trauma: Failure to rescue." Mothers suffered so covertly during this yearly ordeal. Failure to rescue refers to a "clinician's inability to save a hospitalized patient's life when he experiences a complication (a condition not present on admission)" (Clarke & Aiken, 2003, pp. 42–43). The concept of failure to rescue is based on the premise that at times deaths are unavoidable in hospitals. There are times, however, in hospitals when many deaths could have been pre-vented. Failure to rescue has rarely been applied outside of the medical surgical inpatient setting. Beck broadened the use of this concept to childbearing women due to the invisibility of the phenomenon of traumatic childbirth anniversaries. Health care providers, family, and friends failed to rescue mothers during the period surrounding the anniversary of their birth trauma. Mothers hoped that as the anniversary of their traumatic childbirth approached, it would bring some attention to their yearly ordeal that they suffer so covertly from someone: family, friends, or health care providers. Sadly this was not to be. The outcome of the original use of the term, failure to rescue, was a death due to a complication of surgery that could have been prevented. For mothers struggling with the anniversary of their birth trauma, the outcome was not a preventable death but rather unnecessary emotional and physical suffering.

Four themes emerged from the 37 women's stories regarding their experiences of their birth trauma anniversaries (Beck, 2006). The first theme was: "The prologue: An agonizing time." What became apparent was that it was just not the actual day itself that presented difficulties for the women. Weeks, sometimes months before the anniversary some women were plagued with distressing thoughts and emotions. The season of the year and time on clocks were examples of triggers that ushered in this upsetting yearly ordeal. For one mother whose traumatic childbirth had occurred near Halloween, she explained: "There is also a distinct smell of dead leaves in the air that screams, 'October'! Hearing the word, October, and seeing the word in writing gives me chills. When I would see decorations for Halloween, fear rushed through my body" (Beck, 2006, p. 385).

This prologue to the actual birthday/anniversary day was filled with an array of distressing emotions such as fear, anxiety, grief, sadness, and guilt. Terrifying nightmares and flashbacks increased during this time period. The looming anniversary also affected some mothers physically. For example, flare-ups of asthmatic attacks, psoriasis, and digestive problems occurred.

Theme 2 concentrated on the actual day: Was it a celebration of a birthday or the torment of an anniversary? Clock watching consumed part of the mother's dreaded day as it finally arrived. Whenever women glanced at the clock, they would immediately relate it to what was happening at that time during the traumatic day of their childbirth. As one woman shared: "I relived every moment synchronized to the clock. Even today, a clock reading 8:46 will turn my stomach upside down" (Beck, 2006, p. 386). Some women struggled with how to celebrate their child's birthday as this mother who had an emergency cesarean birth vividly illustrated, "I can't stop seeing images of a woman drugged and strapped down and being gutted like a fish. I can't get those or my own images out of my mind. I don't know how to celebrate my daughter's birthday" (Beck, 2006, p. 386).

Fearing that celebrating their child's birthday on the actual anniversary day would detract from what should be their child's special, joyous day, some women scheduled the birthday party on a different day or week. One mother whose son had recently turned 3 years old chose a random day each year to celebrate her son's birthday:

> We made a cake on a random day. I never told my son it was coming up. I bought him things and wrapped them but he doesn't know what they are for. I kissed him and told him before I went to work, "Happy Birthday", but only when he was asleep.
>
> (Beck, 2006, p. 387)

Other women who did celebrate their child's birthday on its actual day needed to physically get away and so planned vacations for the week of the birthday. Some mothers described being "a total faker" during the child's birthday celebration. During her son's birthday party this mom revealed: "I was really empty inside. It felt as though I as looking in at the party from a window. Again I think I was hoping for someone to take me aside and to acknowledge the birth trauma!" (Beck, 2006, p. 386). Failure to rescue was rearing its ugly head not only for this mom but for many other mothers too.

Theme 3 focused on the tremendous toll that surviving the actual anniversary day had on the women. "The epilogue: A fragile state," was the title of this third theme to help bring attention to mothers' need to have time to recuperate and heal their wounds that were just reopened and now were raw. This woman recounted that:

> As hard as I tried to move away from the trauma, at birthday anniversary time I am pulled straight back as if on a giant rubber band into the midst of it all, and spend MONTHS AFTER trying to pull myself away from it again.
>
> (Beck, 2006, p. 387)

The final theme looked at women who had experienced multiple anniversaries: "Subsequent anniversaries: For better or worse." No consistent pattern was found. For some mothers they did see slight improvement with each birthday, as this mom recalled:

> On my son's first birthday I had such a feeling of dread, I only invited three couples that we are friends with because I couldn't face planning a big party. The day of the party, I went upstairs to my dressing room and crawled underneath my dressing table, which sits against the wall. I pulled the bench in front of me so that I was enclosed on all sides in a very small space. I just wanted to stay huddled in there and never leave. I cried for a while, but knew that I had to pull myself together somehow. I did manage to make it downstairs for the party though I secretly counted the minutes until it was over.

This same mother then described her second anniversary:

> We cooked hamburgers and this time I made the cake (my husband had make it the year before). I was determined not to fall apart again. Sadly it was not to be. Although I didn't crawl under the table this time, I again headed to my dressing room. It is the smallest, most private room for me in the house—and sat hunched against the wall shivering under a blanket. A while later I managed to pull myself together and get on with the party preparations. I am more conscious of what went on this time and did enjoy most of it.
>
> (Beck, 2006, p. 388)

Sadly, for some women, they had yet to experience any improvement with subsequent anniversaries. This mom to date had experienced five anniversaries of her birth trauma and painfully revealed,

> I can't believe 5 years later that I feel such strong emotions and that my body responds physically. It is like the birthing trauma and the anxiety, loss, and pain associated with it seems to reside in every cell of my being, with a memory capacity that serves to never let me forget.
>
> (Beck, 2006, p. 388)

The original use of the term "failure to rescue" was the unnecessary death of a patient that occurred as a complication of surgery. The use of the term "failure to rescue" in the anniversary of birth trauma was not an unnecessary death but instead refers to the unnecessary emotional and physical toll it took on women. Quality of life of these mothers took an unnecessary sharp decline as no one recognized this distressing, invisible phenomenon. Four mothers' experiences of their anniversaries of their birth trauma follow. These women had participated in Beck's (2006) Internet study.

Debbie's Story

Debbie's traumatic birth occurred with her second pregnancy. She developed severe preeclampsia and at 24 weeks gestation she had an emergency cesarean birth. Here is her description of her experiences with four anniversaries:

> I have been curious about my feelings about the anniversaries of John's birth for a long time. With my other two children, I feel excitement and joy in the days approaching their birthdays and happiness all of the actual day. With John, the feeling is quite different. I have suffered a lot of guilt because of this.
>
> *John's first birthday.* I was first struck by this on his first birthday. I was filled with a feeling of dread for weeks prior to it. I was also getting conflicting feelings of thankfulness that we had a baby to enjoy a first

birthday with (I hope this makes sense). I planned a big party and was very busy during the day. I noticed later in the year that I was happy about the first anniversary of John coming home from the hospital, more than his actual birthday. In the days approaching his birthday, I kept thinking about the day he was born, going over in my head all of the details. I decided to go online and find some support in the online preemie groups because I just couldn't stop thinking about his birth and the NICU stay.

John's second birthday. It hasn't gotten better as time has gone by. Actually I had a meltdown at about his second birthday. I remember that I was talking to my friend about John's hospital stay or something like that and she turned to me and said, "You realize that I have heard this story three times, right? John is fine. You need to move on with your life." It was then that I realized that I did talk about John's birth to anyone who would listen. Everyone I met knows that I had a 1 lb baby. I was filled with so much embarrassment and shame that I had inflicted my friend with my stories, I ended up crying and apologizing every time I talked to her and this ended the friendship.

John's second birthday was worse because he was doing so well and I just couldn't get over his hospital stay. This is hard for me to talk about but, I started surfing the Internet and going to sites where people had tributes to a preemie that had died. That was it. I spent hours in the evening after the kids went to bed poring over the stories of these little babies that had died. I am not sure what was motivating it. I kept thinking, "Thank you, God, for my sweet baby's life" (I thank God every day for having him. Like I don't want to jinx my luck). Months later, I talked to my husband about it and came to the realization that I was obsessed with this. I stopped going to those sites because it made me feel very depressed.

John's third birthday. For some reason my memories of this aren't as clear. I still remember dreading the day and feeling like a total faker with my smile and feigned excitement. I remember feeling relief after it was over.

John's fourth birthday. This was two days ago. Because of your study, I have been paying close attention to my feelings. As his birthday approached, I have felt depressed and anxious. I take the NICU photos out and pour over them a couple of times a month. I was woken up on Monday morning with John running into my room all excited saying it's his birthday. I of course squeezed him, with a big smile on my face telling him how great being 4 is going to be! But I kind of dragged through the day feeling like a total faker. I told all my coworkers that it was John's birthday and I called him in the middle of the day to see how he was doing on his birthday, but I haven't been able to really work up the joy I have on my other kids' birthdays. I feel very guilty about this and completely ridiculous. We didn't have a party on Monday, only a scoop of ice cream and a candle. We are having the party this weekend.

Right before I went to bed I went into John's room and knelt down beside his bed. I watched him sleep and breathe. Then I put my face in his hair just to smell it. I stayed like that for at least 5 minutes. I thanked God again for my little son's life. John woke up then and hugged me in his half sleep state. Then he gently ran his hands down both sides of my face. I said, "Go to sleep, birthday boy" and he said, "OK, mom." I walked out of his room and into my own. My husband was in the kitchen so I was alone. I took out the little album with the NICU photos and got through about five of them. Then I started to cry. Not just a little, but big sobs (I rarely do this). I cried for 5 minutes or so before my husband walked into the room and put his arm around me. I kept crying. I was trying to figure out why I was crying and all I could feel was grief. Like someone had died. Afterward my husband and I talked. He told me that he cannot even bear to look at the pictures, let alone talk about the day. I felt better, like maybe there is nothing wrong with me. I almost feel like this was a breakthrough of some sort, but I am not sure yet.

I feel very guilty about my feelings like somehow I am cheating John of something, even though he has no clue how I am really feeling. John is doing fine, doing really well. He is healthy, happy, loving, and sweet. Everything I could ask for in a son. Why can't I stop thinking about his traumatic premature birth? I don't want this to define who he is. I would love for this not to be a major part of my life. John's prematurity was what happened 4 years ago. When will it not be a major part of my life? I suffer from PTSD.

Heather's Story

Heather is in her early forties, is married, and has one child soon to be 5 years old. Here are her experiences of the anniversaries of her traumatic birth of her daughter.

Birthdays—what do they mean to you? For me, a birthday prior to the start of the new millennium meant joy, presents, relaxation and celebration. Now it has a darker side to it, a profound depth that I never could have imagined was possible. So what changed? This is the story of how birthdays became the Birth day!

The first birth anniversary was particularly difficult. I had very mixed feelings about celebrating my daughter's birth—for me, what was there to celebrate? What became important to me (indeed all-consuming) was that the birthday should be a technical success, i.e. the food should be good, the guests right and the weather fine. It was, however, not an enjoyable event and I was very emotional. It did bring the whole experience flooding back, the sense of extreme violation by a rough, arrogant male doctor who invaded my space and made me feel disgusting and ruined my inner self. For me, when people ask, what is it like? I say it was as close to a sense of rape without being physically raped. These feelings were vividly present both before and then subsequently. Although they are heightened around the time of the anniversary, they are often with me. The birthday is no longer the celebration of the child but the anniversary of a wrong.

For my daughter's third birthday I decided I didn't want a big party and went for a small event on the beach with my husband, a good friend and my mum and sister. To be honest, this was the best sort of event. It didn't require any sense of celebration and was just a pleasant day out on the beach, something we do anyway. Each birthday the memories become slightly easier to cope with, less intense in memory but there, deep inside.

My daughter's fourth birthday was a children's party and again I focused heavily on getting it right—being successful. I do feel so ambivalent about the whole thing—yes, I want to celebrate the fact she is a gorgeous little girl who survived a particularly horrible birth without any apparent long-term damage. But, on the other hand, each birthday brings back memories of the wrong. It sits as a permanent barrier both in my relationship with my husband and in my sense of attachment to my child. Although this is getting better year by year, I am not sure it will ever really disappear. The reawakening of the birth each birthday does mean I think again about what happened, my role in it, what I could have done to prevent it from happening and my sadness at what was taken away from me. The feelings of having let myself down and allowed this to happen remain with me. The decisions I made that led down the path which led to birth trauma haunt me.

It is not just me that suffers each birthday. My husband is still traumatized by the experience. Neither of us could possibly go through another birth so there is not a chance of having another baby.

This in its turn is another source of confusion—in some ways it would have been nice to have another child, as single children lose out in some ways but I certainly could not go through another birth and the risk of having another similar experience. My daughter will be 5 in June. Yes, I will be thinking again about what happened and again I will approach it with a huge degree of confusion, pain, and ambivalence.

Angie's Story

Angie is married and in her mid-thirties, and has a college degree. She has one child who is now 3 years old. Angie has been diagnosed with PTSD due to her traumatic birth with this child. She is currently under the care of a therapist and receiving EMDR treatment. Angie shared that "PTSD is making a home in my body." Below is her experience with the three anniversaries of her birth trauma.

I have suffered every day for over 1035 days. Every birthday is really an anniversary for the rape. Rape day. My son was conceived from love and born out of rape. I have forgotten nothing. I did not sleep for 2.5 years until I weaned my son and began sleep aid drugs. I'll lead up to what goes through my mind on the days surrounding my son's birthday. I have had to change the date to celebrate to 10 days after the incident/ordeal. The first anniversary I stayed horribly distressed and no mention of a celebration was breached by my husband. I felt terrible guilt that I could not make my son a cake and let him eat it for a video opportunity. I relived every moment synchronized to the clock for 4 days and afterwards for days. I had severe/acute PTSD every day since the birth until this current day but the horror of the numbers falling together a year later and knowing that the people who did this to me don't even know my name or what I have to suffer will be with me for the rest of my life. I don't remember my son's first year. I was hoping that I would just die from self-neglect, all the while everyone told me that I was the best mother they had ever seen. I practiced attachment parenting unconsciously from excessive hyper-vigilance. I tried to compensate and deny the experience in regards to my desire to be the parent I had planned on being while carrying my child inside me for 9 months. I dutifully doted over him constantly but I could not feel anything. I was emotionally numb until the rage hit me before he turned a year old. I openly wished I had not survived his birth. I still feel the same way as the third anniversary approaches.

As the third anniversary approaches, for months in advance I pray that no one asks me what we are doing for my son's birthday. I think of answers in advance. I don't tell anyone the date. I don't attend other children's birthday parties. I am thankful this year that we have relocated and few know us here. Still there is family, insensitive family members, who have no empathy and will probably pass judgment if I can't do it again. My son is getting older and will soon figure out what birthdays are all about. I'll have to just put on my best performance even after changing the day. I've started to lie to him and tell him he was born at home even though I am very visible and open about my experience in order to keep the dialogue going about typical routine hospital births and the devastation to women and their families.

As I am writing this, I am shaking quite a bit and crying. It is now mid-June and the days of mid-August terrify me again. I tried to fast for 52 hours (the length of the ordeal) and retrace and rescript every humiliating, dehumanizing tortuous detail of the trauma in an attempt to reclaim some semblance of personal power but I made it for only 36 hours into the fact before I was sick from dehydration. I was denied food and given inadequate liquids for the entire ordeal while in labor and I couldn't even make it as a purification ritual minus all the stress I had to endure. My labor was 52 hours long. Two days before my son's first and second birthday I am recalling exactly what I was doing and how I was feeling. The entire 2 days before the anniversary I watch the clock and relive all the hell I know that a year or two or three now ago for the first 30 plus hours of labor I was hanging in there, suffering but dealing with the pain virtually alone.

During the anniversary it is still only Saturday evening at 4 a.m. I can't sleep. I know what is to come. I can't escape it then or now. I am there again and it's the day before my son's birthday and I have to think of some way to acknowledge it without going ballistic over every little trivial detail throughout the day. My husband looks as if he wishes he were on another planet for the next 72 hours or more, since life never returns to normal, there is no escape for any of us within this family. The night before I am dreading calls from relatives. I anxiously open cards for our son during the week prior. I pass them to him with a plastic smile and that's all I can muster. I am pleased when he chews them and tears them to shreds with his new teeth. I guess I don't get to display them and toss them in the recycling bin before anyone sees them. I am so conflicted and grief-stricken and full of rage which is grief really, that I can't feel joy and embrace my child's day of birth. I want nothing than to have that experience. To feel that joy. To feel anything other than horrible sadness, betrayal and hopelessness. This is just one tiny aspect of a happy life that has been stolen from my family and me. The list is astounding. Validation from any other soul did not come from anyone for a very long time so I suffered and felt extreme guilt for my feelings regarding his day of "celebration" alone. I am usually unable to sleep most nights but during the anniversary I am conscious of the time of around 4:30 a.m. when I am told by both midwives that the baby is "stuck" coincidentally at the 48-hour labor mark.

The third anniversary just came and went. It was more of the same. No different. I was terrified to go to have a blood test for ovarian cancer. Not because of the risk of cancer, but because of the triggers in that environment. I can't go anywhere near a hospital. I don't watch television as hospital and medical shows are so popular now especially the sad excuses for births on the *Baby Story*. I started a new job and I didn't tell anyone at work and agreed to work an event that evening as well at the museum that I worked at to avoid his birthday. I knew every minute what I was going through 3 years ago, which has not lost its impact at all. The guilt for not having a joyous celebration is no different either. I began the day by bursting into tears on the couch before work while everyone was asleep. The worst of it all is that I am not able to be the loving, patient, even-balanced, open-hearted mother that I would have been to my son and there is no sense of well-being in my family. Realizing how futile, pointless, and useless it is to feel anything, I said, I don't care, it doesn't hurt, let it kill me, it doesn't matter after all. What other conclusion can one come to after 3 years? I read a line in a book I came across: "The Rape of the Twentieth Century, Birth in America" or some sub-subtitle. It read: "as it matters that our children are conceived through rape it matters that they are born through rape." It matters and anyone reading this has the legal and moral obligation to raise the standard of care because the current standard is killing us.

Jill's Story

It's been 5 years today. Five long and racing years since my life ceased to be my own. There is so much beauty and power in being a mother; so much

I live for now. I've found myself in this process of evolution that is motherhood. I've found my life's passion and nothing else could ever hold for me the balance of challenge and reward that makes motherhood the supreme act of humanity that it is.

But the path to motherhood for me was anything but beautiful or empowering. I think of the act of giving birth, the encompassing girth of power and grace. I think of that feeling that I experienced in later births. My womb wrapping itself around me, my body pulsating with power as it moved life into the world. The feeling of a human emerging from me with such an intensity of energy and relief. I think of how I felt afterwards: powerful, strong, accomplished. I believe in the beauty of birth and the continuum that follows. I believe in the maternal forcefield of love and light. I know, in my soul, that it is present every time a life enters the world. But search as I may, I cannot find it there when I became a mother.

I felt sure going in that I was aware, educated, and ready. When my body began the timeless dance toward motherhood, I was anything but. A full day and night from my water breaking, it began. Another night and day passed, I held my first born, and there I sat. Five full years later, I've only begun to be strong enough to recognize this depth of pain, let alone explore it.

The birth of my child should have been a happy time. On his birthday we celebrate his life. This is a hard day for me. There is just so little to celebrate about that memory. While most anything would have been worth bringing this priceless life into my world, the experience is filled with such pain and regret, anger, and sorrow that it's hard to rejoice the day. There's nothing good there for me.

Most of the time, it is just sadness. I think of the day. It comes up in conversation or a memory triggers it. I feel a mixture of happiness that I force because I feel I should and sadness that is far more sincere. I feel terrible that thinking about the birth of my child inspires no real happiness. It is not the child I mourn but the experience that brought him forth. I hope desperately that he never comes to know these things.

I think on the day and I feel a twinge of sadness, a gasp of regret. I think of the technicalities. I recognize it as past. I work to recognize a lesson or purpose in it. I am driven to move on. There is a present child to think on, other births to shift focus to. But late at night, on this anniversary day, that black hole that swirls in my soul opens a crack. I can see past this superficial sadness into a well of heart-breaking pain, remorse, anger, and heartache that I cannot even begin to process. *Not now*, I think, *I must sleep. I must be rested, available, for my children tomorrow. I must have enough sleep to function. Perhaps tomorrow if I get a moment alone.* I think of that shower after the birth. The first time being truly alone. I think of how I clung to the wall, holding on for dear life as I was swept up in a tsunami of pain. It may have been the last time that vortex was opened. *Then when?* I questioned myself. *How long will this live inside you before you can begin to feel it all?*

The truth is, I don't know. It is there. I am a little more aware of it on this date. I smile and take pictures. Sing happy birthday and eat cake. I adore this sweet child. I am so proud of who he is and all the potential that might be. We read the Birthday Book and I ramble off the complex phrases and clever rhymes. I am 1! But underneath it all, the truth shivers. I glance at the time throughout the day. At this point, 5 years ago I was . . .

Here's the problem. None of the memories are happy. At some point it all went gray, then black. I feel queasy to even pull up the memories. I cannot begin to put myself there again, feel the moment I lost it. Where did it go wrong? So much anger, resentment, pain. I wonder if I can put the turn of tables on a certain choice in there. It's not really true, but the tides decidedly turned inside me. As if the moon pulled the tides to change, I am left with ground and broken pieces that once housed life, sitting silent and empty shell indeed.

I don't mean to be dramatic. I tell myself. It all seems petty in the face of the healthy, whole-bodied outcome. *You are ungrateful.* It doesn't help. No degree of logic or rationale can calm the black sea that rages deep in there. I am not yet ready to feel all of that. I can sense the heartbreak that will split me in half. I know the wracking sobs and turning inside out that lies in there. I begin to open to it for just a second before I push it back down again, terrified that it will consume me.

AAArh! The life of my child was marred by the heinous crime of his birth! I am so angry at what we lost. I cannot begin to bring forth words to portray the seemingly endless depth of anguish there. But I can feel the cold tile on my forehead, I can feel my body shake with sobs that come forth with such force that they are soundless. The water is hot on my body and the pain is deep within. I gasp for air. But then I forced it closed. I just can't. Not yet. I am not ready to be ripped in half. The energy left behind leaves me wanting to hit something, but it fades quickly. I am well practiced. I know that one day it will have to be done. Perhaps when they are older and I have that time to tend to me that I dream of now and then. How many birthdays will that be? I need time to be broken. I *need* time to be *broken*.

Clinician's Reaction

In reading the preceding stories, I wonder and ponder about how we are in so many ways a society that shies away from feelings, especially sad, angry feelings. What can we do as health care professionals to "rescue" these women? How can we make sure that their experiences are not ignored, silenced and pushed underground? As Debbie shared with us, she lost a friendship over the need to replay the story of her son John's birth over and over again and how her friend could not listen to her anymore. In many ways, being confronted with her obsessive need to talk about the birth only increased her feelings of guilt and shame, and she had done NOTHING wrong!

Ambivalence is the emotional experience of holding two emotions at the same time, like happiness and sadness. It would be helpful for women to have support and understanding of the process of healing the PTSD, not that it would make the anniversary any less challenging but she may have a gentler feeling of self if she has had the reaction normalized, i.e. it will happen. As you read, over the years some of the intensity diminished but it never went away in the stories shared in this chapter. What is so sad is the amount of internalization, guilt and shame the women verbalized and they had done nothing wrong. They had believed that they could have changed the situation. I do hope that the providers involved in these birth experiences received letters of concern from the women for what happened and their personal reactions. Not that it would have prevented the personal experiences but perhaps the letters would be internalized by the providers to try to change their practice and to be more empathic during labor and delivery experiences. I know I have found in my practice that that has been of some value for some women as they heal from their traumatic birth experiences.

Mother's Reaction

Finding and preserving a safe place, and retreating into it, is a way of steeling oneself as an anniversary comes around. This safe place may be a physical place, e.g., bed, the kitchen or even (more) work, or it may be an altered mental-emotional state for a period of time. For the woman, her emotions may not be simply focused alone on the actual "birth" day, but rather on a catalogue of days which together amount to an "anniversary" billing. Her head may be swirling with vivid and real memories. So be guided by the woman's reactions and what it is all meaning for her. It could be a "this is the day that life changed for me forever." Fear, lack of hope might have been the prevalent state of mind and emotion. Be very attentive to hear and see what is.

On chatting, I would listen and hear what is going on. I would focus on the "good things" that would be of help for her to get through this time. I would never minimize any actions or endeavors played out to survive. Avoidance is unavoidable at this time, so a well-orchestrated program or plan is developed, just to survive. This is perfectly understandable and reasonable, we would say.

Know that the emotions would be strong, if not severe, on the first anniversary, and the following anniversaries may follow a different pathway. Mothers must receive help so that they can shake off this reminder, as "not being the mother you thought you would be or want to be" is in itself an added trauma too. Again, a heart full of hope and the affirmation of supporters will bring the mother through. She must know that she does not walk this path alone.

Conclusion

Cheryl's qualitative research on mothers' experiences of the anniversary of their traumatic birth helps to bring some visibility to this invisible phenomenon.

Clinicians, family, and friends need to be cognizant of the struggles these women may be enduring regarding the yearly anniversary of their birth trauma.

These mothers need to be supported during the time period before, during, and after the child's birthday. We must not fail to rescue these mothers again. The stinging tentacles of traumatic childbirth reach out even further to women as some of them go on to have another child. Chapter 11 focuses on subsequent childbirth following a previous traumatic birth.

References

American Psychiatric Association (2000). *Diagnostic and statistical manual of mental disorders* (4th ed.). Washington, DC: American Psychiatric Association.

Beck, C. T. (2006). The anniversary of birth trauma: Failure to rescue. *Nursing Research, 55,* 381–390.

Clarke, S. P., & Aiken, L. H. (2003). Failure to rescue. *American Journal of Nursing, 103,* 42–47.

Daly, E. S., Gulliver, S. B., Zimering, R. T., Knight, J., Kamholz, B. M., & Morissette, S. B. (2008). Disaster mental health workers responding to Ground Zero: one year later. *Journal of Traumatic Stress, 21,* 227–230.

11 Subsequent Childbirth after a Previous Traumatic Birth

Research findings are beginning to accrue which highlight the chronic nature of posttraumatic stress related to childbirth lasting longer than 6 months after birth. The long-term detrimental effects of traumatic childbirth not only on mothers but also on their relationships with their infants and other family members have been reported (Beck, 2006; Ayers, Wright, & Wells, 2007; Nicholls & Ayers, 2007). This chapter concentrates on summarizing this beginning, pertinent research and also on providing the narratives of two mothers who participated in Beck and Watson's (2010) study of subsequent childbirth following a previous birth trauma.

In a Swedish sample of 617 primiparas when they were 2 months postpartum (Gottvall & Waldenström, 2002), mothers completed a follow-up questionnaire that assessed their experiences giving birth, their satisfaction with their care during labor and delivery, breastfeeding, and their own health, as well as that of their infant. Information regarding the women's subsequent birth and the length of time between the first and second births was collected from the Swedish Medical Birth Registry. Gottvall and Waldenström reported that women who perceived they had a traumatic birth had fewer subsequent children and also a longer length of time to their second baby.

Ayers, Eagle, and Waring (2006) in their UK qualitative study interviewed six mothers who had clinically significant PTSD after birth, regarding the effects of this on their relationships. Time since the birth trauma for this sample ranged from 7 months to 18 years. Women reported a strain in their relationship with their partner and also that their relationships with their friends suffered as a result of their birth experience. Their birth trauma also affected their relationship with their infants. Most mothers admitted that immediately after birth they felt feelings of rejection toward their infants, but over time (between 1 to 5 years) they did bond with their infants. Almost all the mothers shared their fear of childbirth and that their plans for another child had changed due to their traumatic childbirth.

The perceived impact of childbirth-related PTSD on couples was examined in the UK (Nicholls & Ayers, 2007). Six married couples were interviewed separately. Time since the traumatic birth ranged from 9 months to 22 months. All the participants stated that the woman's PTSD affected their relationship with their partner. These effects on relationships included physical relationships (mainly women avoiding sex), communication (avoiding discussing the birth and its related difficulties), conflict, feeling abandoned and loss of intimacy, and barriers to coping. Overall, couples shared that their relationships with their partners were negatively affected.

In Ayers et al.'s (2007) study in the UK, 64 couples 9 weeks after childbirth completed questionnaires regarding the birth, posttraumatic stress symptoms, their relationships and their bonding with their infants. Their posttraumatic stress symptoms were measured using the Impact of Event Scale (IES) (Horowitz, Wilner, & Alvarez, 1979). Parent–infant attachment was assessed using a self-report version of the Bethlehem Mother–Infant Interaction Scale (Pearce & Ayers, 2005) and the couples' relationship with the Dyadic Adjustment Scale (DAS; Spanier, 1976). Five percent of both men and women reported severe posttraumatic stress symptoms. Their PTSD symptoms, however, were not related to parent–infant bonding or the couple's relationship.

Polachek, Harari, Baum, and Strous (2012) conducted a study with 89 new mothers in Israel. One month after birth the women completed the PDS (Foa et al., 1997). Sixty percent of the mothers who developed posttraumatic stress symptoms reported that their previous childbirth had been traumatic compared to 15.5% of women who did not have elevated posttraumatic stress symptoms. Also more mothers who reported elevated posttraumatic stress symptoms after birth stated they did not want any more children due to their birth trauma, compared to women without such symptoms.

One aspect of the chronicity of birth trauma can focus on women's experiences of subsequent childbirth following a previous traumatic birth. What is it like to have to anxiously wait for 9 long months for what is feared the most—the possibility of yet another traumatic labor and delivery? What strategies do women use during pregnancy to cope with their fear? Do women find some healing of their previous birth trauma with this current childbirth or are they traumatized again? These questions were asked of 35 women from the USA, the UK, New Zealand, Australia, and Canada via the Internet (Beck & Watson, 2010). Analysis of these mothers' descriptions of their subsequent childbirth after a previous birth trauma yielded four themes.

Theme 1: Riding the Turbulent Wave of Panic During Pregnancy

This theme revealed the terror, panic, fear, and denial that the women endured for 9 months. Women described the "emotional torture" they suffered: "My 9 months of pregnancy were an anxiety-filled abyss which was completely marred as an experience due to the terror that was continually in my mind from my experience 8 years earlier" (Beck & Watson, 2010, p. 245).

Theme 2: Strategizing: Attempts to Reclaim Their Body and Complete the Journey to Motherhood

Table 11.1 includes a list of strategies women in this study used to help them survive the 9 months of pregnancy while they waited for the dreaded labor and delivery. Figure 11.1 illustrates one such strategy where a mother put a poster up in her home filled with quotes to inspire her.

Another mother shared her successful strategies she used during her pregnancy:

- Writing a detailed birth plan was helpful as it helped focus mine and my husband's mind about what we wanted/did not want. Also it gave us a great tool to give to clinicians to spark a discussion about our options, etc.
- Having a doula was great. My first birth was traumatic not only for me but my husband so having an additional birth partner meant that I could have support from one of them at all times and also that my husband had support too.
- The prenatal yoga helped me bond with my unborn son. So much of my pregnancy was about anxiety of the birth and my feelings I was worried that I would forget that I get a gorgeous (demanding) baby at the end. The

Table 11.1 Strategies used to cope with pregnancy and looming labor and delivery

- Mentally preparing for birth
- Learning birth hypnosis
- Doing birth art
- Writing positive affirmations
- Preparing for birthing at home
- Hiring a doula for labor and delivery
- Celebrating upcoming birth
- Avoiding ultrasounds
- Trying not to think about upcoming birth
- Reading books on healthy pregnancy and birth
- Mapping out your pelvis
- Learning birthing positions to open up the pelvis
- Practicing hypnosis for labor
- Researching birth centers and scheduling tours
- Interviewing obstetricians and midwives
- Exercising to help baby get in the correct position
- Using Internet support group
- Hiring a life coach
- Painting previous birth experience
- "What if?" sheet with all possible concerns and then solutions for them
- "Yes, if necessary/No" sheet for labor of what the mother wanted to happen
- Role of supporters during birth
- Researching homeopathic remedies to prepare body for labor and birth
- Developing a tool kit to help cope in labor
- Developing trust with health care provider

Source: Reprinted with permission from Beck & Watson (2010, p. 246).

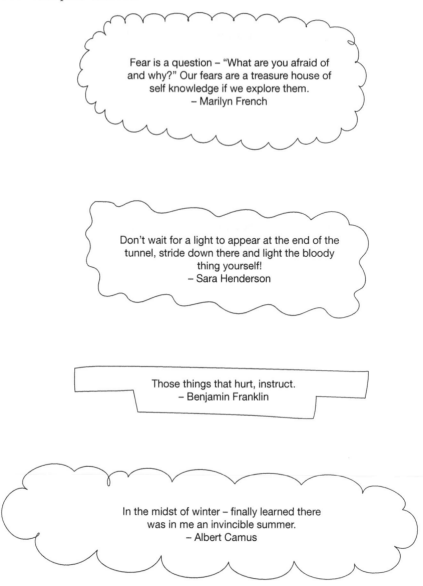

Figure 11.1 A poster of inspirational quotes by one mother

Source: Reprinted with permission from Beck & Watson (2010, p. 246).

yoga classes gave me an excuse to spend time with my unborn baby away from my toddler and husband to focus on him.

• We developed a tool kit to help me cope in labor so that we always had options to try to get through the pain, i.e. hypnobirthing techniques, massage, homeopathy, music, positions, tens machine, water/heat. This was a big issue for me as I would not have pethidine or an epidural so I knew I only had alternative means to get me through.

- Building up trust with my doctor, etc. really helped me as I felt that they were on my side and it meant we didn't worry about asking hundreds of questions or asking for time to make decisions as they understood our situation.

Another mother shared:

- I read a book about natural birth around the world by Sheila Kitzinger and as much other information as possible about natural birth the way it "should be."
- I did a lot of writing about what I wasn't happy with the first time around and what I could control to change this next time around.
- I researched a midwife that had the same philosophy as me—active and natural childbirth—and who I felt comfortable with to be supportive and caring.
- I worked on a folder with my life coach to prepare for the birth. This included:

    - Stretching exercises
    - Exercise plan
    - "What if" sheet with all my possible concerns then solutions for them
    - "Yes, if necessary, No" sheet for the labor of what I wanted to happen
    - Preterm possibilities sheet
    - Role of supporters during birth
    - Calendar to schedule preparation, i.e. when to exercise, days for "me time." Work and other commitments, when to start homeopathic remedies, etc.
    - Research on homeopathic remedies to help with preparing my body for labor and birth.

Theme 3: Bringing Reverence to the Birthing Process and Empowering Women

For 75% of the sample, their subsequent childbirth was described as either "a healing experience" or at least "a lot better" than their previous birth trauma. For those women, their confidence increased in themselves as women and as mothers. When asked what it was that made their subsequent birth a healing one, women shared that:

- I was treated with respect, my wishes and those of my husband were listened to. I wasn't made to feel like a piece of meat this time but instead like a woman experiencing one of nature's most wonderful events.
- Pain relief was taken seriously. First time around, I was ignored. I begged and pleaded for pain relief. Second time it was offered but because I was made to feel in control, I was able to decline.

- I wasn't rushed! My baby was allowed to arrive when she was ready. When my first was born, I was told "5 minutes or I get the forceps" by the doctor on call. I pushed so hard that I tore badly.
- Communication with labor and delivery staff was so much better the second time. The first time the emergency cord was pulled but no one told me why. I thought my baby was dead and no one would elaborate.
- Ultimately I was treated with respect, dignity, and compassion. In my previous birth I was made to feel like a production line and that took away the magic that I had dreamed of for those 9 months.

(Beck & Watson, 2010, pp. 246–247)

Women shared that they had a strong sense of control and felt like they reclaimed their bodies during their empowering subsequent birth. Their birth plans they had prepared during their pregnancy were honored by the labor and delivery staff. These women felt respected and cared for. They felt they were truly listened to by the physicians and nurses this time around. The obstetrical staff actually communicated with the women throughout labor and delivery.

Eight of the 35 women opted for homebirths since they feared the high level of medical intervention in the hospital setting. For 6 of the 8 women, their homebirths did fulfill their dreams of a healing subsequent birth. Mothers who did experience healing subsequent births warned, however, that nothing will erase the memory of their prior traumatic birth.

Even though it was an enormously healing experience, the expectations I had were unrealistic. What I went through during and after my first delivery cannot be erased from memory. If anything, with this second birth being so wonderful, it makes dealing with my first birth harder. It makes it sadder and me angrier as before I had nothing to compare it to. I didn't know how different it could be or how special those first few moments are. I didn't fully understand what I had missed out on. So now 3 years later I find myself grieving again for what we went through, how I was treated and what I missed out on.

(Beck & Watson, 2010, p. 247)

Other mothers admitted that their subsequent healing births can never change the past:

All the positive, empowering births in the world won't ever change what happened with my first baby and me. Our relationship is forever built around his birth experiences. The second birth was so wonderful I would go through it all again, but it can never change the past.

(Beck & Watson, 2010, p. 247)

Theme 4: Still Elusive: The Longed-For-Healing Birth Experience

Two of the women who opted for homebirths went on to experience yet another traumatic birth as they needed to be transferred to the hospital via an ambulance. One of these women revealed:

> When the ambulance arrived, I felt rescued. I have never been so grateful that hospitals exist. The blue light ambulance journey was terrifying and I was in excruciating pain. By this point I was trying to detach my head from my body, as I had done years earlier when I was being raped.
>
> (Beck & Watson, 2010, p. 247)

Another woman in Beck and Watson's (2010) study who needed to have another emergency cesarean birth due to fetal distress described how devastated she was at "failing again":

> I was still only 3 cms. and the baby's heart rate was looking very worrying. It wasn't recovering between contractions anymore. I was whisked into surgery immediately and given a second emergency c-section. I just cried. I reacted badly to the epidural and my blood pressure dropped to 80/30. I kept fainting and throwing up. I thought I was going to die. When my baby was pulled out of me, I couldn't bear to look at him. I had failed him. I just cried. All I could think about was the fact that this had been my nightmare and it was happening all over again. I wanted to die. I had failed as a woman. I felt sick. I was kept in recovery for 12 hours because my blood pressure wouldn't rise and they were worried that they had cut my bladder during the surgery. When being discharged from the hospital, I went home in tears. We came down in the hospital elevator with a couple who had had their baby 6 hours earlier. She was smiling. She didn't look tired. She was in a pretty sundress. I looked like I had been in a car crash. I had a catheter attached to my leg for another 5 days. I had totally failed. I was living my nightmare. It wasn't fair.

Thomson and Downe (2010) also explored women's experiences of a positive birth after a prior traumatic birth. Fourteen mothers were interviewed and analysis of their birth stories revealed these women changed the future in order to change the past. Four themes described their process: (1) resolving the past and preparing for the unknown; (2) being connected with their caregivers; (3) being redeemed; and (4) being transformed. A positive birth helped women resolve their guilt, distress, and self-blame related to their prior traumatic birth. Women shared that this redemption moved them from a "state of dis-grace to a state of grace." What must be noted, however, was the mothers' memories of their earlier traumatic births were forgiven, but not forgotten.

A subsequent childbirth following a previous traumatic birth provides health care providers with a perfect opportunity to help traumatized women to reclaim their bodies and complete their journey to motherhood. Pregnancy provides a golden opportunity for clinicians to help mothers recognize and help deal with unresolved traumatic issues from a prior birth trauma. Women who are multiparas should routinely be screened during pregnancy for posttraumatic stress symptoms. Discussion with mothers of their prior labor and delivery experiences should be an essential component of prenatal care.

Necessary referrals for mental health follow-up can be made if necessary for therapy. Some types of therapy that can promote the healing of traumatic birth are: cognitive behavioral therapy, mindful cognitive behavioral therapy or eye movement desensitization reprocessing (EMDR) treatment. Women who have suffered prior birth trauma can be encouraged to use some of the successful strategies employed by the mothers in Beck and Watson's (2010) study of subsequent childbirth after a prior traumatic birth. Subsequent childbirth has the potential to either heal or retraumatize mothers, which places the responsibility on clinicians to tip the scale towards empowering women with a healing subsequent labor and delivery.

Two stories follow from Beck and Watson's (2010) study. The first story is one of a subsequent childbirth that was yet another traumatic birth. The second story was one of a healing subsequent labor and delivery.

Nancy's Story

Nancy was in her mid-twenties and had had an emergency cesarean birth with a postpartum hemorrhage $2^1/_2$ years earlier. She was misdiagnosed with postpartum depression after that first birth. Six months after the birth of her second child, she was correctly diagnosed with PTSD due to childbirth. The story below is Nancy's story of her second pregnancy, labor and delivery experiences which were subsequent to her first traumatic birth.

Nancy adamantly wanted to have a VBAC (Vaginal Birth After Cesarean) homebirth with her second baby. She did manage to have her homebirth but this subsequent childbirth was not a healing experience at all, as she suffered a postpartum hemorrhage which necessitated a terrifying ambulance ride to the hospital and medical procedures. Here is the rest of Nancy's story in her own words.

> Following my first traumatic birth, I was petrified of sex. Unfortunately, my husband felt that sex was a vital part of our marriage, to the extent that we fought over it continually following the birth. I yielded despite how disgusted, terrified, and agonized I felt, only because I did not want to lose my husband. We used birth control religiously (even obsessively) but it did not change my feelings about the act—it was something I did mechanically because I felt I had to.

I remember the exact moment I realized what was happening. I was on my lunch break at work, sitting under a large oak tree, watching cars go by my office, talking with my husband. I suddenly knew . . . I am pregnant again! I remember the exact angle of the sun, the shading of the objects around me. I remember looking into the sun, at that tree, at the windows to the office thinking, "NO! God, PLEASE NO!" I felt my chest at once sink inward on me and take on the weight of a 1000 bricks. I was short of breath, my head seared. All I could think of was "NOOOOOOOOO!"

Somehow I finished working that day, picked up my daughter, and went through the motions of an entire weekend. I remember only that my husband brought me a pregnancy test the day of our fifth anniversary. Two days passed since that afternoon at work. I took the test and crumpled over the edge of our bed, sobbing and retching hysterically for hours. I was dizzy. I was nauseous. I was sick. I could not breathe. I thought my chest would implode. I had a terrible migraine. I could not move from the spot where I had crumpled. I could not talk to my husband or see our daughter. I felt torn to pieces, shredded as shards of glass.

Eventually I willed myself from that place and went back to work. I felt immense waves of fear, anxiety, panic, and terror as my first birth flooded through me in such detail and with such intensity that I felt as if I were experiencing it again. I was depressed, enraged, and hysterical. I felt helpless, hopeless, paralyzed, and frighteningly alone. I felt like I was going crazy because my emotions were so much, so overwhelming, so consuming. Fortunately I was very, very physically ill during the beginning of my pregnancy and the physical illness consumed my energy. I had little energy to function, let alone to face what was actually occurring. I forced myself to keep working because it provided an escape. I woke up, went to work, came home, and went to bed.

After a couple of months passed and I started to experience some relief from the physical symptoms of pregnancy, my husband decided that this might be our opportunity as a couple to have the birth we had wanted with our daughter. We started researching birthing centers and scheduled a tour. I felt an intense sense of dread, fear, and panic and did the best I could to continue to distract myself with work and my daughter rather than having to speak with my husband or admit to him that I was not sharing his optimism about the possibilities of this birth. All my feelings were still there but buried because I did not dare share them. I knew that what I was feeling, thinking, and experiencing was not normal, that it was too much, too overwhelming, too intense, but I could not express it or put it into words. I thought I was wrong, crazy, or weird.

At the birthing center we learned that our State did not allow VBACs in medical facilities including birthing centers. I felt crushed and the weighted sensation I had been experiencing only increased. That visit confirmed all my fears and made the dread and panic worse. I refused to do anything further related to researching birthing facilities. As the pregnancy progressed and I felt physically stronger, I insisted that I would have an unassisted homebirth. My husband did not feel that an unassisted homebirth was safe. He was uncomfortable with the idea of my giving birth at home without a midwife present. I was furious with him. Finally, I got online and found pages of research on the safety of homebirths, gave them to my husband, and scheduled an interview with a midwife who did homebirths. She was also a paramedic, which I thought might ease my husband's fears. He did not like her and I didn't care for her either but she was the only one in the area. We filled out the paperwork that day because I informed him that he could choose this woman or I would have the baby on my own without anyone present, including him, if need be. That assertion, rather than helping me to feel better, made me feel more isolated and crazy.

We began having prenatal visits with the midwife about 4 months into my pregnancy. The visits involved very little—some nutritional counseling and very brief well checks. I had provided her with the medical records from my first birth and my own written description of my experience of the birth. I also expressed to her that this birth HAD to be different. I felt relatively at ease with her indirect involvement and willingness to allow me to determine what prenatal care would occur.

I felt a bit more at ease as I began doing yoga and using the Hypnobabies© program. It helped tremendously with the out-of-control feelings, decreasing them and releasing some of the negative emotions. It kept the emotions of fear, dread, and panic contained, at least, for several months. When these emotions began to increase, I told my midwife who told me that it was normal and paid no more attention to it, despite my sense of urgency and insistence that what I was experiencing felt and seemed far from normal. I felt completely unheard and angry. During the two months before the birth I stopped working and spent 95% of my day doing yoga or listening to the Hynobabies© tapes in an attempt to avoid panic. I called my husband and friends numerous times a day just to have something to do as a way to avoid feeling consumed completely by my thoughts and emotions. I walked. I paced. I exercised. I went shopping. I wrote letters to the baby. I wrote in my journal. My skin was crawling.

My labor started a week past the projected due date. I woke up that morning having a sense that something was different and experiencing contractions that felt quite a bit more intense. By 11 a.m. I called my husband and told him to come home. I felt a very complex mix of joy, of dread, of sheer panic, of "I wonder if I can make it through this." My contractions grew stronger it seemed by the minute. My husband made it home in 30 minutes and took my daughter to a friend's home. I got in the birthing tub/pool in our bedroom. The water made a miraculous difference in how I was feeling emotionally, psychologically, and physically. As long as I was submerged in it up to my neck, the contractions were bearable, and I felt calm, confident, and competent. If I tried getting out of the tub, I spiraled in the complete opposite direction emotionally, psychologically, and physically. Somehow for me the water made all of the difference in how I felt. Out of the water I was in tremendous pain and felt immense panic and fear. From 12 noon until about 8:30 p.m. I stayed in the water, drank water, snacked, and talked with my husband between contractions. I felt relieved at how the labor was going, though I was beginning to drain of energy. Then the contractions started coming on top of each other, leaving me little time to breathe or to regroup. I began feeling very, very afraid and asked my husband to call the midwife.

When the midwife arrived, she did a quick check of everything and announced that I was well on my way to 8 cm. She and her assistant prepped for delivery in another room then stayed in the room with us as I began to push. When I did, I felt very uncertain, nervous, and frightened, particularly when the midwife stated she was unable to find the baby's heartbeat and started insisting on me moving, changing position, and on checking my vitals and the baby's heartbeat more often. I concentrated as much as I could on pushing and I remember very vividly looking at the midwife. I was completely frightened saying, "Can someone help me, please? I don't know if I can do this." The midwife offered some quick pointers for pushing and then went back to checking for the baby's heartbeat WHILE I WAS TRYING TO PUSH!!! I was infuriated with her for this and moved her away with my arm. Then she began stating very loudly that she was growing more and more concerned that she could not find the baby's heartbeat, that we needed to get the baby delivered ASAP, that I needed to get into different positions, that if I didn't push faster/harder and get the baby out, we were going to have to look at transporting to the hospital, that she was considering calling EMS.

The midwife gave me oxygen and went on and on and on about how critical and dangerous things were getting for the baby while I was pushing . . . VERY loudly. I was terrified and furious and adamant that we were NOT going to the hospital. Rather than listen to my body and push, when I felt it was time to push, I pushed as hard and as fast as I could, struggling to catch my breath and to remain even remotely calm as she continued insisting that the baby had to come out immediately. I was shaking and horrified. And then the baby began to crown and she started whispering to her assistant. They insisted I move into a position I was not comfortable with and away from my husband, so that they could both reach me. I was at this point too tired and too involved in pushing to disagree and they physically moved me mid-push anyway. As the baby began to ease down I felt this tremendous pressure, as though I were being ripped apart and then the baby was in my hands (my husband told me later that the midwife literally grabbed the baby and tore him from me as I pushed). He was somewhat blue and the cord was wrapped around him numerous times. I stood there holding him crying, rocking him in my hands, calling his name and pleading with him to be OK. Calling his name over and over as they worked around my hands and got the cord off of him and the assistant took him away from me as the midwife and my husband carried me to the bed. I started to feel sick and woozy, shaking, and having a really hard time staying "with it." I expressed this to the midwife and explained I was really, really terrified. Then I began passing out. I was completely horrified and was panicking, having trouble breathing, felt like a huge weight was on my chest. I felt EXACTLY like I had following my first birth when I was hemorrhaging severely in a life-threatening manner and had to receive pints of blood. I tried to tell the midwife and couldn't make the words form. She asked my husband if she could start an IV and told him she would probably have to catheterize me. I passed out again. When I came back, my arms and legs felt like they weighed 50 pounds. I passed out another three or four times. She catheterized me. Then they started collecting my things and told me they were calling an ambulance and left the room. I kept calling for them, horrified, not knowing what was going on or if they even could hear me. My husband and baby were not in the room either. I was terrified. Finally, the assistant came and talked with me for a moment about what was happening. I kept passing out. Then the ambulance arrived. I was loaded into the back of the ambulance, shaking, horrified, freezing, dizzy, feeling sick, taken from my husband and baby. I heard the midwife tell the EMT in a complete panic/rage that my BP kept crashing and that she couldn't get me stabilized. They shut the doors to the ambulance and I could see my husband plead with the EMT, crying, to please take care of me and not let anything happen to me. He assured my husband I would be just fine and he would take care of me and shut the doors. I told the EMT I didn't think I could take any more. He told me I'd be fine, that he would make sure I was safe, took out the IV the midwife had put in and started a new one. Nearly immediately I started to feel less sick, dizzy, woozy, and "out of it." I begged the EMT to do something to help me through the ride to the hospital (I had no medication of any type at that point including over-the-counter meds and I was in tremendous pain. I was so scared I thought I would die from the fear alone.) He sat and held my hand and promised me he'd take care of me. He also gave me a very small dose of morphine. I begged him to make sure that they put me to sleep before any of the doctors or nurses came anywhere near me at the hospital. He assured me he would do as I was asking and kept telling me that I was OK and that he would make sure nothing would happen. He talked to me the whole way to the hospital (30 minutes) and I felt slightly calmer during the ride until we got there.

As soon as we reached the hospital, and I saw my husband, I began pleading with him to stay with me and to make sure I was put to sleep before I had any interaction with hospital staff before they touched me. The doctor talked to my husband at the end of the bed and they gave me some type of medication and wheeled me to the OR where I made them promise me multiple times I would be put completely to sleep and that I would feel nothing and know nothing of what happened. Then I could hear fuzzy voices talking about the procedure, that I was receiving countless stitches, a third degree tear (really a fourth degree tear), and then I was with my husband again and they were trying to get me to nurse because my son had not eaten. It had been hours. My husband explained that I kept waking up during the procedure in the OR, that I had so many stitches they didn't count them, and that they had given me some type of pain medication and anti-anxiety medication because I was freaking out so much. I insisted on getting up to use the bathroom because I was going home. They made me eat something first, then let me use the bathroom, and finally let my husband take me home. There was blood everywhere, covering everything at our house and the birthing tub was still there. My husband took me to our bedroom and removed what he could as quickly as he could.

Amelia's Story

Amelia's story provides an insider's view of a subsequent childbirth following a traumatic emergency cesarean birth. Her second birth

> was amazing in that I felt that she had been born the way she was meant to be and my body birthed her beautifully. I wouldn't say it healed my first birth, but was a lot better and seemed right, which meant a lot to me and I'm happy that she had a gentle introduction to the world, not like her brother had.

Amelia realized that she had virtually no chance of a VBAC natural birth in a hospital setting. She found a midwife who did homebirths. Amelia also hired a doula to provide additional support during her labor and delivery. Amelia's labor started on her due date. In her own words, she described her homebirth:

> I played my hypnosis CDs and selection of music my sister had prepared for me and rocked on all fours on my soft lounge and labored gently for several hours, sometimes falling off to sleep. At dawn I could hear our hens laying eggs outside the lounge room window amidst lots of squawking. I could empathize with how they were feeling. While my family slept, my dog kept a vigil by my side. I was coping well although the surges were about 5 minutes apart and getting slightly more intense, requiring me to breathe and vocalize through them.
>
> Throughout the afternoon the surges gradually became more intense, yet seemed to stay 5 minutes apart which I was grateful for. I phoned my doula and midwife in the late afternoon to advise them that things were moving along now. We agreed that I was still managing for the time being and I would keep them posted of any changes. I think it was about an hour later that I decided I wanted them both there and called them back and they made arrangements to come over. I continued to labor mostly in my bedroom by leaning on the floor with my upper body rested on the bed.

I seemed to like being in a folder position, perhaps it helped my uterus contract. My midwife arrived shortly before my doula. My attendants dimmed the lights and I continued to labor under candlelight with my music playing. I was finding it hard to get into a comfortable position so I decided to hop into the bath. I felt very relaxed in the bath and was able to lie on my side. When later kneeling, I could grab the sides of the bath with all my strength. I was feeling an urge to push and tried my hardest to keep my vocalization low but it often ended in a screech. My doula would say to me that I was safe.

My body was doing an amazing amount of intense work to mold my baby's head. I am thankful for the time in the bath as I feel it served to help mold my baby's head to move through my pelvic floor. My mind was doing an amazing job too to keep me focused and holding myself together during a very challenging time. I was thankful for the constant support of my birth attendants. While still in the bath, my surges were causing me incredible pain and I felt I was at the end of my tether. I eventually got myself out of the bath and sat on the toilet seat through a surge. I leant into my doula's shoulder as she crouched on the floor. The physical support was very helpful for me. Once out of the bath, my midwife offered to do a vaginal exam to see if there was anything holding things up. I was more than ready to have some guidance at this point in time and felt spurred on. I had a couple of surges on my way to the bedroom. I had a vaginal exam and it was pretty painful yet very encouraging to know that there was no anterior lip. Being upright and even laying on my back, I felt helped my daughter descend as she moved her body away from the front of my pelvis to a better aligned position.

I stood leaning into the change table in my bedroom and rocked my hips from side to side. My doula suggested placing one foot at a time on a step. I could feel my baby descending and it felt amazing to know that she was coming out. Still she seemed to be taking her time and I was ready to meet her. I asked where she was at and my midwife suggested I feel for myself but I just couldn't bring myself to touch anything below my waist. Through each surge she came down a bit more and started to stretch the perineum. She was still "in the bag" and had membranes over her face which were pulled away. A few more surges and she was out and between my legs.

I glimpsed at her through half-closed eyes and could see that she was pink and she had started to cry. All was well. I held my daughter and my midwife helped me to get comfortable with cushions and a blanket. I was feeling shaky and took some homeopathics offered by my midwife and had a lovely cup of sweet tea and jam on toast. My baby cried for a minute or two as if telling me her birth story and crawled up my body and found my heart and left breast. My heart swelled with so many emotions—love, joy, happiness, pride, relief and wonderment. The flood of newborn hormones was amazing. She was perfect in every way and I was so proud of what she and I had done. All the planning, preparation, determination, faith and hard work had come to fruition. I had my baby in my arms and she was healthy and content. Neither she nor I had been exposed to drugs. She was born at term. She had not been separated from me, allowing breastfeeding and bonding to commence immediately and I was fit and able to care for her adequately.

My husband and I examined the placenta, which had come out about 10 minutes after my daughter was born. The cord had stopped pulsating and my husband cut it. My son was mesmerized by his little sister as if comprehending that she was a little person. All four of us fell asleep in our family bed and my daughter and I continued feeding throughout the night.

Clinician's Reaction

Each of these stories triggers responses for me as I read them, especially Nancy's story as I ponder what it would have been like for her to have a therapist who was able to support her and her process during that second pregnancy. So much of the desire to correct the experience can indeed lead to re-traumatization as well as shame, blame, guilt and sadness. In so many ways it is the process of trying to get pregnant as well as the pregnancy that can help bring home the point that we cannot control anything but ourselves and how we perceive our experiences. I know with the women I have worked with, in subsequent pregnancies after a traumatic birth, we spend many sessions dealing with what one can control and what one cannot. In both of these women's stories they did that. The women did not want to have babies in a hospital setting. They did their homework to find the midwives and doulas to guide them through their births yet as we read, there were two very different experiences. Could anyone have predicted the outcomes? NO. But how could we have in essence, softened the blow? Nancy had a postpartum hemorrhage with this birth as she had with her first birth. She was terrified and when the situation appeared to be reoccurring, her birth experience was similar to her first birth and I am not sure that she had the emotional resources to help her.

It is so important that health care providers be cognizant of individual women's experiences so that the nursing care plan that is developed during the second or subsequent pregnancy is viewed as an experience that could re-traumatize. So how can we, as health care providers, facilitate a different experience for the woman we are caring for?

Suggestions that the women provided in Cheryl and Sue's study are very useful in helping to provide the women with some semblance of control; as I mentioned, there is little control over the process of birth, it will happen. The goal is to provide women with the tools, skills, mental strategies and support to work with the birth process and know that they did the best that they could do. This is the key role for empathic holding and interpersonal relationships. It is critical that nurses push to be able to provide care to laboring women on a more consistent basis, i.e. in the room working with the woman and her partner. Perhaps the old nursing practice model of "primary care" needs to be brought back to the labor and delivery suites? This was the model where one nurse was assigned to one patient for the birth experience, and stayed with her. This has become the role of doulas, which are not provided by hospitals but need to be hired by the woman and her partner to attend and assist with the birth process. In many ways I feel they have taken over a role that nursing used to have and is not adequately provided in most American hospitals today due to staffing numbers, budgetary restrictions and changes in insurance reimbursement rates.

Based on these stories and other women's experiences that I have had the privilege in my clinician practice to hear, there are a few care plan aspects that I would recommend:

- *Antenatal assessment*: Information must be obtained from the woman at her first prenatal visit regarding her previous birth experiences. As we know, there is often secrecy and shame surrounding stories of birth trauma. We need to provide women with safe places to share their stories and not fear recrimination or judgment when she tells her story regarding her perceived birth experience. They will need to be encouraged to tell their stories in as much detail as possible when you ask them as part of the assessment. The assessor (i.e. the nurse) needs to encourage description and memories of the previous birth experiences. It is also helpful to ask women what they would like to have different from the previous birth and what can we do, as health care providers, to help facilitate the birth experience for her? In my practice, I will work with the women to develop lists of questions that they want to ask the health care provider and we will process strategies to ask and obtain valid information. I will also offer to call their providers so that we are all on the same page and collaboration will take place. I have, at times, been in attendance at the birth as a support person for the woman and her partner. It is my objective to be an additional support person for her but not take the place of her primary nurse. I do have history of teaching childbirth classes as well and find it a privilege and an honor to be invited into the birthing room as a guest of my client.
- Development of a birth plan that can be discussed antenatally with health care providers. All too often when a health care provider hears that a woman has a birth plan, there is a preconceived transference in that this "woman is going to be controlling and hard to work with." I also remember hearing from colleagues about birth plans, how it will probably all go wrong now that she has a plan. There can be a countertransference issue between the nurse and the patient regarding birth plans. Clinicians need to remember that this birth plan is a way to feel some sense of control. It is in essence a key starting point for discussion as no birth is the same as another. However, if the woman feels that there can be discussion, negotiation, collaboration and flexibility, and that the health care team will work with her and her goals and objectives, she feels seen, heard and validated. Remember it is the woman's perception of the experience that can lead to symptoms of posttraumatic stress.

Mother's Reaction

Women are powerful and resilient. Once the cascade of emotion has lessened after the news of pregnancy, then trust her to know herself. Often PTSD sufferers have a clear distinction between life before the traumatic birth and life afterwards. Therefore, listen, listen, listen . . . with your eyes, your ears and not your mouth. Work with her. The need for support is paramount; ask what she already has in place and work with this. If, however, there is a lack of strategies and no other professionals are involved, then put your thinking cap on, think outside the box and gently suggest possibilities. You are not abandoning her, but rather strengthening her position. This is all about emotional equilibrium for her. Help her to put in place strategies that will help during the pregnancy, during the labor and birth and also for the first few weeks. Many are "list" makers. Breaking down their needs into the immediate, tomorrow, next week or "can wait." Writing such thoughts by hand is very therapeutic. A skilled counselor will indeed be able to work with her, for the past, present and future.

Therefore good support is like a rainbow, arrayed in many colors. In a TABS conversation, it would be "tell me what you are already doing to get through this." Also say, "you are not alone and you can survive." The birth itself can be for many a healing experience and for others just the knowledge of getting through and going forward with the new life is enough. Support in the weeks and months following the birth is important, as is just "hearing" what it is she is communicating. Be a positive partner for her and her family throughout this time.

Conclusion

This chapter focused on the more chronic nature of posttraumatic stress following birth, particularly on women's experiences of subsequent childbirth after a previous birth trauma. In Chapter 12, Jeanne describes a case study from her clinical practice that illustrates the assessment and treatment of this aspect of chronic posttraumatic stress.

References

Ayers, S., Eagle, A., & Waring, H. (2006). The effects of childbirth related post-traumatic stress disorder on women and their relationships: A qualitative study. *Psychology, Health and Medicine, 11,* 389–398.

Ayers, S., Wright, D. B., & Wells, N. (2007). Posttraumatic stress in couples after childbirth: Association with the couple's relationship and parent–baby bond. *Journal of Reproductive and Infant Psychology, 25,* 40–50.

Beck, C. T. (2006). Anniversary of birth trauma: Failure to rescue. *Nursing Research, 55,* 381–390.

Beck, C.T., & Watson, S. (2010). Subsequent childbirth after a previous traumatic birth. *Nursing Research, 59,* 241–249.

Foa, E.B., Cashman, L., Jaycox, L., & Perry, K. (1997). The validation of a self-report measure of posttraumatic stress disorder: The Posttraumatic Diagnostic Scale. *Psychological Assessment, 9,* 445–451.

Gottvall, K., & Waldenström, U. (2002). Does traumatic birth experience have an impact on future reproduction? *BJOG: An International Journal of Obstetrics and Gynaecology, 109,* 254–260.

Horowitz, M. J., Wilner, N., & Alvarez, W. (1979). Impact of Event Scale: A measure of subjective stress. *Psychosomatic Medicine, 41,* 209–218.

Nicholls, K., & Ayers, S. (2007). Childbirth-related post-traumatic stress disorder in couples: A qualitative study. *British Journal of Health Psychology, 12,* 491–509.

Pearce, H., & Ayers, S. (2005). The expected child versus the actual child: Implications for the mother–baby bond. *Journal of Reproductive and Infant Psychology, 23,* 1–15.

Polachek, I. S., Harari, L. H., Baum, M., & Strous, R. D. (2012). Postpartum post-traumatic stress disorder symptoms: The uninvited birth companion. *Israeli Medical Association Journal, 14,* 347–353.

Spanier, G. (1976). Measuring dyadic adjustment: New scales for assessing the quality of marriage and similar dyads. *Journal of Marriage and the Family, 38,* 15–28.

Thomson, G. M., & Downe, S. (2010). Changing the future to change the past: Women's experiences of a positive birth following a traumatic birth experience. *Journal of Reproductive and Infant Psychology, 28,* 102–112.

12 Case Study 2: Anne

Anne, a 41-year-old, came to my office for an evaluation. She was the mother of three children: two girls and a boy. At our first meeting, she described that she had been feeling "depressed, sad, and crying at the drop of a hat. I get in my own way." She described that these emotions felt different to her in that during most of her life she just would get through whatever she felt that she had to and move along. She was concerned now in that things were not getting any better and in fact, "my feelings are now getting in the way of my life and the care of my family."

She had been married to the same man, Dan, for 13 years and is on leave from her own business. She gave birth to her second daughter 6 months ago, and has a 4-year-old daughter and a 2-year-old son. She states: "I don't feel like I can go back to work . . . something changed after this birth . . . I don't know what is going on . . . I am just so nervous, can't sleep, and I always feel scared."

I explained to her that my evaluation process was based on my basic philosophy that all aspects of our lives—genetics, life events and reproductive events—impact not only our psychology but our physiology, and that in my assessment/evaluation I would be collecting information pertaining to those domains of her life. She sat back on the couch and appeared to be calm and eager to talk. We began with the genetic/family history. What this information would provide would be the potential for genetic underpinnings of mood and/or anxiety disorders, her vulnerabilities.

Anne began to describe that, as far as she knew, her mother did not have any medical problems but indeed had had some periods of depression. She did not know if her mom had ever been treated for depression but she would ask her. She did feel that her mother was a bit "introspective" and maybe even shy. Anne described that she had a "good relationship" with her mother; in fact, she was watching the children so she could be at this appointment. According to Anne, her father was "another story." She described him as a source of "trauma" in her life. He was highly educated and emotionally abusive. "He was unpredictable in his rage, and he is and was scary." She did not believe that he had ever been diagnosed or treated for any emotional disorders. "You know, though, how it is with brilliant people. They get away with a lot because of their intelligence and their contribution to their fields." She went on to describe that her dad was an academic and had been on the faculty of a university for most of her life and was currently retired. Her parents were divorced and she stated that that had happened when "I was a senior in high school." Her father does not live close by and she has limited contact with him.

Anne had two older brothers. Mark was 47 and according to Anne, he was "doing well." She stated that he was happily married, lived in New Jersey with his wife and their two children. She knew that he had a history of depression but had been treated for that although she did not know what medication he had been taking. Her brother Steven was 44 years old and single. She said that she felt he had a mood disorder but that to her knowledge he had never been treated for any psychiatric illness. She described him as "strange in his social behavior" and mostly moody. He lives in the Midwest and works for the federal government. She shared with me that he rarely comes east but does communicate regularly with their mother.

I asked Anne to tell me more about growing up with her father as she had described him as the "source of trauma" in her life. She verbalized that she felt she had been emotionally abused by her Dad with his rage attacks. He never apologized and just acted like he was right and the rest of the world was beneath him. She described that she would never know what to expect with her father. "He could be all smiley and interested and then he would switch into aggressive, hostile and belittling." I asked if she would say that he had mood swings: times when he would be "fine" and then times when he was aggressive. She felt that he had a bipolar disorder but was never diagnosed. "He would never go to a psychiatric person. He did not believe in psychiatry." She went on to tell me that her maternal grandparents were "wonderful people" and maybe her grandmother had some depression but nothing "bad," while her paternal grandparents were eccentric and the grandfather was an alcoholic. So in the first aspect of our assessment I had learned that Anne had a genetic propensity for mood and anxiety disorders from her immediate family of origin.

The next area to assess was her life events and her experiences of them. Anne went on to describe grammar school as "good." She could not recollect any significant problems. "I went to a private grammar school, had nice friends, liked school and got good grades." High school was another story for Anne.

She described that high school was okay but that during her freshman year she "tanked." She describes becoming "disinterested in academics, loved being with friends, moved into an 'existential' time of my life. I was reading all the time, philosophers, thinkers, etc. I was bored by high school reading." She recalls that in high school was when her parents were having significant conflicts and her father was more rageful and aggressive. Her brother Mark had gone away to college and Steven had graduated but was not in college yet. "He was at home, not working, just hanging out." She believes that she was getting more depressed but did not share that with anyone. She felt she was going more into herself, although "everyone thought I was fine." She explained to me that she attempted suicide as a consequence of feeling so depressed and dark.

The cuts were superficial, but I did get admitted to a psychiatric hospital for a week. The truth is, I really liked being at the hospital. I was away from my family. There was only one problem. I had a very aggressive therapist who reminded me of my father and it wasn't until after *this* birth that I began to remember how bad that was . . . I was afraid of that therapist and wouldn't talk to him about anything. They diagnosed me with an adolescent adjustment disorder and sent me home but I was to continue to see that therapist.

She verbalized she began to "just feel that adults let you down" and that she had to take care of herself and be responsible and just wait to get away from these "adults."

She graduated from high school and has not looked back. She would summarize that it was a time of distrust and when she learned not to depend on adults for anything. "When I turned 18, I decided I had to create my own life. It was scary and terrifying but I was, in essence, fighting for my life." While all of Anne's friends went off to college, she decided to get a job so that she could become independent and not rely on anyone but herself. Over the next few years she earned money, worked in various positions: research assistant, child care worker, non-profits, etc. Anne then decided that she wanted to go to college and was ready. She went back to school and finished in about 5 years. She studied liberal arts and was considering becoming a teacher. She liked children and wanted to help them because she felt there were not very many people around to help her when she was a child. She continued her personal interest in philosophy and focused much of her reading in women's studies and psychology. She continued her education to obtain a doctorate and was a consultant in the area of early childhood curriculum design. She had her own business which she had started when she had gotten married.

I wanted to have the flexibility to combine work and family. It has been very successful and I have two people who work for me now which is why I am able to take this time off. I have no idea when I am going to go back, I just feel so overwhelmed.

Anne went on to tell me that she met her husband while she was in graduate school. "He is kind, gentle and adores me. I adore him and we have an excellent life, I feel like I hit the lottery when I met him." Anne's husband Dan is a business executive. He is "very supportive and an active father. He is really such a great guy. He is very worried about me now." Anne has a nanny to help with the children as Dan travels a lot for his work. "I want to go back to work as I love what I do," but she feels that she is not emotionally balanced. "I am so emotional and don't always feel in control of myself or my emotions."

The next area to assess, based on the Earthquake model (Figure 12.1), was her reproductive system. She got her first period when she was 12 and did not remember having any problems. She described taking birth control pills in her twenties and denied any mood changes on them. Anne's first pregnancy was planned and much anticipated. The first trimester, she described, was nausea every day, all day. When she moved into the second trimester, the nausea subsided and it was a "good pregnancy." She described a "terrible labor." Her labor was described as long in the early stages. "My first contraction was as painful as the last one, and after 3 to 4 days of that type of labor, I had a c-section." She had a baby girl, who weighed about 8 pounds and she described that the cesarean birth was due to her "failure to progress." Anne verbalized feelings and experiences pertaining to this birth with sadness and what felt like frustration. Her breastfeeding experience, "which I really wanted to do," was filled with conflict and feelings of insecurity. "I had a pediatrician who just kept pushing formula. I think I had baby blues then because I was weepy and just felt a bit conflicted at times about what I was doing." She described that she did join a mothers' group which was a good thing for her. She was able to learn from other women and received some validation for her feelings of sadness about having the cesarean as well as support for her breastfeeding. She went on to describe the conflicts she felt then regarding doing what was right for her versus what others were telling her to do, especially regarding feeding her daughter.

> I did finally breastfeed full time and that was really important to me after the cesarean birth. As I think back on it now, I had so many feelings of loss, sadness and anger about that whole experience about "failing to progress"

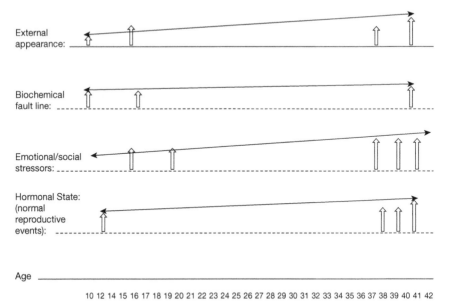

Figure 12.1 Anne's Earthquake Assessment

Source: From *Women's Moods* by Deborah Sichel and Jeanne Watson Driscoll © 1999 by Deborah Sichel and Jeanne Watson Driscoll. Courtesy of HarperCollins Publishers.

but when the feeding got better, I just pushed along, which is how I live my life . . . just do it.

One year postpartum, Anne experienced a miscarriage "at about 10 weeks. It was so sad. We were excited about the pregnancy even though we didn't actively plan to get pregnant that soon." She talked about the grieving she experienced after the miscarriage and how she felt she had dealt with it. About a year later, she became pregnant. During this pregnancy, she experienced a lot of nausea and vomiting in the first trimester. She verbalized how she was happy to be so sick because it made her "really feel pregnant" as she was afraid of another miscarriage in those early weeks. Anne shared with me that she was really set on having a vaginal birth with this pregnancy and secured the key people on her care plan team to help with that planned outcome. She hired a nurse midwife with whom she felt she had a good connection after searching and interviewing many health providers.

Her second and third trimesters were uneventful and she took classes for experiencing a vaginal birth after cesarean (VBAC) and was working hard to prepare for that experience. When she went into labor at 39 weeks, it was in the evening so they called her mother to come and watch her 2-year-old daughter.

> She is very close to my mother so I felt great that she was with her as I was not sure what the outcome would be although I was so geared up for a vaginal birth after a cesarean. I was doing everything I could to be prepared for this baby's birth.

The labor was long and tiring but Anne did have a vaginal birth after her first cesarean.

> It was great. I was able to push him out and I was feeling so proud of myself. Then when I got home, I felt pretty blue. Dan had to go back to work and I was home with two children: a 2-year-old and a new one, fortunately my mom was able to help me out a lot.

She described that she moved right back to her usual coping skills of "just do it" and eventually "I believe that time heals."

She continued her reproductive history story but sharing with me that she and Dan had wanted a third child so they had not used birth control after the second baby and "when we got pregnant we were both excited." She had interviewed nannies when she was pregnant as she had learned through experience that she needed more help when Dan went on business trips and her mom was getting older and couldn't commit to regular times. Anne had felt that she would have her own "village" for her family and they were fortunate in that their income allowed them to have this support system and they had room in their house for a live-in person.

Anne described that this last pregnancy was a bit harder in that she was more tired and did indeed have the first trimester nausea. It was, however, "the birth that has totally pushed me over the ledge." It was "horrific and now I just can't get myself to feel better." She had planned to have another vaginal birth and had hired the same midwives and health care team that she had with her second baby and had had such success. "I felt I had a great relationship with the midwives and I had a huge amount of confidence in my abilities and theirs. Unfortunately, this was the birth from hell."

Anne began to narrate her story.

> I was 40 weeks and went to the midwifery office for my weekly checkup. They found the baby's heart rate was very fast and they were not sure why. They felt since I was 40 weeks that it would be a good thing to induce me and get this baby born.

She recalls that she was admitted to the hospital. Again, "thank goodness for my Mom who was able to move into our house to take care of my other children as the nanny that we had hired was not going to start for another month."

Anne remembered that she was in the birthing room feeling "very scared and anxious." She was not sure what was being triggered in her but she did not feel like herself. "I was very nervous. They started an intravenous and were hydrating me as they felt I was a bit dry. All of a sudden, I couldn't control anything anymore. I was scared." She describes that there was

> one nasty nurse taking care of me. She wanted me to lie flat so she could watch the fetal monitor tracings or something. I also had a very strong feeling that there was an animosity between this nurse and my midwife as the conversations were terse and short and it just felt stressed in that room.

Anne continued to describe her birth as she looked off into space, sat up straight and gradually she began to cry and her breathing increased and she just looked different to me. I was paying close attention as I realized that her sharing this story was a trigger to her emotionally and I wanted this process to be gentle and safe for her. She was explaining how when she was in the birthing room, with the intravenous in her arm, the midwife examined her, and she was 3 centimeters. There were low-level contractions going on and the baby was responsive but the heart rate was still "fast." The decision was made to add a small dose of pitocin to the intravenous to see if that would help pick up the strength of her contractions.

> I remember thinking to myself, I really have no say in this whole damn thing . . . I felt I was between a rock and a hard place . . . baby with fast heart rate, don't know why, 3 centimeters, 40 weeks gestation. So much of my reading has led me to believe that with induction there can be an

increase in the need for a cesarean and I wanted a vaginal birth. My midwife knew this. We had been together for years. Was this going to have a good outcome?

I did know that often when the technological aspects of labor are introduced into the experience that I was perhaps descending down the slippery slope to a c-section. I had done my reading. I am an intelligent person and was now anxious, doubting myself and feeling like I had no power. I was scared.

The pitocin did indeed trigger the labor and when that started, she was thinking,

This may be okay. I was hoping my body would follow the pattern of my second birth and we would be having a vaginal birth and be home in 2 days . . . was I wrong . . . the descent into hell was just beginning but I wasn't aware of the totality of the experience at that point.

She went on to explain that she was experiencing contractions that were strong and regular and things were moving along so that eventually she was fully dilated and ready to push.

Then something happened. My nurse midwife had this look on her face and all of a sudden she runs out of the room and I am not sure where she went. I had no idea what was going on, I had started to push and for me that felt great, however, what I then learned as she came back into the room with the doctor was that my baby's heart rate was changing on the fetal monitor. Now I could feel my blood pressure go up and my fear move from a 6 to a 10. The pushing process became emergent. I was being told to push her out, I was so afraid that she was not going to be alright so I was pushing like my baby's life depended on it. The midwife described that there was meconium and that she could feel the cord around her neck. The pediatricians were called. When my daughter was born, she was rushed over to the warming table where I figured they were suctioning her as well as doing some respiratory things to her. Dan went over and for some reason the look on his face changed drastically . . . it now looked like they were doing CPR on my baby and I now thought she was dead. All the attention was on her and I am yelling to someone, anyone, to tell me what was going on but no one was even acknowledging that I was there.

My husband was standing over there looking at her and then back at me. He was as white as a ghost. She was not breathing. There was no crying. It was so quiet. I remember thinking, I am not going to make this. My baby is dead. Then I heard a cry, more like a scream and I just began to sob and shake.

The baby did begin to breathe on her own, and from that point seemed to be okay.

They did have to give her some antibiotics as she had swallowed some meconium so she had to go to the NICU on a regular basis for the intravenous medication but she was alive and seemed fine but I kept looking at her, holding her, praying for her. I was a nervous wreck. Oh, and her heart rate was normal. They are still not sure what that was all about with the elevated heart rate . . .

The baby continued to do well but Anne did not. Here she was in my office, 6 months postpartum and could not shake the feelings of sadness, depression, rage, anger and disappointment. She was breastfeeding well and "doing okay with the other children, but I do not feel like myself, I feel like I have lost myself somewhere." I asked Anne to tell me more about what she was experiencing at this time with regard to symptoms. She was anxious all the time.

> I am not comfortable being alone with the children. I am afraid that I am going to lose it. I get so easily irritated. I cry if you look at me funny. I cannot sleep, keep having nightmares that she is dead, and I am just watching her die. At times I feel like I am just not here. I am off in another world. I am not connected to anything. I am here but I am not. Anxiety is present all the time; sometimes I feel like I am going to die. I can't breathe and I get so nervous.

She goes on to say:

> I was fine before this birth. Why can't I get it back together and "just do it," that was how I functioned before? I am used to working hard and moving forward. I learned that long ago people let you down but you just keep going forward. It is not working anymore. I am tired and scared. I don't think I am ever going to feel any better. My husband is scared too as I have been the one who manages the household and I am like a little kid now. I don't want him to go to work or leave me alone.

She had been searching online and had been visiting the TABS (www.tabs. org.nz) website regularly. She considered that she was having posttraumatic stress after this birth experience. "It is like this was the worst . . . three strikes and you are out!" PTSD is an anxiety disorder that indeed can occur in women postpartally. Women describe nightmares, flashbacks of the horror that they experienced. Other symptoms of PTSD are fearfulness, hyper-vigilance, depression, disturbed sleep, anxiety, headaches, etc. Very often when women have experienced traumatic births they will try, as Anne had, to just move past it, to bury the experience and try to live life in the present. However, as more recent studies have shown, there have been some biochemical changes in the brain as a result of the dramatic fight or flight experience of the trauma birth. These dysregulations cause many of the symptoms that are described by Anne.

As we had learned in her assessment, she also had a vulnerable biochemistry to depression and anxiety secondary to her genetic heritage and her own life experiences so we would be working on how to come upon the care plan to help her as she healed from these experiences.

After this assessment, I shared with Anne that I did indeed think she had experienced posttraumatic stress disorder after the birth but also the interpersonal relationship issues (issues with her midwife and trust) of these experiences were also disappointing and upsetting. She described that she felt depressed, anxious, and vulnerable, easily irritated, although she is sleeping okay and her appetite is fine. She doesn't feel like herself and she cannot shake the feelings. In the past she had felt that she had a high level of resiliency but now she was feeling like she was "drowning."

> I did all I could to get the right team. They disappointed me. I feel like they all let me down and now they all want me to be happy and they can go on their merry way. My midwife has called many times and wants to process the events of the birth but I am still so angry at her for abandoning me and not standing up for me . . . that nasty nurse took over and then the doctor had to deliver the baby and it was just a mess . . . then I am trying to get help and no one is helping me to get better.

We processed the information she had shared with me. I described the issues pertaining to postpartum depression and PTSD, and we went over how her feelings were indeed important and real. I also went on to discuss the use of medications to quiet some of the biology, especially the anxiety and shortness of mood, so that she would feel a bit more in control. I do believe that talk therapy can indeed heal biology but that at times medications need to be part of the care plan, especially in the case of new mothers who don't have any luxury time. They have to be present in the work of raising a family. These early years are critical to the emotional development of their babies and children and they need to be emotionally available.

We discussed the up to date research with regard to breastfeeding and medications as well as the fact that her daughter was 6 months old and was eating some solid food, had a highly functioning liver to metabolize the medications. We discussed the classes of medication that we could use and the approach of titrating the dosage slowly starting at a very low dosage. I was a bit concerned regarding the questionable bipolar history in her family and the use of antidepressants which is another reason why we would be dosing the medications at low dose and moving up slowly. We developed her NURSE Plan (© Sichel & Driscoll, 1999), to include the following at the first session and we would assess and adjust the plan at each session.

- *Nourishment and needs:* As described above, I suggested the use of an antidepressant to help Anne with her anxiety and her depression symptoms. She was unsure and we would continue to discuss it at each session.

We went over her nutritional intake. She was taking a daily multivitamin, calcium, and vitamin D. We discussed small, frequent feedings as a way to keep her blood sugar in balance and avoid symptoms of hypoglycemia. She shared with me that she was conscious of maintaining her hydration and only had one cup of coffee per day.

- *Understanding:* She agreed to come for regular therapy where she could process her experiences as well as integrate those experiences. She readily accessed online resources and did feel that her best friend was readily available for support.

- *Rest and relaxation:* Anne had a nanny. So we talked about ways for her to have some rest time in the day. She had planned to go back to work but secondary to how she had been feeling she was delaying that for a few more months. So we went over sleep hygiene: regular bedtime, no television in her bedroom, regular waking times.

- *Spirituality:* Anne had a strong faith although did not belong to any formal religious organization. She also had a history of meditation and doing yoga which she planned to re-engage in.

- *Exercise:* Anne described that she walked with the children to the park a few times a week but that she did not have a formal exercise plan. She did have a treadmill in her home and was planning to use that at least three times per week.

At this session, after much discussion, Anne decided to try sertraline, a selective serotonin reuptake inhibitor anti-depressant medication. So we went over the medication, the dosage plan and the potential side effects. She would begin on 12.5 mg. per day for 4 days and then increase by 12.5 mg. every 4 days. She was encouraged to call with any questions and we made an appointment for the next week. Anne was indeed dealing with a posttraumatic stress disorder secondary to the birth, as well as being in some ways re-traumatized by the angry nurse (triggering responses she had with living with her dad) and the alterations in the interpersonal relationships that had occurred over the past months. My hope was to promote healing for Anne both psychologically and physiologically.

At our next meeting, Anne shared with me that she had not started the medication as she was not completely comfortable with the idea of medications and breastfeeding although she had been doing a lot of research online regarding the treatment plan. I supported her process as she became more comfortable with the idea of taking medication. I have found that this is a major decision for women in my practice. It requires lots of processing, information, support, and education.

The next week Anne came in for our session and she shared with me that she had taken 12.5 mg. of sertraline. She had begun the medication 2 days ago and was already feeling less anxious and "better." She spent a lot of time in that session describing and wondering why she felt a little bit better already.

At the next meeting, Anne was up to 50 mg. of sertraline. "I cannot believe how much better I feel. I am not sobbing and I feel less anxious." She went on to describe that she was now feeling anger at the relationship with her midwife and felt like a major relationship had been disconnected. She described how she felt abandoned and similar to her first birth experience and even growing up. In so many ways, I feel that therapy after birth can be such a corrective experience for women to do the work of processing their lives and moving into an empowered sense of self with authenticity and voice.

In our work together over time, Anne's symptoms of sadness, irritation and anxiety began to recede, and she felt that she was doing well with herself and her relationships with her husband and children. She was still preoccupied with the abrupt termination of the relationship with her midwife and we spent many sessions processing those events in relation to her other life events and ways to strategize in the future. Medication-wise we slowly moved the dosage up to 150 mg. per day and finally she felt that a dose of 175 mg. per day seemed to be the best to manage her symptoms and she was not experiencing any side effects.

Our therapy work focused on healing from the trauma of the birth and the issues of altered interpersonal relationships with other women in her life. At the anniversary of her daughter's birth she was able to write a letter that she mailed to both her obstetrician and her midwife. She shared with them her experience of the birth and the postpartum experience and hoped that they would pay attention to their interpersonal skills in caring for other women in their practices. She felt that that helped her with closure and "I am hoping that they will read and understand how important it is in their work to be in relationship with the woman. We are in the bed!"

Anne gradually weaned from the medication after about two years and described that she felt back to herself, but maybe more like a "new self." She went back to her consulting practice. She and Dan were happy with their family and when last I spoke with her they did not want to have any more children.

Reference

Sichel, D., & Driscoll, J. W. (1999). *Women's moods: What every woman must know about hormones, the brain, and emotional health.* New York: HarperCollins.

13 Selected Treatment Methods for PTSD

In reviewing the literature pertaining to the specific treatment of PTSD secondary to birth trauma, there are limited data. In this chapter we will briefly discuss the methods that were reported as well as share the narratives from the ongoing study conducted by Cheryl and Sue on mothers' experiences of eye movement desensitization reprocessing (EMDR) treatment.

Debriefing

Debriefing is a structured intervention which is intended to serve as a primary prevention to decrease symptoms of acute stress reactions, in this case, to traumatic childbirth. Debriefing can consist of the following seven phases: introduction, description of traumatic event's facts, thoughts, emotions, symptoms, teaching, and a re-entry phase which provides the person with an opportunity to ask unanswered questions and to develop a plan of action (Mitchell & Dyregrov, 1993). The efficacy of postpartum debriefing for posttraumatic stress symptoms has been studied in three randomized controlled trials. In all three studies debriefing did not result in a significant decrease in women's posttraumatic stress symptoms (Priest, Henderson, Evans, & Hagan, 2003; Kershaw, Jolly, Bhabra, & Ford, 2005; Selkirk, McLaren, Ollerenshaw, McLachlan, & Moten, 2006).

In Priest et al.'s (2003) study in Australia, 1745 new mothers were randomly assigned to either the control group (n = 870) or to the debriefing intervention group (n = 875). Mothers in the intervention group received one standardized debriefing session in their hospital rooms prior to being discharged from the hospital. Women were followed at 2, 6, and 12 months postpartum using the Impact of Event Scale-Revised (Weiss & Marmar, 1997). No significant differences were reported between the groups regarding their level of posttraumatic stress symptoms.

Also in Australia, Selkirk and colleagues (2006) examined the effect of a midwife-led debriefing session in mothers within 3 days postpartum. Some 149 women were randomly assigned to either the debriefing treatment group or to the control group. Data were collected at 2 days, 1, and 3 months postpartum using the Impact of Event Scale (Horowitz, Wilner, & Alvarez,

1979). There were no reported significant differences between these two groups.

The third study was conducted in the United Kingdom with 319 women who had given birth to their first child by an operative delivery (forceps, vacuum, or emergency cesarean birth) (Kershaw et al., 2005). Women were randomly assigned to the control group or to a community midwives-led debriefing at 10 days and 10 weeks postpartum. The Impact of Event Scale (Horowitz et al., 1979) was completed by the mothers. The debriefing session did not make any significant difference in posttraumatic stress symptoms between the two groups.

Cognitive Behavioral Therapy

Cognitive behavioral therapy (CBT) has been one of the most studied interventions for PTSD in the general population (Institute of Medicine, 2012). CBT is a combination of behavioral and cognitive interventions. The behavioral component focuses on decreasing maladaptive behaviors and increasing adaptive ones. This is achieved by modifying antecedents and consequences and by introducing behavioral actions that lead to new learning. The cognitive component's goal is to modify maladaptive cognitions or beliefs. CBT focuses on problem-focused interventions that are based in learning and cognitive theories (Craske, 2010). Ayers, McKenzie-McHarg, and Eagle (2007) reported two case studies of women with postpartum PTSD and their treatment with cognitive behavioral therapy (CBT). In both these cases CBT was effective in the treatment of the mothers' PTSD. No other studies were located that investigated the efficacy of CBT in PTSD secondary to childbirth.

EMDR

Eye movement desensitization and reprocessing (EMDR) is a treatment strategy that was developed by Francine Shapiro, PhD, in the late 1980s. She found, when using eye movements while on a walk in the park, that the negative emotions she was experiencing in response to her own distressing memories appeared to go away. She wondered if the eye movements had a desensitizing effect on the emotions. She went on to use this technique with others and it became clear to her that the eye movements alone did not create thorough therapeutic effects, so she added it to other treatment elements and developed the standard treatment that she has called Eye Movement Desensitization (EMD) (Shapiro, 2001). Over time, Shapiro continued to develop and test her methods changing the name in 1991 to Eye Movement Desensitization and Reprocessing (EMDR). This name change reflected the cognitive and insight changes that occur during the treatment and to identify the information processing theory that she developed to explain the treatment effects (Shapiro, 1991). Tables 13.1 and 13.2 describe the EMDR protocol.

Table 13.1 Protocol for eye movement desensitization and reprocessing

Stage	Contents
1. Client history	Biopsychosocial evaluation, assessment of current & past medical status, family & childhood history, & presenting problem
2. Preparation	Developing a therapeutic & trusting relationship between patient & clinician, explanation of the theoretical background & actual steps in EMDR
3. Assessment	The patient visualized the target incident and formulates a negative cognition (NC) about herself related to the traumatic experience. Subsequently, she formulates a positive cognition (PC) she would like to believe about herself, and quantifies this on a scale from 1 to 7 (validity of cognition, VoC). Then, the patient describes the emotions associated with the target event and scales the disturbance on an 11-point scale (subjective units of distress, SUD). Finally, she is asked to scan her body for the location of sensations of distress.
4. Desensitization	While the patient focuses on the distress she experiences, bilateral stimulation is applied for several seconds to minutes (depending on the patient's reaction). Subsequently, she is asked to clear her mind and describe what thought or feeling comes to mind. Several sets of bilateral stimulation are repeated until she repeatedly reports similar thoughts and the subjective units of distress is 0.
5. Installation	The positive cognition is revisited in relation to the original disturbing image, and its validity of cognition is rated. Sets of bilateral attention are applied until the positive thought is experienced as being totally valid (6-7 on the validity of cognition scale).
6. Body Scan	Patient closes her eyes, concentrates on the target experience, and mentally scans her entire body. If sensations are reported, short sets of bilateral stimulation are applied until the sensation subsides or a positive feeling is experienced.
7. Closure	Explanation of the session by the therapist, including guidance on dealing with uncomfortable feelings after the session.
8. Reevaluation	Reevaluation takes place at the beginning of the following session.

Source: Reprinted with permission from Stramrood et al. (2012, p.72).

Two studies have been published on the effectiveness of eye movement desensitization and reprocessing (EMDR) treatment with women who are suffering from posttraumatic stress disorder secondary to childbirth. EMDR treatment for posttraumatic stress after childbirth was first reported by Sandstrom and colleagues (2008). Four women participated in their pilot study in Sweden. One woman was pregnant at the time and the other three were not pregnant. Their before and after treatment design also included follow-up 1–3 years after EMDR treatment was finished. Posttraumatic stress symptoms were measured using the Traumatic Event Scale (TES) (Wijma, Soderquist, & Wijma, 1997). All four women reported their posttraumatic stress symptoms had begun at

Table 13.2 EMDR procedural outline

Explanation of EMDR: "When a trauma occurs, it seems to get locked in the nervous system with the original picture, sounds, thoughts, and feelings. The eye movements we use in EMDR seem to unlock the nervous system and allow the brain to process the experience. That may be what is happening in REM or dream sleep—the eye movements may help to process the unconscious material. It is important to remember that it is your own brain that will be doing the healing and that you are the one in control."

Specific instructions: "What we will be doing often is a simple check on what you are experiencing. I need to know from you exactly what is going on, with feedback that is as clear as possible. Sometimes things will change and sometimes they won't. I may ask if something else comes up; sometimes it will and sometimes it won't. There are no 'supposed tos' in this process. So just give feedback as accurately as you can as to what is happening, without judging whether it should be happening or not. Let whatever happens, happen. We'll do the eye movements for a while, and then we'll talk about it."

Stop signal: "If at any time you feel you have to stop. Raise your hand."
Establishing appropriate distance: "Is this a comfortable distance and speed?"
Presenting issue: "What incident would you like to work on today?"
Image: "What picture represents the worst part of the incident?"

Negative cognition (NC): "What words best go with the picture and express your belief about yourself now?" (Have client make the statement in the form of an "I" statement in the present tense. This must be a presently held negative self-referencing belief.)

Positive cognition (PC): "When you bring up that picture/incident, what would you like to believe about yourself now?" (This must be a present desired self-referencing belief.)

Validity of Cognition (VOC) (for PC only): "When you think of that picture/incident, how true does that (positive cognition) feel to you now on a scale of 1 to 7, where 1 is untrue and 7 is totally true?"

Emotions/feelings: "When you bring up that incident and those works (negative cognition), what emotion(s) do you feel now?"

Subjective units of distress (SUDs): "On a scale of 0 to 10, where 0 is no disturbance or neutral and 10 is the highest disturbance imaginable, how disturbing does it feel to you now?"

Location of body sensation: "Where do you feel it (the disturbance) in your body?"

Desensitization: (I'd like you to) bring up that picture, those negative words (repeat the negative cognition), notice where you are feeling it in your body, and follow my fingers."

1. Begin the eye movements slowly. Increase the speed as long as the client can comfortably tolerate the movements.
2. Approximately every 12 movements, or when there is an apparent change, comment to the client, "That's it. Good. That's it."
3. It is helpful to make the following comment to the client (especially if the client is abreacting): "That's it. It's old stuff. Just notice it."
4. After a set of eye movements, instruct the client to "Blank it out" and/or "Let it go and take a deep breath."
5. Ask: "What do you get now?" or "What are you noticing now?"

(Continued)

Table 13.2 (Continued)

---

6. If the client reports movement, say, "Stay with that" (without repeating the client's words). The client should be reporting a 0 or 1 on the SUD scale before doing the installation.

Installation of positive cognition (linking the desired positive cognition with the original memory or image):

1. "Do the words (repeat the positive cognition) still fit, or is there another positive statement you feel would be more suitable?"
2. "Think about the original incident and those words (selected positive cognition). From 1, completely false, to 7, completely true, how true do they feel?"
3. "Hold them together." Lead the client in an eye movement set. "On a scale of 1 to 7, how true does that (positive statement) feel to you now when you think of the original incident?"
4. VOC: Measure the VOC after each set. Even if the client reports a 6 or a 7, do eye movement again to strengthen, and continue until validity no longer strengthens. Go on to the body scan.
5. If the client reports a 6 or less, check appropriateness and address blocking belief (if necessary) with additional reprocessing.

Body scan: "Close your eyes; concentrate on the incident and the PC, and mentally scan your body. Tell me where you feel anything." If any sensation is reported, do EM. If a positive/comfortable sensation, do EM to strengthen the positive feeling. If a sensation of discomfort is presorted, reprocess until discomfort subsides.

Closure (debriefing the experience): "The processing we have done today may continue after the session. You may or may not notice new insights, thoughts, memories, or dreams. If you do, just notice what you are experiencing. Take a snapshot of it (what you are seeing, feeling, thinking, and the trigger), and keep a log. We can work on this new material next time. If you feel it is necessary, call me."

Source: Reprinted with permission from Shapiro (2001).

childbirth (between 3–7 years earlier). After the initial treatment, all four participants had a decrease in posttraumatic stress symptoms especially for intrusive thoughts, avoidance, and numbing of general responsiveness. In the follow-up 1–3 years after EMDR completion, it was revealed that for three of the four women there were still beneficial effects of the treatment. For one woman, however, her symptoms recurred at the same level as before treatment.

Stramrood et al. (2012) reported using EMDR treatment with three women during their second pregnancy. Each woman had suffered with posttraumatic stress symptoms after the birth of their first baby. With their first births, one woman had an emergency cesarean birth, another woman had a second degree laceration due to a shoulder dystocia birth, and the third woman had pre-eclampsia. The EMDR treatment during their second pregnancies decreased their posttraumatic stress symptoms, decreased their stress, and increased their confidence regarding the upcoming birth. Even though all three women went on to experience complications with their second births, they all reported having positive experiences.

There have been limited studies that have focused on the management of PTSD due to childbirth in contrast to the number of studies conducted with non-childbirth PTSD. In a literature review of studies that examined the effects of different interventions on posttraumatic stress due to childbirth, Lapp, Agbokou, Peretti, and Ferreri (2010) concluded that the results from the limited number of studies investigating treatment of PTSD specific to traumatic childbirth are similar to results from the non-childbirth PTSD literature. Debriefing is inconclusively effective while EMDR and CBT may improve posttraumatic stress symptoms but randomized control trials are needed before any firm conclusions can be made.

A comprehensive review of treatment for PTSD in military and veteran populations was undertaken by the Institute of Medicine (2012). Even though this thorough assessment of research focused only on military and veteran populations, it is an excellent resource for clinicians who treat PTSD patients in other populations such as women whose PTSD is secondary to traumatic childbirth.

Mothers' Narratives of Their EMDR Treatment

Ten mothers participated in Beck and Watson's qualitative study of women's experiences of EMDR treatment for their posttraumatic stress symptoms due to birth trauma. Here are some quotes from a few of these mothers which summarized their treatment experiences:

- I do know that the EMDR took the sting out of the trauma. The power was knee-capped.
- EMDR helped me reprocess my traumatic birth memories and feel more empowered. Although my memories are still present, they no longer have the devastating impact on me as they once did.
- All in all, I did EMDR for about 6 months and it helped me tremendously. It's not that my memories or feelings about them are gone. But they are less excruciating and they don't haunt me on a daily basis.
- I highly recommend EMDR to anyone suffering from PTSD. A competent EMDR therapist can not only help you resolve your issues, but she can empower you to reshape your trauma.

Women undergoing EMDR treatment focused on their traumatic childbirth memories in order to allow them to unblock and experience them again briefly so that they are reprocessed in a positive way. One mother who participated in our research on EMDR treatment had experienced both talk therapy and EMDR treatment. She compared these two treatments for her PTSD due to birth trauma in the following way:

> If I had to pinpoint what is so different between traditional talk therapy and EMDR, I would have to say based on the experiences I've had with it (which have both been to help me cope with traumas of traumatic childbirth), I think the EMDR definitely provides much faster and longer-

lasting relief from the anguish, depression, and continuously retraumatizing thoughts. Upon my completion with the EMDR process it's as if the emotionally devastating components of my experience that made me burst into tears constantly and feel hopeless, had been processed in a way that I now had a new understanding of what was so upsetting to me and I was able to put it in a place within my mind where it would be manageable. Prior to EMDR that would not have been possible. I also think it would have taken a VERY long time through traditional talk therapy to help me get to the same point that literally one or two EMDR sessions helped me to arrive at. For example, I cannot imagine how I would have coped with the sense of failure, depression, and disconnect I was feeling about the birth of my son and also dealt with my chronic abdominal pain from my c-section, had I not had the EMDR sessions when I did. I don't think I could have handled both.

If I had to summarize the EMDR process, it's an emotionally charged one that will require you to dig deep down and face emotions, images and thoughts that are truly devastating. Who would want to do that? No one, right? However, it is a quick and very effective tool to help us deal with traumas that if we opted for traditional talk therapy alone, would take multiple sessions and probably months to sort through. So with that said, who wouldn't want to accomplish a faster healing period if something is truly causing us deep emotional anguish and negatively impacting our lives! I highly, highly recommend EMDR for women who have experienced traumatic childbirth. My experience has been that prior to EMDR the images, thoughts, and emotions that were devastating to me kept playing over and over in my mind like that of a CD that keeps skipping. Whether that's my "sticky brain" or not is irrelevant, that was what was happening for me. As you can imagine, when these images, thoughts, and feelings keep replaying, they continue to retraumatize. I found that the only way to unstick them and allow the CD to keep spinning was to process these emotions, thoughts, and feelings through EMDR. Once I partook in this process I not only learned more about what was really bothering me but I processed this information in a way that allowed me to understand it and put it in a place that was manageable.

Another woman had both cognitive therapy and EMDR treatment. She compared the two therapies in this way:

EMDR was absolutely the reason that I was able to get through my PTSD. When I was going to the cognitive therapist, I just found myself constantly retriggered through the questioning of my trauma, talking about my trauma, and never really resolving the pieces of my trauma that would send me into panic. EMDR and my EMDR therapist caused those triggers to dissolve through the act of rewiring those bits and pieces. Those "stuck" neural pathways that always seemed to cause panic.

During one woman's cesarean birth she couldn't breathe through her nose. Her mouth and throat were too dry and she felt like she couldn't breathe through her mouth either. She asked the anesthesiologist for help but he ignored her. After she got home from the hospital she started having nightmares about not being able to breathe during the surgery. She would wake up with panic attacks. This mother described some effective tools her EMDR therapist gave her to use when she was at home. Here are three of those tools:

1   *The Four Elements Tool.* My therapist got out a bag of stickers and asked me to choose one and put it on my phone. I chose a sparkly pink fish. She explained it was to remind me I had this tool. The sticker is genius. I always have my phone in my hand so I always see the sticker. It also reminds me of all my tools. She said when I forget it's there, it's time to change the sticker. I love the fish. I haven't forgotten about it yet.

    (a)   Earth—things in the room, notice what sounds I hear.
    (b)   Air—from my abdomen to my chest, breathe in for 4 seconds, hold for 4 seconds, out for 4 seconds.
    (c)   Water—water switches on a relaxation response, notice if I have saliva in my mouth, think of a lemon, chew gum or drink tea. When you're anxious or stressed, your mouth dries and shuts off your digestive system. This was huge for me because I think that's what happened during my C-section when my mouth was too dry and I couldn't swallow.
    (d)   Fire—light up the path of my imagination; bring up my safe place imagery while doing earth, air and water. Use a butterfly hug to tap in positive feelings.

2   *Staying in your Window of Tolerance* (not trying to push too hard or avoid). I was afraid to drink water because I realized I couldn't breathe and swallow at the same time. I couldn't drink water or even think about it without thinking about my C-section and the surgery room. My therapist asked me to describe how I drank it. I told her I had to hold the glass for a while and take deep breaths first. Then I gulped it down as fast as possible to get it over with. I tried to drink as much as possible so I didn't have to do it again for a while. It was hard to breathe.

    She explained staying in your window of tolerance, setting small manageable goals, not doing more than I can tolerate and not avoiding it altogether. She does this thing with her arms where she shows you what it looks like. I don't know how to explain it but it's AWESOME. I always remember it. She brought me a very small bottle of water, 4 or 6 ounces, and asked me to take a sip. Then another sip. She asked me what I noticed. I noticed it was a lot easier to drink this way and easier to breathe. I thought about this every time I needed water. Soon I was able to drink without feeling panic about the surgery. Then without thinking about the surgery at all.

    I love this tool. I use it all of time. Now I think about everything in terms of "taking a sip of water."

3   *Container.* This is a thought-stopping technique. For future tripping, "what if?" thinking and things outside of my control. I was doing a lot of this. She asked me to think about a container with a lock and describe it to her. I was only 2 or 3 weeks postpartum. I thought of a Diaper Genie. She asked if it had a lock. It didn't so I had to visualize a lock and describe it to her. If it's something outside of my control, I stop the thought and lock it away in the Diaper Genie.

The following are four narratives from the participants of Beck and Watson's ongoing study regarding the experiences of EMDR treatment for PTSD secondary to birth trauma.

Taylor's Story

Taylor was diagnosed with PTSD due to the physical and emotional complications she experienced as a result of her traumatic emergency cesarean birth. Taylor had been fully dilated and pushed for over 4 hours. Her obstetrician told her that if the baby did not come out after 3 more pushes, then she would be having a cesarean birth. The following description is in Taylor's own words. She wanted to provide the details of her traumatic birth to set the stage for her EMDR experience:

> When the vacuum and pushing combo didn't work, I watched my doctor take her gloves off and pack up her tools and she said, "That's it, we're done, you're having the c-section." I cried my eyes out all the way to the OR. All I could think about was all the work I had done to mentally, emotionally and physically prepare for a vaginal delivery. Now, vaginal birth, the one thing I had feared the most in my life but also worked SO hard to become comfortable with, was no longer a possibility, and I felt like I had completely failed. The c-section hurt a lot. I had an epidural and it should have only felt like lots of tugging/pulling but overall, it felt like someone had sawed me in half and was digging for gold in my insides. I yelled out a lot but just kept hearing that it shouldn't hurt that much and all I should feel was the tugging. Clearly no one cared that it felt way worse than that. Unbeknownst to my husband and I, the baby had moved so far down the birth canal when I had pushed, that he had to be physically shoved back up into my abdomen and even still he was wedged pretty tightly in there. The baby had his arm over his head which was the reason he could not come out vaginally. They almost had to break his arm in order to get him out!
>
> In addition to physical complications, I experienced emotional ones as well. Soon after I came home from the hospital, I began to feel very sad and found myself crying much of the time at the drop of a hat. I was very upset about how the delivery had gone, my wound infection and was struggling to come to terms with all of it. I was also exhausted and sleep-

deprived. Given how my labor had concluded, I was also struggling, feeling like I hadn't really even given birth to my own baby. It basically felt like I just laid there while he was cut out of me. I started to notice a feeling of disconnect between the world around me and my perspective on my place in it and knew I needed to seek help from a therapist. I have struggled with both depression and anxiety in my early twenties and knew the signs that would warrant my seeking assistance. Overall, my recovery from childbirth has been a really long and difficult road. What should have been such a joyous and special time in my life turned out to be one of the most painful, scariest and uncertain.

Taylor then went to a therapist who diagnosed her as having PTSD due to trauma she had endured in childbirth. Her therapist suggested EMDR treatment. Here is how Taylor described her EMDR treatment:

My therapist asked me to spend the time in between the next session reflecting on the thoughts and experiences that I found particularly troubling and we'd address them through the EMDR. My therapist used the tripod structure with the red light that moves back and forth. She asked me to track the movement of the lights with my eyes. I found that just watching the movement of the light as it goes back and forth helped me to relax a bit and it's almost as if I don't even have to think that hard of the images or thoughts that are causing me emotional discomfort. They just simply come to my awareness as I watch the light's movement. Then once the light is stopped and I talk about what came to mind it's almost as if that thought helps lead to the next thought and so on and so forth.

The following are the thoughts and feelings I remember addressing in EMDR:

- I was devastated that I could not complete a vaginal delivery. Since I could not get my baby out in the final three pushes with the vacuum, I felt like I had failed at the childbirth process. I felt the weight of the world on my shoulders when I remembered the doctor telling me I only had three more chances and then we were done. The way I heard it was "Three more strikes and you're out!"
- Since I had to have the c-section, I did not feel like I had actually given birth to my daughter. While mentally I knew that I had, emotionally it did not feel that way.
- Since I had to stop breastfeeding due to the infection, I also felt like I had failed in that area as well.

Through EMDR I experienced a great emotional release and I realized all of the feelings and thoughts listed above. Prior to EMDR I don't know that I would have been able to identify all of these thoughts and feelings and known truly what was causing all of my distress. I believe that the process of EMDR allowed me to fully explore and process these thoughts and feelings and once that occurred, I no longer felt emotionally stuck. I felt like I could put these feelings away in a place that was manageable and think about them differently. I moved from a place of feeling like a victim to recognizing the successes and positive contributions I made to the childbirth and childrearing process.

Overall, EMDR has been an incredibly helpful and powerful tool. It has provided me with a great deal of relief in coping with past traumas, anxiety related to labor, and most recently with PTSD related to childbirth. I am not sure how long it would have taken to recover from such a depressing and traumatic experience but know that without EMDR it would have taken a lot longer. EMDR allowed me to experience an immediate release that made it possible for me to delve deeper into my thoughts and feelings without breaking down and feeling like I couldn't handle them. While it has only been 6 months since all this occurred, and I still think about what happened, it does not consume me, nor does it feel unresolved. It is still unpleasant to think about, but I do know that I had successes in labor, and I most certainly do not feel like I failed in any way during the labor or delivery. Most importantly, I did give birth to my daughter.

Lisa's Story

Lisa was diagnosed at 6 months postpartum with PTSD due to birth trauma. The therapist suggested she try EMDR therapy and referred her to a colleague. Here is Lisa's description of her EMDR treatment in her own words:

At that point I was pretty open to anything but when I read about EMDR online, it sounded a bit bizarre. I began EMDR at about 9 months postpartum. At that point I was still reliving my traumatic birth and postpartum complications daily, although an antidepressant had certainly eased my symptoms. My therapist asked me to remember the scene of my daughter's traumatic birth. The fresher memories that I had about lying in the delivery room helpless when they told me that the baby was in the wrong position (face up) and in distress brought up more intense emotions. As I held the pulsing electrodes and remembered how I felt that day, I shook (the same way I shook lying on the table). I cried. I felt nauseous. I rocked back and forth a little like I was on a roller coaster. I could visualize, as instructed, the sights of the room and in particular the very concerned look on the nurse's face as she watched my baby's vital signs on the monitor. I remembered how they shoved an oxygen mask over my nose and mouth with no explanation. I felt like my baby was not going to make it and I wasn't so sure I would either. I recalled how powerless I felt when I could not feel any more contractions, could not feel myself pushing, and could not get the baby out. I imagined how the doctors ran around the delivery room chaotically and, with my permission, used forceps to deliver my son. I remembered the sound of silence. The most excruciating noise I had ever heard. And then, thankfully the sound of crying. "Is he okay? Is he okay?" because for a few minutes I didn't see him at all and I was not allowed to hold him right away. I recalled a nurse saying to me callously, "Those had better be tears of joy!"

After we walked through all of these memories, my therapist then had me replay the scene but this time with much more sympathetic doctors and nurses, less chaos, and a less complicated delivery. I replayed it and had more encouragement from dialogue with the medical staff. They told me what was happening every step of the way. After it was over (we may have done this in two different sessions), I felt more empowered, as if I had actually given birth to my son instead of having him ripped out of me in a fourth grade science experiment gone wrong. I remembered that I helped to create him. I carried him for 9 months and I was THERE for the moment he arrived and I have been there for him ever since. I felt much more empowered as I somehow incorporated this confrontation into my memory. When I opened my eyes, I felt much better about the entire memory. I know that in reality it did not play out that way but somehow the memory now is more complete in my mind and easier to process emotionally.

Laurie's Story

I started EMDR treatment because of the trauma I had experienced during the birth of my daughter 9 years earlier. It worked wonders for me. The experience had moved into "normal memory," and I now have no stress when I think about what happened. During my EMDR sessions my therapist used a small machine that had two little paddles. I would hold one in each hand and they vibrated alternatively. This facilitated the REM function for me. I did this throughout the entire session.

The first session we had involved my birth experience and it was distressing. I held the paddles and went over the memory of the moment when I thought I was going to die over and over again in my mind. Remembering that was very hard. It was difficult to do because it was like going through it all over again, remembering the sights, the smells, the sounds, the feelings, the thoughts, etc. When the session ended, I was stressed. My therapist helped me with a relaxation exercise before I left which helped relieve the anxiety.

The second session was much different. My therapist suggested trying to think of something that would help my distress with that memory. I began going over the moment in my mind, I was lying on the operating table and I couldn't breathe. Then all of a sudden, I imagined myself today being present with myself then, so there were two of me: the past self and the present self. The present self knows that I did not die and that everything was going to be okay eventually. The past self did not know that. So I imagined my present self comforting my past self, stroking her hair, and telling her that everything was going to be alright. I just started to cry. It was such a comforting thought. I spent a good 10 minutes just dwelling on that because it was so soothing. My therapist was very pleased with my creativity and the progress I made in just a few minutes.

Then my therapist brought up the fact that I didn't get to hold my baby until after I woke up. I told her how empty I felt after he was born. I went to sleep pregnant and woke up not pregnant. I just kept thinking, Where is my baby? He's gone. I wanted him back inside me but he was right there in my arms. I just couldn't make the connection. I felt ripped off and so incredibly empty. She suggested that I imagine myself in the operating room again and having the doctor give the baby to my present self. So I imagined my present self watching my son being born, then the nurses wrapping him in a blanket and handing him to me. I began to cry again. I never had that feeling of joy. It had been stolen from me but I was able to reclaim it for myself. I kept imagining my present self holding my newborn son and crying, and I let myself heal. Then in my mind I brought my present self and my past self back together at the moment when I woke up in the recovery room from my c-section when I got to hold him for real. Oh my, what closure. The tears I cried that session were tears of healing, joy, and release. I never realized how wonderful healing could be. I can truly say that I have brought joy to the memory of my son's birth that was never there before. I would recommend EMDR to anyone who has experienced trauma.

Katie's Story

Katie's traumatic childbirth involved post dates, induction, long labor, failed epidural, dislocated hip, face presentation, forceps delivery, third degree laceration resulting in permanent fecal incontinence, and postpartum hemorrhage. After suffering with posttraumatic stress symptoms for a year and a half, Katie finally sought treatment for her mental health. She begins her story saying that "EMDR was, at first, very strange. I had never heard of anything like it, never seen it done, and could only explain it to others as a sort of hypnotism without falling asleep." Katie's EMDR sessions usually lasted between 2 and 2½ hours.

My therapist started each session by asking me to talk about my week, any triggers, any good things/bad things, what was going on. We then determined if my week was going to guide the EMDR therapy, or if I wanted to work on another trigger. I would then be given the choice of the tappers, headphones, or both. Next I would create a statement about how I felt, how true it felt to me, and the emotions surrounding that statement. My anxiety level was measured and numbers were assigned to that statement. An example of one such positive statement is: "I can get over this, I can trust my mind to know what to do, and I will be able to get over (whatever trigger we were going to work on)." I would then state how true this statement was and how much anxiety it gave me. Usually, statements at the beginning of a session were totally untrue and anxiety was at a very high level. By the end of the session, I usually could see that the statement was true, and my anxiety was lessened. It was amazing to me each time that my mind could process that during the session to truly answer affirmatively that I was less anxious and more positive in my outlook in getting rid of my triggers.

EMDR therapy started and was guided by my therapist. Often, I was given time to think and the associations in my head were encouraged to be spoken aloud. My therapist would engage in cognitive interweave in an effort to help me understand the thoughts, sights, and sounds associated with certain triggers. During sessions if I was stuck, or perseverating on a certain point, or being triggered too much (having extreme unmanageable anxiety/fear/grief during the session), my EMDR therapist would point out insights ("Do you think you could be thinking this, because of this?" , "Does it make sense that this could mean this?" , "When people have this visual, an archetype of it, it usually means this, does this apply to you?"). All of this interweave helped me make sense of my session and allowed unmanageable triggers to become both manageable and dissipate through-out session(s).

Finger tracking was done in an effort to dispel the associations of the triggers with trauma. I was encouraged to feel, cry, grieve, laugh, and do whatever came to mind. During sessions, I experienced fear (although controlled by my skilled therapist), sadness, grief, anger, relief, joy, elation, as well as a sense of accomplishment, pride, and control. Towards the end of the session, I revisited my statements and assigned numbers regarding my anxiety, the trueness of statements, and my emotions. I was never encouraged to leave until I felt well enough to walk out the door.

Clinician's Reaction

The stories of Taylor, Lisa, Laurie and Katie again remind us of the perceptive reality of the woman and how she interprets the experience. Her perceptive reality is critical and ideally needs to be assessed in the immediate postpartum phase. It is very helpful to have the new mother discuss, describe, and share with health care providers how she experienced the birth. This does not mean that it will prevent PTSD secondary to birth trauma, as we learned from the studies using debriefing as a treatment strategy but rather allows her to be, in my mind, validated in her experience. I would think that most people have feelings that surface when they are told that what they experienced did not occur or that the person who was witnessing it denies the individual's truth. All too often the assumption is made that "how I see the world, is the way everyone else does" and as we have seen in reading the narratives of the women, there is nothing farther from the truth. I am always struck with how hard it is for people to listen to another's story without commenting, judging, or analyzing, but in essence just listening. The promotion of therapeutic relationships is based on establishing rapport and trust. For many women the birth experience is quickly pushed away by others as "over" and it is now time to move on to care of the baby. Yet if the mother is not present in that mother–baby relationship, i.e. she is focused on self and safety and survival, there is little that can be done. New mothers need to be seen as having lived through an amazing experience and heard as to how that experience was experienced by them. Once the baby is born, we cannot forget to ask them how they are feeling rather than move into the interrogation regarding the baby's care and concern: Did he eat? Does she need a new diaper, etc.?

EMDR appears to have excellent results in the treatment of PTSD secondary to birth trauma. I am sure we will see more research in the future, validating this as a primary treatment method.

Mother's Reaction

It is important and essential to conclude one's therapy session, whether it be EMDR, CBT or any other treatment, feeling safe. One might feel tired or emotionally drained, which is of course usual, yet for a PTSD sufferer the "safe place" is paramount. Entrusting one's trauma memories to another person is necessary, but as it should be only to a skilled and qualified person, being sure of the skill of the practitioner is vital. The results of taking this step are well worth it, despite how hard it is to be treated and to revisit aspects of one's traumatic experience. However, even making the initial call for support, often telling their story to a complete stranger, is itself a huge step—the sufferer is already on their way to recovery. As they have done that, they have it in them to regain (mostly) who they once were. Everybody's treatment will be individual, and worth the time, care and energy taken to obtain it.

Conclusion

As can be seen from the literature reviewed in this chapter, studies pertaining to the specific treatments of PTSD secondary to birth trauma are limited. We described briefly debriefing, cognitive behavioral therapy, and EMDR treatment methods. The chapter ended with the narratives from the ongoing study conducted by Cheryl and Sue on mothers' experiences of EMDR treatment. In Chapter 14, another case study from Jeanne's clinical practice is presented to illustrate her treatment methods used with this patient.

References

Ayers, S., McKenzie-McHarg, K., & Eagle, A. (2007). Cognitive behavior therapy for postnatal post-traumatic stress disorder: Case studies. *Journal of Psychosomatic Obstetrics & Gynecology, 28,* 177–184.

Craske, M. (2010). *Cognitive-behavioral therapy.* New York: APA Books.

Horowitz, M., Wilner, N., & Alvarez, W. (1979). Impact of Event Scale: A measure of subjective stress. *Psychosomatic Medicine, 41,* 209–218.

Institute of Medicine. (2012). *Treatment for posttraumatic stress disorder in military and veteran populations: Initial assessment.* Washington, DC: National Academies Press.

Kershaw, K., Jolly, J., Bhabra, K., & Ford, J. (2005). Randomised controlled trail of community debriefing following operative delivery. *British Journal of Obstetrics & Gynaecology, 112,* 1504–1509.

Lapp, K. L., Agbokou, L., Peretti, C. S., & Ferreri, F. (2010). Management of post traumatic stress disorder after childbirth: A review. *Journal of Psychosomatic Obstetrics & Gynecology, 31,* 113–122.

Mitchell, J., & Dyregrov, A. (1993). Traumatic stress in disaster workers and emergency personnel. Prevention and intervention. In J. P. Wilson, & B. Raphael (Eds.). *International handbook of traumatic stress syndromes.* New York: Plenum Press.

Priest, S. R., Henderson, J., Evans, S. F., & Hagan, R. (2003). Stress debriefing after childbirth: A randomized controlled trial. *Medical Journal of Australia, 178,* 542–545.

Sandstrom, M., Wiberg, B., Wikman, M., Willman, A. K., & Hogberg, U. (2008). A pilot study of eye movement desensitization and reprocessing treatment (EMDR) for post-traumatic stress after childbirth. *Midwifery, 24,* 62–73.

Selkirk, R., McLaren, S., Ollerenshaw, A., McLachlan, A. J., & Moten, J. (2006). The longitudinal effects of midwife-led postnatal debriefing on the psychological health of mothers. *Journal of Reproductive and Infant Psychology, 24,* 133–147.

Shapiro, F. (1991). Eye movement desensitization & reprocessing procedure: From EMD to EMD/R—a new treatment model for anxiety and related trauma. *Behavioral Therapist, 14,*133–135.

—— (2001). *Eye movement desensitization and reprocessing: Basic principles, protocols, and procedures* (2nd ed.). New York: Guilford Press.

Stramrood, C. A. I., van der Velde, J., Doornbos, B., Paarlberg, K. M., & Weijmar Schultz, W. (2012). The patient observer: Eye movement desensitization and reprocessing for the treatment of posttraumatic stress following childbirth. *Birth: Issues in Perinatal Care, 39,* 70–76.

Weiss, D. S., & Marmar, C. R. (1997). The Impact of Event Scale-Revised. In J. P. Wilson, & T. M. Keane (Eds.). *Assessing psychological trauma and PTSD.* New York: Guilford Press.

Wijma, K., Soderquist, J., & Wijma, B. (1997). Posttraumatic stress after childbirth: A cross sectional study. *Journal of Anxiety Disorders, 11,* 587–597.

14 Case Study 3: Sheila

Sheila comes into my practice complaining of "anxiety, shortness of breath. Sometimes I feel like I am having a heart attack and I am just so nervous and scared." She is a 37-year-old married woman. She was referred to my practice by her obstetrician. Sitting on the couch in my office, she appears as tense and tightly held together. She had already taken out a few Kleenex from the box on the table between us in the office. I sat back in my chair and asked Sheila to share with me what she had been experiencing that led her to call and make an appointment with me.

She went on to tell me that she had had her second baby about 2 months ago and had not been doing "too well since." She went on to wonder out loud if she wasn't depressed after her first one even though she went back to work about 3 months postpartum. With this postpartum, she explained that "I cannot get my act together." She went on to describe symptoms of severe anxiety as well as fears and concerns that something bad was going to happen to her. "I keep thinking, I could get a major infection or some disease and I am going to die." She feels that she can cry at the drop of a hat and just doesn't feel like she is "coping at all." "This is not who I am. I am competent and can go with the flow. I am not sure what is going on with me now."

I asked Sheila to share with me the story of her second pregnancy and birth experience as she seemed to imply that the symptoms began after this little baby was born. "This was my second pregnancy; I was expecting it to be fine, as I did not have any trouble with my first pregnancy." Sheila described that she was over a week late with this baby and was ready to give birth. "I was on time with my first one so I did feel a bit anxious as the days were going by the due date." She described how she "finally" went into labor and headed to the hospital where she then encountered the "epidural from hell."

I asked Sheila to back up a bit on her story and give me more information about the days leading up to the birth. Sheila was 10 days late when she went into labor. "I was feeling very comfortable, yet was so happy to be getting this show on the road." Upon admission to the labor and delivery unit of the hospital, she learned that she was about 4 centimeters. She knew that she wanted an epidural as she had had a good experience with that type of anesthesia with her first birth. "I had had an epidural with my first so I knew I would be comfortable shortly and as I said I was feeling pretty good and excited to be finally having this baby." Sheila spoke about how the anesthesiologist attempted at least seven times to insert the epidural catheter into her back. "I thought I was going to die." Sheila narrated how she had sat as still as she could on the side of the bed but after four or five attempts she experienced "excruciating pain" and said that she could not move her head or neck.

> I felt as though everyone that was talking sounded like Mickey Mouse. There were changes in my hearing . . . they kept telling me everything was fine, but it wasn't! They ended up giving me a spinal as he couldn't get the damn epidural into the right spot . . . seven attempts . . . can you believe that?

As she described the experience, her hands were shaking. She was obviously very tense and tight as she moved closer into the cushions on my couch. Sheila continued to have severe head and neck pain and shared with me that she ended up with a cervical collar around her neck as she moved into the pushing phase of her labor.

Sheila further described that on her first day postpartum she had the worst spinal headache. "It was the worst experience." She expressed profound sadness as she went on to describe how she felt that she did not get any support from her obstetrician for the epidural episode. "He never brought it up." She did not get any acknowledgment or apology from the anesthesiologist for the seven attempts and the ultimate spinal.

> It was like it was my fault. It was the worst to have lived through that experience and to basically feel invisible. No one acknowledged that they had screwed up. The message that I was given was that the baby was fine and that we needed to move on . . . move on . . . can you imagine . . . it was disgusting.

She went on to share that there was one nurse who was extremely caring and supportive to her and her experience.

> If it wasn't for that postpartum nurse . . . she really encouraged me to get the spinal patch to help with the spinal headache. That really did help the headache. I felt so much better after I had that done. My headache was so bad, Jeanne; I couldn't even hold my baby. I would complain to the doctor and I basically felt like I was being considered as a hysterical female. My gut feeling is that there was air in my neck secondary to the seven attempts at the epidural, but no one wanted to go there.

Sheila continued her story of unexpected outcomes during the postpartum phase. She had been breastfeeding her baby who then developed a gastro-intestinal infection with severe diarrhea and had to be admitted to the hospital.

I had to stop breastfeeding. It was too hard to pump, feed, worry, and anxiety about my other child. She ended up on special formula as her gastro-intestinal system had really suffered from whatever she had had . . . diarrhea, antibiotics, hospitalization. I tell you, Jeanne, it was like being in the twilight zone. What else could go wrong?

At 2 months, her baby was doing much better, gaining weight and had been tolerating the special formula. She felt that basically everything was better, but she didn't feel any better. She felt anxious and obsessive, "I keep thinking something else is going to go wrong, for the inevitable other shoe to drop."

I asked Sheila if she would provide me with some information pertaining to her family history and other aspects of her life (see Figure 14.1). I needed more information to help me formulate a diagnosis and a nursing care plan. Sheila sat back on the couch, took a drink of water and she appeared to be in a more relaxed psychological place. She began to tell me about her family.

Sheila came from a family of four and was the second child, first daughter. She had two brothers and one sister. Her mom was a stay-at-home mother and her dad was an engineer. She felt that her mother had a lot of anxiety and focused all her attention and concern on her children. "We are her life." Her dad was described as even-tempered, hardworking, and involved as a father. She did not feel that there were any significant issues from her upbringing. Her siblings were employed and married with families of their own. She did not know of any history of mood and/or anxiety disorders. She had known both of

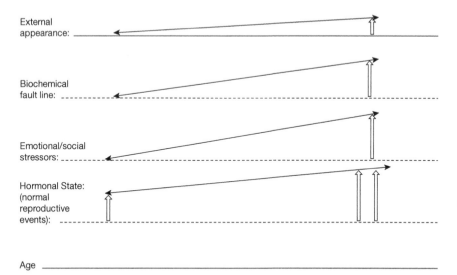

Figure 14.1 Sheila's Earthquake Assessment

Source: From *Women's Moods* by Deborah Sichel and Jeanne Watson Driscoll © 1999 by Deborah Sichel and Jeanne Watson Driscoll. Courtesy of HarperCollins Publishers.

her sets of grandparents and that they were mentally stable and had died of natural causes. She did not have any family history of alcohol or substance use. "No one smokes in my family or in my husband's." She described feeling very close to her siblings, even though they lived in other states, and she spoke with her sister a lot. "She has been extremely supportive to my mental state as has my husband, John."

Sheila's life history was then described. She told me she was the oldest daughter and did feel that she took on a major mothering role to her brothers and sisters. She did not have any significant memories of childhood either good or bad. "I liked school and we lived in the same house and neighborhood my whole life. I would say I am the responsible one of all my brothers and sister, maybe because I am the first girl?" She went on to describe that she felt she had always been resilient, had good problem-solving skills and had always felt authentic and real. "I have a lot of friends and acquaintances; I love my family and my career. I do not understand 'why now', why do I feel so bad?"

She was a teacher and had hoped to go back to work that month but she was having problems with anxiety. "I think I am having panic attacks, and when I was talking with my boss, she told me to take a few more weeks. I have been teaching in the same school system for over ten years so they are really great and understanding." I asked about a history of anxiety and she responded that she did not feel she was an "anxious" type. "I have always been a responder with good coping skills, I am usually always in charge and tend to be the one who supports and takes care of others." She described that she felt her nutrition was okay, although "I am probably eating too many cookies at this time. I just grab anything and really have not been paying attention to my nutrition, but the kids are eating fine." She had continued taking her prenatal vitamins; "I had refilled that prescription in my early postpartum weeks." She describes that her sleep has been different in that she "can't shut off my brain. I keep ruminating about the what if scenarios. I am afraid something bad is going to happen and I have no control over how I feel." She did not feel that she was getting "good sleep" and indeed felt "exhausted" most of the day. "I find I can get very short with Danny, my 3-year-old, especially by the end of the day, and he is doing so well with his adjustment to the baby. I feel so bad when I get irritated with him and sometimes yell."

Sheila described that she continued to keep her coffee decaffeinated since the pregnancy and did not smoke cigarettes nor drink alcohol at all. She denied thoughts of suicide and did not have any harmful thoughts about her husband or her children. "I just don't want to keep feeling like this."

As we sat together, I shared with Sheila that I felt that she was experiencing a posttraumatic stress response to her birth experience, principally the traumatic epidural experience. As our evaluation meeting was coming to an end, I shared with Sheila some of my thoughts regarding her treatment plan. I felt that it might be helpful to initiate the use of medications to help quiet her biology so that she could feel less anxious, get a better night's sleep, and feel calmer through the day. We talked about the use of clonazepam as an anti-anxiety agent that works relatively quickly, lasts about 5 to 6 hours and would, hopefully, decrease her feelings of anxiety and the ruminations in her head. She did not seem to have any problems with the idea of using the clonazepam. I shared with her that I would be prescribing 0.5 mg. and she could take it 2 to 3 times per day, in the early morning, mid-day and at bedtime. We went over the side effects and I answered any questions that she had at the time. She had heard of clonazepam from one of the women at work who took it for anxiety. We also began to discuss the use of antidepressants which are also helpful with anxiety and do not have the dependence issue attached to them that the anti-anxiety agents do. I stated that we would try the anti-anxiety medication to start and re-evaluate at our next meeting. I developed the following NURSE Plan at this first meeting:

- *Nourishment and needs*:
  - Adequate protein intake; short, frequent meals of protein high foods (yogurts, sliced chicken/turkey; cheddar cheese; string cheese, etc).
  - Fluid intake: 6–8 glasses of water per day
  - Medications: Klonopin (clonazepam) 0.5 mg. by mouth. One at bedtime, one in the morning and one in the middle of the day if she felt that she needed it. We also spoke about breaking the pill in half to take 0.25 mg. if she felt the 0.5mg caused her to be too sleepy. Her husband would be home from work tomorrow so it would be a good day to begin this treatment and assess her response.
  - Vitamins: continue her prenatal vitamins; add 3000 mg. of Omega 3 fatty acids (fish oil), Calcium and Vitamin D.

- *Understand*: I recommend weekly therapy sessions so that she could have a safe place to share her thoughts/feelings and we could assess the impact of the medication on her symptoms.
- *Rest and relaxation*: I was hoping the using the clonazepam at bedtime would help her to get to sleep sooner and diminish the rumination that she described occurred prior to falling asleep. We also spoke about taking a rest when all the children were down for naps in the afternoon and perhaps getting a babysitter to help in the afternoons.
- *Spirituality*: Sheila described a strong spiritual connection and felt that she had hope that she would get better and she was glad that she had come to meet with me and get connected.
- *Exercise*: We spoke about taking the children for a walk in the morning. There was a possibility that she would talk with John and get to the gym maybe three times a week, and we also talked about jump roping in the garage when John came home from work as a type of aerobic exercise.

So Sheila left my office that day with a NURSE program and an appointment for the next week as well as my card with phone numbers to call if she had any questions and/or concerns.

The next week Sheila came into my office. "In many ways I feel better, in that I am able to get to sleep at night without the worry that I had last week, that clonazepam really works." What Sheila had not expected was that since she had shared with me the birth experience she was now feeling more angry and upset. She began to describe the pain that she had experienced after the attempts at the epidural.

> I had 8 hours of severe labor with severe head and neck pain. I was crying a lot, and I felt weak in my leg and my arm . . . no one thought that was related to anything, but where did that come from? All I wanted was to have an epidural. I had had one before with no problems. . . . seven attempts and such pain . . . do you know when I went for my 6-week checkup and complained about the weakness in my arm and leg, they sent me to a neurologist to rule out multiple sclerosis. Where did that come from? He did not think I had MS but no one wants to correlate the seven attempts at the epidural to any of these complications . . . the medical system can make you go crazy.

As we sat together, we were trying to strategize a plan that would help her feel empowered and authentic, in that what she experienced was indeed real to her and needed to be validated by the medical team. She was worried that if she set up an appointment to talk about her birth experience that they "would think I was crazy, a nut case." I shared with her that there was no rush and that as she and I worked together it was my hope that she would indeed feel her power to write and talk to the medical team about her feelings and her experiences. She just needed some time right now to feel in control of the situation and that I would support her in this process of healing.

We decided at that second session to add some antidepressant to the medication plan of care. We added a low dose of sertraline. At the next session, Sheila felt that she was having a positive response to the sertraline. "I do feel less anxious and I don't feel like I need to take the clonazepam three times a day, so I have been taking one half in the morning and one whole tablet at bedtime. I definitely sleep better now." Our plan for the next week was for her to increase the dose of sertraline to 50 mg. per day as she was not having any side effects on the 37.5 mg. that she was taking now. We made an appointment for next week.

At this fourth session, Sheila was very upset. She had an exacerbation of the anxiety/panic symptoms. She had to go to the hospital for an appointment, the hospital where she had given birth, and she experienced "flashbacks" the night before.

> I was terrified; my heart was beating so fast. I was shaking. I couldn't even go in, and so I canceled the appointment. I went home and I couldn't stop crying. Thank goodness John was there and I could just fall apart in his arms. What happened to me?

My impression was that just being near the hospital triggered the trauma response. She described flashbacks the night before, she was remembering the birth experience and being at the hospital and her stress response system went into overdrive. She had a physiological response to the potential return to the scene of the birth, "but Jeanne, now I feel hopeless, how am I going to get better?"

As we processed the events, we talked about increasing the sertraline, and focusing her healing. I suggested some calming strategies: focused breathing, prayer/meditation, etc. So the plan was now re-adjusted: increase the sertraline to 75 mg. per day, use the clonazepam as needed to help with the anxiety that had come back. She was also going to sign up for yoga class that they were offering at the gym. John was described as very supportive to the idea and had reassured her that he would be home from work in time for her to go at least three times a week. We agreed to meet the next week and again she was reassured that she could call me if she had concerns/questions.

At our next session, she was feeling calmer and had had a good week. She was tolerating the sertraline at 75 mg. and we talked about increasing the dose to 100 mg. per day and we would leave it at that dosage for a few weeks and reassess her symptom presentation, if any later in the month. She described that she was only taking ½ tablet (0.25 mg. of clonazepam) at bedtime and felt "pretty good" through the day. She was considering going back to work and had it all arranged with the day care to bring the baby next week. Her other child had been attending day care regularly. She had a day care arrangement with a family day care provider who watched only children of teachers so she had her children home in the summer and they were in day care during the school year. "My day care provider is fantastic. She is not only the provider but she had become a friend. My son loves her and I have no problem leaving the baby with her . . . I am in many ways so much more ready to go back to work." We went over her NURSE Program being cognizant of the "back to work" plan.

Over the next few weeks, Sheila symptomatically felt better and did return to teaching. She had a bit of anxiety the first week but that resolved and she made a gentle transition back to full time teaching. She was sleeping through the night with only a rare use of clonazepam at bedtime.

At about 5 months postpartum, Sheila began to talk again about what she felt she needed to do to inform the health care providers of what the experience had been for her even though they had failed to validate the experience. In so many ways, this behavior can be infuriating when the sufferer experiences someone telling you that you don't feel the way you do. I have very strong feelings about perceptive reality and that the way a person experiences an event is their experience and needs to be respectfully heard and validated. Health care professionals need to hear how their words and behaviors can impact others; all too often, there is a sense of informality that does not endorse nor respect the patient and their experience. Being a nurse psychotherapist has really impacted me with regard to the power of words and how we have no idea how another interprets the words unless we seek clarification and validation.

Although Sheila was feeling "so much better," she would at times wake up with anger about what had happened to her at the birth of her second child. She wanted the providers to know how she felt but she is worried that they will consider her a "nut case" or an "angry bitch." In many ways, she could be the "good girl" and just "pretend that it was nothing." As she had shared with me earlier in our sessions, she was used to being in charge and taking care of others. She wanted to write a letter to the professionals and let them know that their behavior did indeed have an effect on her and her postpartum experience: physiologically and psychologically. "I know as a teacher, I would want to know if I had impacted someone positively or negatively." Perhaps, in some ways, writing this letter and sharing her feelings would be taking care of her! She was feeling betrayed.

> I am a nice person. Why did they do that to me? I know they were pressured and there is stress with the procedure . . . I felt people did not take care of me . . . did not keep me informed. I felt when I was in pain, it was only the nurse who came in to talk to me . . . the doctor stayed out . . . and anesthesia stayed away . . . I felt as though I had to hang tough. Devalue the amount of pain that I had . . . thought if I was a good sport . . .

Sheila started to cry now as she continued, "this birth experience . . . this whole process took my confidence away." Sheila continued to share her process and I sat supporting, validating, and encouraging her with empathy and presence. At the end of the session, we went over what had gone on, tweaked the NURSE program with focus on yoga, meditation (which for Sheila was praying) and practicing being mindful. There has been significant increase in research concerning mindfulness and the effect on the biochemistry of stress and trauma (Ogden, Minton, & Pain, 2006; Siegel, 2011). Sheila was very comfortable using breathing strategies to quiet her sympathetic and parasympathetic nervous system. She had been a student of yoga prior to this traumatic birth and had been going back to her yoga classes, so she felt very positive about this strategy.

Things were going along relatively smoothly over the next few months, until a friend of Sheila's was diagnosed with ovarian cancer. Sheila began to experience an exacerbation of her anxiety/panic symptoms as well as ovarian pain. This horrible news had re-triggered in Sheila her fear of the unexpected, her fear of death and the "what if?" worst scenarios. In response to this trigger, she increased her sertraline to 125 mg. per day and did use some clonazepam again. I felt that a concrete thing that could be done to help her anxiety was to have a consultation with a gynecologist and maybe even a pelvic ultrasound to rule out ovarian cancer. I discussed this with Sheila but she did not want to go back to her own gynecologist/obstetrician because she still had not met with him to discuss the birth trauma and she felt that would make her too anxious. So I suggested a colleague of mine and with Sheila's permission I called the physician and shared Sheila's story and concerns. My colleague agreed to meet with Sheila. They had an excellent consultation with a pelvic ultrasound that demonstrated to Sheila that she did not have any growths on her ovaries. This intervention was corrective for Sheila. She felt I had listened to her, validated her concerns/worries, and we had been proactive. She was relieved and her symptoms of anxiety went back into remission.

Sheila now felt ready to do the healing work of writing a letter to the anesthesia department at the hospital, talking with her obstetrician and then writing a letter of thanks to the postpartum nurse. We spent a few sessions processing her letter, editing, moving it from pure rage to the deliberate sentence structure that made her point and spoke from her voice regarding how she felt and how she experienced the birth. She felt empowered by this exercise. We also processed the potential of response and non-response. She felt that it was important closure for her and that she would feel "done," in some way. She had made an appointment with her obstetrician and we did some role play in my office with various scripts so that she felt prepared and ready.

She mailed the letters and went to the appointment with her obstetrician. Fortunately, he was able to listen to how she felt, respected her process and her narrative and apologized for not stepping in sooner and advocating for her. Sheila felt it was an excellent meeting and felt that their relationship had been re-connected and she felt very proud and happy with regard to her process. When Sheila's baby turned 1, she was able to process the anniversary and put, what she called "closure" on the trauma. She continued on the sertraline until she was about 18 months postpartum when she wanted to discontinue the medication as "I feel so much better." She weaned from 125 mg. of sertraline by decreasing the dose by 25 mg. every 2 to 3 weeks. This gradual wean allowed her time to feel confident in herself and her weaning process. We terminated our relationship at that time and Sheila knew that she could come back to my practice if she ever needed that.

Sheila and her story again reminded me of the resiliency of the woman's soul/spirit and the critical aspects of validation of experience. As I said before, as health care providers we need to pay attention to our words and be sure that we adhere to the primary rule, "first do no harm."

References

Ogden, P., Minton, K., & Pain, C. (2006). *Trauma and the body: A sensorimotor approach to psychotherapy*. New York: W.W. Norton & Company.

Sichel, D., & Driscoll, J. W. (1999). *Women's moods: What every woman must know about hormones, the brain, and emotional health*. New York: HarperCollins.

Siegel, D. J. (2011). *Mindsight: The new science of personal transformation*. New York: Bantum Books Trade Paperbacks.

15 Fathers and Traumatic Childbirth

In this chapter we turn our attention to fathers and their experiences of being present at their partner's traumatic births. First in this chapter the research regarding fathers and traumatic childbirth is reviewed. Following this are narratives of fathers who participated in Cheryl and Sue's ongoing research study.

Five studies investigating PTSD in fathers have been published. In Norway, 81 fathers of a healthy baby completed the Impact of Event Scale (IES; Horowitz, Wilner, & Alvarez, 1979) and the General Health Questionnaire (GHQ-28; Goldberg & Hillier, 1979) at three time intervals: 0–4 days, 6 weeks, and 6 months after birth (Skari et al., 2002). PTSD-like symptoms were operationalized as an intrusion score ≥20, avoidance score ≥20, and hyperarousal score ≥2. Eighteen percent of the fathers reported moderate to severe intrusive stress. Two fathers reported severe avoidance symptoms and 3% of fathers experienced hyperarousal symptoms.

In New Zealand, 21 fathers participated in a phenomenological study of their experiences of posttraumatic stress following childbirth (White, 2007). Four themes emerged from the qualitative data: (1) It's not a spectator sport; (2) It's about being included; (3) It's sexual scarring; and (4) It's toughing it out. Fathers in this study shared with the researchers that they felt alienated as they sensed they were perceived as spectators rather than participants. Men also described that they felt excluded in the childbearing process as they were not acknowledged as a vital component of the family unit. Fathers reported intense distress, both psychological and physiological, during sexual activity as this triggered memories of the traumatic birth. Lastly, the men shared that suppressing emotional distress during labor and delivery led the fathers to experience shame, humiliation, and helplessness.

In a study conducted in London, 5 percent (n = 3) of 64 men reported severe PTSD symptoms of intrusions and avoidance at 9 weeks after birth (Ayers, Wright, & Wells, 2007). The Impact of Event Scale (IES; Horowitz et al., 1979) was used to measure traumatic stress symptoms. Results of a multiple regression on sets of variables that best predicted PTSD symptoms revealed that "something going wrong and emotions during birth" were the strongest determinants. Ayers et al. (2007) reported that PTSD due to childbirth was unrelated to parent–infant bonding and the couples' relationship.

In another study, 199 men in the UK were asked 6 weeks after their partners' delivery of a healthy infant to complete the IES (Horowitz et al., 1979) and the Post-Traumatic Stress Disorder Questionnaire (PTSD-Q; Watson, Juba, Manifold, Kucala, & Anderson, 1991; Bradley, Slade, & Leviston, 2008). Analysis of the PTSD-Q scores revealed that 6 fathers (3%) reported clinically significant intrusion symptoms, 1.5% (n = 3) clinically significant avoidance symptoms, and 11.1% (n = 22) hyperarousal symptoms. None of the fathers were fully sympto-matic of PTSD but 23 men (11.6%) experienced clinically significant symptoms on at least one of the three dimensions of PTSD. Using scores on the IES, 2.5% (n = 5) of the fathers experienced clinically significant intrusions level and 1.5% (n = 3) achieved a clinically significant level of avoidance symptoms.

In the UK, 212 couples completed the Impact of Events Scale (IES; Horowitz et al., 1979), the PTSD-Q (Watson et al., 1991), the EPDS (Cox, Holden, & Sagovsky, 1987), and other questionnaires measuring trait anxiety, social support, and attachment (Iles, Slade, & Spiby, 2011). Partner's support and attachment were also examined in relation to posttraumatic stress symptoms and postpartum depression during the first 3 months after birth. Couples completed this battery of tests within the first week postpartum and also at 6 weeks and 3 months after birth. Men's trauma symptoms were found to predict their partner's posttraumatic stress symptoms.

Beck and Watson are conducting a qualitative study on fathers' experiences of being present at their partners' traumatic birth. Nine men to date have participated over the Internet study. Men were recruited through a notice placed on Trauma and Birth Stress' (TABS) website. Helplessness was the theme that came out loud and clear from the men's stories. The experiences of four fathers from this study are now highlighted in this chapter.

Robert's Story

Robert, a Maori father in New Zealand, recalled his wife's traumatic birth that had occurred 15 months earlier. His wife had been diagnosed with PTSD due to this childbirth. He described that his wife was overdue and needed to be induced. After pushing for a couple of hours with the fetal heart rate dipping, the obstetrician decided to do a high forceps delivery. His wife tore badly. The rest of Robert's story is in his own words:

> Blood began gushing. Everyone began running around and I was pushed to the side, handed my baby and told to sit in the corner. Blood was everywhere and they threw a bucket under my wife to help catch it all. My wife went unconscious and it was later told to us that she lost over 2.5 liters of blood. It was like something out of a horror movie. I thought my wife was going to die.
>
> My wife had to spend the next week in the hospital getting transfusions and was very upset over not being able to hold our darling wee girl until hours after the birth. During this week my wife attempted breastfeeding

and found it near impossible to do while attached to all the machines and being so wasted from almost dying.

This experience was terrifying and I can't believe it happened to us. When my wife went unconscious after birth I truly believed she was going to die and to be in that room was the most scared I have ever been. It was crazy!!!! I sat there with our new baby watching as the doctors worked to save my wife and I was helpless. I've not felt that helpless before. I just didn't know what to do. During the week in the hospital after the birth, I had to keep going over the trauma as my wife didn't remember anything. That was hard.

Curt's Story

Curt, a father from the USA, recalled his fear, terror, and helplessness as he watched his wife hemorrhage on the delivery table during her cesarean birth 4 months earlier. His wife was fully dilated and had been pushing for $3^{1}/_{2}$ hours. His following story vividly portrays in detail his wife's harrowing birth of his son and his response to that experience:

My fears are building. At some point my wife's blood pressure plummets. It dropped from the 170–180 over 110–120 to approximately 40 over 25. My wife is pale, and in and out of consciousness. There is a crew of medical professionals hovering around her as the anesthesiologist began pushing medications to try and raise her blood pressure. My concerns are way out of whack. My mind is freaking out. I am beginning to lose control. I am yelling on the inside. LET'S JUST DO A C-SECTION!!! I CAN'T DO THIS!!! I NEED TO KNOW YOU ARE GOING TO MAKE IT!!! WHY DID WE DO THIS IN THE FIRST PLACE!!!

Four hours . . . 5 hours . . . We are still in the same place we were 4 hours ago. Nowhere! I cannot deal with this much longer. My wife is still trying to push. It is very apparent to me and I believe the doctor realizes the same thing. The baby is not going to make an appearance this way. Something more has to be done. LIKE A C-SECTION!!! I know my wife wants to give the baby every opportunity to be born healthy, but I do not want to lose my best friend in the process. My wife is told by the doctor that they will try suction, if that does not work, we will have to get the c-section. YES!!! It is about time someone is using their head. I am a nervous wreck. I want it to be over. I want to see the suction fail and throughout the process I am begging inside that the suction fails. First try, my wife pushes like a champ, the suction pops off. Second try, again she pushes like only my wife could, the suction pops off. The doctor tells us it is time for the c-section.

My wife is wheeled away, I am walking behind. I feel some sense of relief. I mean, we are heading into the operating room. This will be over in a matter of minutes. They make a cut, pull out the baby, we cry, they stitch and off to recovery. Well, that plan went to hell. I was given garments to put on over my clothes. I had to sit outside the OR while nurses and doctors walked by me, never saying a word. It was a very lonely experience. When I was finally led into the OR, I saw my wife strapped down to a table, with a curtain blocking her torso. She had all the same tubes sticking out of her, but for some reason this was comforting to me. I felt like, now this will be over and we can begin our new lives. I made light of everything, taking pictures of her and her thermometer taped to her forehead.

The procedure begins; I can hear the doctors and nurses discussing bar-b-que. It was going to be as easy as I presumed it was. I hear my wife speaking with the doctors about what is going on, but I am just happy that I am going to have my wife safe. The baby is not even a concern up until the point the doctor holds him over the curtain and I see his little face. What had I missed out on all these months? Why had I feared the process? I have a beautiful baby and my wife is safe. I had nothing to worry about. Why did I waste my time stressing? I can see a team of nurses working to clean my son and ensuring he is healthy. I lean over and kiss my wife. "Happy Birthday Sweetheart," was all I could utter.

The anesthesiologist leans over and tells me I can get up and stand by the scale to take pictures. I walk over and stand by the scale. I can feel myself grinning from ear to ear. This was the best feeling in the world. I am the luckiest husband and father in the whole world . . . "You either need to sit down or leave the room!" sternly shouts the doctor. Suddenly all my fears come rushing back. I know when something is not right. And this was not right. I quickly walk back to the seat adjacent to my wife's head. The anesthesiologist leans over and apologizes. I am just trying to get a grip on what is going on. I hear the door to the OR fling open and see four individuals quickly rushing into the room. The conversation between the doctors and nurses has ended. I am looking over at the area in which they are working on my baby. I look back at my wife; she has just asked the doctors if they were having trouble stopping the bleeding. She was told they were. I was certain that I was going to be raising that precious little boy all by myself.

I turned back to my wife, she was very pale and her eyes were struggling to stay open. She went lifeless. Her blood pressure had dropped once again and she was no longer conscious. A nurse brought my son over to me, just as my wife was regaining consciousness. He was so small and delicate. His face was so perfect with his mommy's nose. I leaned over with our baby so his mommy could see him. I remember my wife's only concern was that our son had a good suck. Through all this, she was still more concerned for her baby than for herself. The anesthesiologist took my camera and snapped a few photos of all of us. I wanted to make sure there was at least one of my son and his mommy, just in case. The anesthesiologist released one of my wife's arms, so that she could touch our son. I saw huge tears roll from my wife's eyes as she reached out for her son. To me, I knew this was her acknowledgement of her final moments with him and her sorrow that she will not be there for her son as he grew. I was counting the moments. I heard more individuals coming into the OR. They knocked the screen back, to make room for the extra people that just came rushing in.

I had been aware that a newborn was only presented to the father for 5 minutes or so. Then they would take the baby back to ensure he stayed warm. Five, 10, 20, 30 minutes came and went. I still had my son. I knew something was not going right. I heard a doctor ask what else they had that would stop the bleeding and clot. Then I heard someone run out of the OR. A couple of minutes passed and that person came running back into the OR. I was sitting near the suction jug and could see all the blood that had been removed from my wife's stomach. My toes were numb from forcing them into the floor as I tried to maintain my composure. I did not want to be removed from the OR, especially not now. I felt myself weeping uncontrollably. I was replaying all the movies and television shows I had seen in the past that ended like this. The happy couple that was to give birth to their baby, something goes wrong and the husband is left with a baby and a dead wife. "THIS ISN'T SUPPOSED TO HAPPEN TO ME!!! My baby never made a sound, never cried. He might have if he had known his mommy might pass away.

Over an hour had passed and I still had my baby in my arms. My wife was still alert and I began to hear a different chatter from the other side of the screen. I was beginning to believe everything was going to work out. But I still had my doubts; shortly after our doctor came around to our side of the curtain. She told my wife about the surgery and said she would be by in the morning to see how she was doing. I was asked for the baby and handed him off to one of the nurses. I told my wife I did not want to leave her side.

We made it into recovery. I spent the next few minutes crying uncontrollably. I could not get it together. I could not understand what I was feeling. Any thought of what had just happened threw me back into an emotional nightmare. I found it hard to sleep that night.

My wife told me that I needed to get out of the hospital and go home to check on our dog. I drove to the house, crying all the way there and all the way back. It occurred to me what my issue was. I was grieving. I was grieving the loss of my wife. The reality of her loss became so real the past night, that it was as if it actually occurred. I came to this conclusion, because it was the same loss and pain I felt when my mother passed away. Even though my wife did not die, I came to accept the fact that I had lost her. I accepted that I was going to be a widower father and I would have to explain to my son that night how strong and brave his mommy was. How much she loved him and how she would have given anything to ensure he was healthy and happy, including the life that she inevitably gave. Thankfully this will never happen. I will never have to have that talk with our son. I will, on the other hand, have to endure the pain of that evening, every time I think of my son's birth and my wife's strength as a mother.

Patrick's Story

The preterm birth of twins at 27 weeks gestation sets the stage for this next story of a New Zealand father's experience witnessing his wife's traumatic birth. Even though it had taken place two years prior, Patrick vividly recounted the horrifying details. Helpless, he felt like a "spare part observer." Both he and his wife since have been diagnosed with PTSD following his twins' preterm birth. Here is his story in his own words:

> I will never forget the horrible feeling of dread when the mobile rang at 4 a.m. My wife was in the hospital desperately clinging on to keep the twins inside at they ticked past 27 weeks gestation. Only a dramatic development would have caused her to call me at home at that time . . . and so it was, the waters had broken and the twins were on their way (ready or not).
>
> The journey to the hospital for the birth of our only children was not supposed to be like that—a worried, upset feeling of team failure. The pregnancy had been a nightmare from start to finish and here I was racing in to hospital with all the fears available to an imminent father of 13-week premature twins. Would they survive? If they survived, would they have disabilities like brain damage, sight issues, developmental issues later on? Wouldn't it be a blessing if they were to be disadvantaged that they just quietly pass? Yes, I actually thought that as the traffic lights at 4 a.m. presented no lawful barrier.
>
> When I arrived, I saw my wife with a resigned look of failure on her saddened face. Alas, the smaller twin had broken her waters and that meant emergency cesarean delivery for both of them. Within 4 hours, we were in the delivery theater feeling incredibly scared in the same way you do as a child on the way up on your first roller-coaster ride . . . you were committed and no turning back now.
>
> I donned all the protective clothing essential for a major operation. The screen went up and our obstetrician arrived and with the screen went all those beautiful father-to-be thoughts and wishes for cutting the cord and holding my babies as they made their way into our world. I was to be confined to the non-business end to comfort my wife and try to encourage her through the procedure.
>
> The babies were born and immediately required resuscitation and so began their horrifying 3-month journey of utter dependence on modern science to keep them alive long enough to give them a chance. My wife wasn't even allowed to see the girls. They were removed to the recovery room and she was left to be stitched up and prepared for her own recovery. I was allowed to travel through the hospital with the twins in their trolleys and saw for the first time how pitifully small and helpless they were; I had to leave my wife in the good hands of the medical team; we were separated again, but this time even worse for her was the fact that her babies were detached too. I cannot begin to imagine how my wife really felt in the whirlwind of that early Friday morning . . .

In the NICU the pediatric team worked hard with all manner of things as they hooked up this and inserted that, intubated here and resuscitated there. I was like a spare part observer—all these people fussing with things all around my twins' tiny bodies. The girls were just 900 grams and 910 grams when born. It was an enormous shock to see them lying there. I was there for about 20 minutes before I was finally allowed to touch the extension of my flesh and blood. The twin that went on to be named Shannon curled her delicate fingers around my little one and momentarily opened her swollen eyes—that was a moment I will treasure forever. I knew at that precise point through a moment of intense clarity, that if she died, which part of me almost certainly expected, I would at least have had that moment to cherish for the rest of my days. It was so personal; it was so human; it was so beautiful that finally I was able to weep.

My attentions immediately turned back to my wife whom I knew must have been weeping somewhere in solitary elsewhere in the hospital. The medics completed the insertion of horrible tubes into Janet's belly button and took a Polaroid for me just before her face disappeared beneath the C-Pap contraption that was to support her breathing for the next 8 weeks. I had a sorrowful picture to take back to my wife so that she could see what we had produced.

I found my wife emotionless, in shock. The girls were here and, short of our love, were out of our hands and direct help. We hugged and wept—our nightmare version of what is supposed to be a couple's most amazing event was over . . . and another one was just about to begin.

Andrew's Story

"Hurt, angry, sadness, helpless, cheated, and resentful" were the words used by Andrew to summarize how it felt to remember his wife's traumatic birth 3 and a half years earlier when she gave birth to their stillborn daughter. In Andrew's words:

> I am on an island watching my wife drown and I don't know how to swim.

> The moment when the word "death" was uttered from the perinatologist will be etched in my mind forever. I remember the coldness of both the nurse and the doctor when they uttered that word. I remember being numbed by a shock that went way beyond my emotional abilities. I like to think that I have a firm handle on my emotions. I am not afraid to share my feelings with myself, those close to me, and especially my wife. Yet I am just now able to begin my introspection and, hopefully, healing and resolution. I am coming to terms with her death every day but afraid that I did more damage by appearing strong when I never was.

> I don't remember the drive to the hospital. The revelation was at the Perinatal Office. The next moment I remember was in the hospital room

watching my wife argue with her OBGYN that was recommending we go home to wait for the induced labor of our dead child. My wife basically said they were going to do a c-section now. The OBGYN finally acquiesced.

I remember the silence and coldness by the medical staff during my daughter's delivery except for one of the male nurses who turned to me and said: "You would be amazed how often this happens." I remember holding my wife's hand feeling her emotional paralysis. I remember that I forgot who I was. That it didn't matter. I was going to be a father. She was our first so that transcendence of fatherhood turned to a transcendence of horror.

I remember the medical staff coming in asking if we wanted to view our daughter's body. We said no but I later changed my mind that evening which was the right decision. I will never forget holding her. She was beautiful and nothing was wrong with her except she was dead. I was supposed to be there for my wife. To be strong. To be the rock for her grief, her horror, her loss—the worst thing that could happen to a mother and yet as I said before,

I am on an island watching my wife drown and I don't know how to swim.

I not only do not know how to swim but I was drowning myself. But I am a man. I do not need help—John Wayne, you know. I was fooling myself at the expense of my wife and myself. Also, a man does not know the grief of losing a child as he has not carried that child in the womb for 9 months, so he has no clue to the devastation. I do not disagree with that statement. But, my baby was still my child. My loss is just as relative. And my grief is just as intense but is dismissed as the context of a man's role in the birth is secondary, therefore so is his grief.

Lastly, the system doesn't even recognize your child as a human being with a piece of paper that states "birth certificate." The state issues a "certificate of fetal death." The lack of human life recognition is yet another slap in the face regarding how America and the health care industry treat the loss of your child.

Clinician's Reaction

These stories brought tears to my eyes and my breathing was faster, these poor men. The heartfelt narratives that these men chose to share show the depth and the emotional trauma that affects people living through these experiences. What can we do as health care providers to provide a therapeutic holding experience for these families during the trauma experience as well as after? What role is there for a person in the operating room with a major traumatic event to be the emotional support for the husband/partner/father? I know we cannot predict these birth experiences but I wonder about a triage team model that could be implemented if needed when the birth becomes a traumatic event?

Mother's Reaction

I held my breath as I read these fathers' stories and I honor them for so bravely recalling their experiences. And I think of how many more could be carrying the weight of such untold emotions, and, given the chance (or is it permission?), would also benefit from the telling their story. TABS has always said it is a family having a baby, and all may need to be given a voice. Traumatic birth is devastating and now with the coming home, the fathers will be dealing with the aftermath, most likely trying to hold things together and giving little thought to their own interpretation of what happened before their eyes. They too experienced the traumatic birth. It is known that health professionals are given opportunity to debrief—I say YES to a skilled person extending such conversations to the entire family unit, who will be present. Fathers will start talking.

References

Ayers, S., Wright, D. B., & Wells, N. (2007). Symptoms of post-traumatic stress disorder in couples after birth: Association with the couple's relationship and parent–baby bond. *Journal of Reproductive and Infant Psychology, 225,* 40–50.

Bradley, R., Slade, P., & Leviston, A. (2008). Low rates of PTSD in men attending childbirth: A preliminary study. *British Journal of Clinical Psychology, 47,* 295–302.

Cox, J. L., Holden, J. M., & Sagovsky, R. (1987). Detection of postnatal depression. Development of the 10-item Edinburgh Postnatal Depression Scale. *British Journal of Psychiatry, 150,* 782–786.

Goldberg, D. P., & Hillier, V. F. (1979). A scaled version of the General Health Questionnaire. *Psychological Medicine, 9,* 139–145.

Horowitz, M., Wilner, N., & Alvarez, W. (1979). Impact of Event Scale: A measure of subjective stress. *Psychosomatic Medicine, 41,* 209–218.

Iles, J., Slade, P., & Spiby, H. (2011). Posttraumatic stress symptoms and postpartum depression in couples after childbirth: The role of partner support and attachment. *Journal of Anxiety Disorders, 25,* 520–530.

Skari, H., Skreden, M., Malt, U. F., Dalholt, M., Ostensen, A. B., Egeland, T., & Emblem, R. (2002). Comparative levels of psychological distress, stress symptoms, depression and anxiety after childbirth—a prospective population-based study of mothers and fathers. *BJOG: An International Journal of Obstetrics and Gynaecology, 109,* 1154–1163.

Watson, C. G., Juba, M. P., Manifold, V., Kucala, T., & Anderson, P. E. (1991). The PTSD interview: Rationale, description, reliability and concurrent validity of a DSM-III based technique. *Journal of Clinical Psychology, 47,* 179–188.

White, G. (2007). You cope by breaking down in private: Fathers and PTSD following childbirth. *British Journal of Midwifery, 15,* 39–45.

16 Trauma and Birth Stress (TABS)

Sue and Ralph Watson

The history of TABS is the story of the remarkable success of a group of post-partum posttraumatic stress disorder (PTSD) survivors. They supported others affected by the condition, and encouraged the health sector in New Zealand and elsewhere to minimize the occurrence of this condition, if possible, and reduce the suffering of women affected by it. As a result, many other women were helped, and their suffering better understood and treated. In the 13 years that TABS was active, it substantially achieved that purpose. TABS has stepped back, but its achievements remain.

Beginnings

Four births, in 1991, 1992, 1993 and 1995 respectively, laid the foundation of TABS. For Narelle, Toni, Sue and Carolyn, the births of their children were, to put it simply, "Traumatic," and did *not* bring joy. Narelle, Toni and Carolyn had mishandled deliveries, while for Sue, defective care before and after birth combined with "bad luck." In the following months and years, these women each waged prolonged battles for their sanity in the face of misdiagnosis of their distress and a lack of effective support from family and friends. In time, each was diagnosed with postpartum PTSD and successfully received treatment. Their experiences meant that they could not leave the matter there; surely, each was not the only one affected. If other women were also struggling, they too needed to know about the diagnosis and the available help, a way forward for recovery, and to regain their former selves.

Little Treasures Magazine is a New Zealand parenting magazine. It encourages reader contributions, not least in its "Letters" section. In that section, the following letter appeared in early 1998:

PTSD SUFFERER

My labour and delivery were a nightmare. I required forceps and wasn't properly anaesthetised. My intention is not to tell my 'horror story' but to highlight my struggle after the birth to hopefully help anyone who may go through the same.

Physically I healed quickly but mentally I had a long struggle. Early months were taken up just surviving my newborn. I began having flashbacks of the delivery, reliving the pain. I withdrew, lost all self-confidence and gradually I lost my temper until I began to lose control. I felt trapped in someone else's body. I believed I was such a bad person. I was terrified when left alone with my baby in case I lost control. I couldn't concentrate, couldn't make decisions and hated waking to face a new day. I caught myself imagining how I'd have a serious accident so that someone would have to take care of me. My husband remained supportive despite my behaviour and yet I felt very alone in my turmoil.

My GP referred me to Maternal Mental Health. They referred me to a psychotherapist who diagnosed me as having Post Traumatic Stress Disorder and finally I received treatment. PTSD is a stress disorder brought about by an intensive traumatic event.

Seven months later I have regained my self-confidence. My husband and I are very much in love and we enjoy our 2 yr son so much! My point is this: Depression following childbirth is NOT necessarily Post Natal Depression. These symptoms are similar but the treatment differs.

PTSD Survivor.

Reprinted with permission from *Little Treasures Magazine*

In the May edition of *Little Treasures Magazine* another letter appeared:

SURVIVOR

I am another Post Traumatic Stress Disorder survivor (Feb/Mar 1998). I had a long and painful first labour overseas and the hospital staff were unsupportive. After that, any reminder of birth gave me flashbacks, sweaty palms, racing pulse and feelings of terror—and there were plenty of mentions of birth as I am a doctor and went back to work quite soon. I thought I was going mad and my husband thought I was just being silly. Our relationship deteriorated drastically.

Finally, when the baby was a year old I took myself to a psychotherapist who put paid to the disabling flashbacks with psychodrama.

We re-enacted the traumatic event and inserted some positive and supportive memories. It worked like magic! So then, when someone mentioned birth, instead of flipping into panic, I would remember the supportive reply. It was like going into deep meditation.

Survivors are troubled by depression, flashbacks and anxiety attacks long after most people think they should have 'gotten over it'. It is important to talk about the trauma, often going over it many times, but the problem is that some friends and family just don't want to hear!

If this happens, find someone else and keep talking. The bravest thing you can do is ask for support and a listening ear. Midwives, Plunket Nurses and GP's are good, but some are better than others.

I will be a contact person to form a support group if one is needed and doesn't exist already. Write to me.

Narelle

Reprinted with permission from *Little Treasures Magazine*

The first two writers (Toni and Narelle) were from Auckland, the largest urban center in New Zealand. With the co-operation of the magazine, more letters were exchanged, some coming from elsewhere in New Zealand. Narelle was a medical doctor, and Toni had contacts with the Maternal Mental Health organization, and belonged to Plunket, an organization dedicated to promoting the post-natal welfare of mothers and children. In addition, the psychologist who had treated her supported what the women were doing. Sue and Carolyn, also from Auckland, were among the first people to respond, each bringing networking experience and contacts. Sue was active in SANDS (Stillbirth and Newborn Death Support: her first baby had died), while Carolyn, as a mother of twins, had contacts in the Multiple Birth Association, and was also training to be a childbirth educator.

Initially, the women circulated photocopied articles about postpartum PTSD. This was by post, as many households did not have Internet connections, and most articles were only available in print. Narelle was instrumental in sourcing and circulating these articles; she had access to professional journals, and could identify articles about postpartum PTSD as they appeared.

Stepping Out

New Zealand has a strong tradition of self-reliance. These women were no exception. With support for their efforts initially coming only from those who had helped them and others who had immediately recognized PTSD as a feasible diagnosis for some forms of post-natal distress, they realized that they primarily had to look to themselves to progress their concerns.

As trust grew, the women decided to meet. In July 1998, seven women met at Narelle's home. While their children played, they talked about their PTSD. They told their stories, unchallenged and uncorrected, their experiences and feelings really heard. It was good. It was safe. They were able to tell their stories without the hearers recoiling in horror or embarrassment. It was their understandings, their perceptions that counted, not the "objective clinical" facts that their files recorded. The women gelled. They agreed on confidentiality.

They agreed to form a PTSD support group to make the condition of PTSD known.

The women formed a committee. Sue was the Chairperson. Another woman from outside Auckland, Karen, also agreed to be part of the committee. The group opened a bank account under the name of "Post Partum PTSD Support Group." Meetings were held and minutes were taken.

The group had two aims. First, it wanted to support people suffering from postpartum PTSD. Second, it wanted to raise the profile of PTSD as a diagnosis for post-natal distress, so that other women would not face the same delays in diagnosis and delivery of effective treatment.

It did not look to build a nationwide organization, or claim to represent those suffering from postpartum PTSD. It wanted simply to "get the word out" about postpartum PTSD. None saw the group's work as a route to paid employment or otherwise achieving their personal goals. The group existed for others.

As more women contacted the group, a wide range of needs was apparent. Toni, Narelle and Sue had already received successful treatment for their PTSD, but many contacts were only beginning to become aware of what they or their loved ones were confronting.

The response was simple. "You are not going mad. This is not your fault. This is something that can happen to anyone. You are not alone. We have suffered from it too. Recovery is possible. It is worth the effort and journey." These first words of support were often the most helpful and reassuring that the contacts had heard for a long time, and the first to ring true. Following that, referral to practitioners who offered treatment for PTSD was often the next step, though some only wanted to talk.

From January 1999, the group held two monthly support meetings for mothers who wished to talk, one in the morning, the other in the evening. Attendance at these meetings fluctuated. While participation in some support groups arises from circumstances and conditions that are either permanent or long-term, this group considered diagnosis of PTSD as a signal that something could be done, not as a sentence to prolonged or even permanent suffering. While on-going support via email and phone was available, prolonged dependency on the group was not envisaged. Support meetings ceased to be a strategy.

It was out of these meetings that TABS acquired its name. The women were considering various options when another woman commented how the group was keeping tabs on each other. This immediately suggested itself as a name fitting neatly with the group's focus: Trauma and Birth Stress.

In the years ahead, most support was by email and phone. Initially TABS was mostly first contacted between 10 to 18 months after the traumatic birth, but over the years that time-frame shortened, with contacts coming within 7 days of the traumatic birth. In this scenario, TABS advised mothers and health professionals alike that mothers should "stick with and communicate with their maternity carer," until the mandatory 4 to 6 weeks of state-funded post-natal care had passed, to consider their situation then and if necessary immediately contact the mental health system.

Communicating

To promote awareness of PTSD as a postpartum mental illness, the women first turned to their existing contacts: their family doctors, and those who had cared for them during the period when trauma occurred. Through Sue's contacts in SANDS, TABS had contacts in the obstetric, neo-natal and social work departments in the local hospitals. The usual strategy at this stage was to forward copies of articles, but the limitations of that prompted TABS to publish its own materials. These took three forms: newsletters, handbooks and brochures.

Newsletters

To maintain contact with sufferers and supporters, the women decided after a few months to issue a newsletter. The first, published in November 1998, contained information about PTSD, advice for self-care, and information about available support, as well as the following story:

> My name is Karen. I am married and have a one-year-old daughter called Madeline.
>
> Before Madeline's birth, I spent the last 6 years working for a small firm specialising in tax and accountancy. A job which I have enjoyed but isn't really my desire in life. My real dream is to become a midwife, something I am passionate about. I work 3 days per week at my tax job, study and do work at a hospital helping run the parent/baby swimming classes. It is my favourite part of the week and it is impossible to leave without grinning from ear to ear! The rest of my time is spent with M, and now at the age of one, she has finally worked out that she has a say in things!
>
> My own experience of PTSD began with the birth of my daughter. I had a perfect pregnancy and loved it. My problem is that I am strong-willed when it comes to setting goals and this time I set the unachievable. And needless to say I was setting myself up for a huge fall. The sheer ferocity of labour shocked me. I could not move, I felt paralysed with fear and worst of all, I couldn't take part in my labour. I let it consume me. The drugs are something I will never forget, way up there with the scariest parts of my life. An epidural, threats of a cesarean, countless nameless faces doing examinations, it all broke me. I felt like an observer, and acted the same way. Where was this woman who could handle it? 24 hrs later (and a ventouse extraction and an episiotomy), my beautiful baby was born. The events prior were put temporarily on a shelf to deal with later!
>
> Hindsight is a wonderful thing. But time did provide the answers, and they were so simple. I had put too high an expectation on myself, that the only way to give birth was the natural way. I had not left myself contemplate the alternatives. I realised that I had not failed at giving birth, I had failed myself. However painful it was for me to reach the stage

> where I accepted this, I would not change it for the world; it had taught me such a lot and I am a stronger person for this.

The women collaborated in compiling these newsletters, which they published quarterly. The effort involved in producing these newsletters was substantial. Initially, as none of the women had Internet access at that stage, they either mailed or hand-delivered articles to each other. The newsletters were produced on PCs, printed and photocopied in bulk, before being mailed. The printed newsletters only ceased when TABS's website was published.

Handbooks

The newsletters contained a small portion of the available information. Individual articles might feature one or more aspects of PTSD and its treatment, but no systematic presentation of the information was available. Moreover, an article that was useful for health professionals would not necessarily be helpful for mothers.

The response was to develop two handbooks: one for health professionals, and one for mothers and their supporters. Some of the material appeared in both booklets. However, the health professionals' handbook contained technical literature, along with citations and additional references designed to assist readers who wished to read further. By contrast, the mothers' handbook was less technical. Self-help and self-care were important features, as were coping with PTSD and seeking help.

Both handbooks were available for purchase at a price set to cover costs and contribute to the funds of TABS. The newsletter advertised these, and they were available for purchase at TABS presentations. Sales were steady, often with health professionals buying a copy of each. Even after their content later appeared on the website, the convenience of hard copies meant that some continued to be sold.

Brochures

The need for a simpler form of communication was also apparent. Only TABS contacts received the newsletter, and likewise only contacts and audience members were in a position to buy the booklets. An attention-getter, and a cheap, convenient and easily distributed option, was necessary, something that would resonate with mothers and their supporters, be picked up and read, perhaps leading the reader to contact TABS or embark on her own path to wellness.

Bad Birth Experience was the first publication. It briefly described the symptoms of postpartum PTSD. It identified sources of available help. It gave contact details for TABS, first the postal address, then the email addresses and website details as email and the Internet became more widely available. After some years, the brochure was retitled: "Troubled by your birth experience?"

Troubled by
your birth experience?
TRAUMA AND BIRTH STRESS
Do you suffer from . . .

Flashbacks	Nightmares
Irritability	Avoidance
Panic Attacks	Anger issues
Hypervigilance	Mood swings
Difficulty sleeping	Numbed emotions

Difficulty concentrating?
You may be suffering from Post Traumatic Stress Disorder (PTSD).

PTSD is the psychological term for a set of reactions anyone may experience when something traumatic, scary or bad has happened to them. And of course these reactions may be caused by a difficult pregnancy or as a result of events that have occurred during the early post natal period and/or childbirth.

These events may cause the mother to fear for the life of her baby and/or for her own life, or fear for the integrity of her body. The mother's response may be one of intense fear, helplessness or horror. Or the events may trigger memories of earlier or childbirth traumas which have remained unresolved.

Symptoms of PTSD might not emerge for 3, 6, 9, or 12 months after the troubling birth experience or much, much later, but once they emerge are very difficult to live with or control.

The Way Forward . . .

Unlike Post Natal Depression, PTSD will NOT go away if left untreated. Therefore professional help is advised.

Where to get help?

- Pregnancy Help Inc
- Maternal Mental Health
- A Social Worker
- Plunket Nurse
- Trauma Counsellor
- Your Ante Natal Educator
- Your LMC involved in that birth
- Self Care/Family Support.

A good place to begin, is to tell a trusted friend or family member who will support you in your journey to recover from your trauma symptoms.

For more information, see the TABS website which contains a vast array of information for the community.

www.tabs.org.nz

A note from Tabs—Trauma and Birth Stress . . .

This pamphlet is written for the express purpose of alerting the community to the symptoms of PTSD and is NOT intended as a diagnosis. Should any of this information be applicable to the reader, then professional help is recommended quickly!

TABS is NOT a health provider or mental health service, but is an organisation of mothers educating the community and supporting mothers.

PO Box 18 002, Glen Innes, Auckland

Naturo Pharm is proud to support TABS in its work.

> Homoeopathy is a natural, non-drug therapy that aims to promote good health by stimulating the body's own natural healing ability. The remedies are highly diluted, natural substances and can be used to assist a number of common problems and ailments.
>
> Naturo Pharm is a New Zealand-owned homoeopathic remedy manufacturer producing a comprehensive range of remedies distinguished by smart blue and white packaging. These remedies are at health stores and pharmacies nationwide.
>
> www.naturopharm.co.nz

TABS distributed these brochures widely. Almost all psychiatrists throughout New Zealand, many midwives and every branch of Plunket, New Zealand's nationwide support agency for new mothers and infants, have received copies of the brochure, as well as many medical and community centres.

TABS is not aware of the full reach of these brochures, but many contacts came after distraught mothers and their supporters found them. On one occasion, Sue by chance met a woman from the southernmost part of New Zealand, two and a half days drive from Auckland, who had found the brochure, read it, recognized her need, and had sought and received appropriate help without contacting TABS. How often similar events have occurred is unknown, but it is unlikely that this was the first or only time that it has happened.

The brochures have also been the most enduring means of communication. Printed newsletters ceased with the launch of the website, and the publication there of the bulk of the content of the booklets reduced demand for them. However, despite the visibility of the site through leading Internet search engines, there remained a need for printed matter to catch the eye of people not actively looking for help on the Internet.

Presenting

It was soon apparent that there were opportunities for the women to present their stories and message to groups of health professionals. The first presentation was on 3 December 1998, when the women spoke to a group of midwives, maternal mental health workers and childbirth educators at a nearby base hospital. To illustrate the presentation, they use acetates and an overhead projector—not dropping slides and keeping them in order were the biggest immediate concerns. The audience was excited and very vocal when question and answer time arrived. The women then knew that they were on the right track. Presentations were never easy in the early days, but with sound guidance from experts in PTSD, they were always successful in looking after themselves, and did not "re-trigger" themselves.

Further invitations followed. In March 1999, the women held a two-hour session on the topic, where a psychologist who treated postpartum PTSD in his practice was the featured speaker. The continued interest delighted the women.

The next connection was with the New Zealand College of Midwives. The College was cautious when TABS's material arrived, but meeting the women allayed its fears: they perceived them not as an angry, bitter or vengeful group, but simply as mothers telling their stories. The College recognized that the women wanted to smooth the paths for others, in particular to warn against the all-too-common identification of trauma as depression.

The first main encounter with the midwifery community as a whole was at the biennial conference in the Waikato in July 1999. They negotiated a place in the trade area on the basis that they "stayed put and bought our own sandwiches." They were very warmly received. Conference attendees took their literature, and gave cash donations—the women's efforts were surely appreciated. Most important was the 40-minute presentation by Sue and Nimisha, a midwifery educator met through SANDS, who came to be a longstanding supporter of TABS. Sue told her story and Nimisha provided a midwifery perspective. The audience was supportive and the presentation was well received; the women now had confidence that they were more than capable of communicating their message.

The next significant contact was the result of Toni's efforts. The women were granted some time to present at a maternal mental health workers workshop in Auckland in May 2000. Three TABS members attended and presented. That they were making an impact was very evident when, in the midst of sharing their stories, a psychiatrist stood up and gave them $40.00 on the spot—"to help them on their way." This doctor also assisted TABS by inviting it to present as consumers at the Marcé Society meeting in Christchurch in 2001, an opportunity that led to TABS's interaction with Professor Cheryl Beck.

Presentations were always to health professionals or community groups. While women who had suffered postpartum PTSD often attended, they did not present to audiences of affected mothers; for them, recovery rather than information was the priority.

Feedback from these presentations showed strong interest in another mode of presentation: for TABS to run its own teaching and information events. This was a challenge for TABS; while they could present a full range of information on PTSD, they were all relative latecomers to the field, so how could they give such events a high enough profile to ensure their success?

Study Days

Toni led the efforts for the first Study Day. For previous presentations the women had engaged the support of health professionals already known to them. However, for the first Study Day, the presenters included Judy Crompton, an English midwife generally credited with being the first writer to consider PTSD as an explanation for some types of postpartum maternal distress. They had contacted Judy previously, and had become aware that she was going to visit New Zealand. They therefore invited her to speak at a Study Day they were organizing, and she accepted.

The day was a success. The involvement of Judy Crompton and the caliber of the other presenters made the event a satisfying one for all who attended. More importantly, TABS had established an independent presence as a contributor on the subject of maternal mental health.

As Seen on TV

In mid-2001, Sue received a call from Dr Sara Weeks, a psychiatrist specializing in maternal mental health who had treated her. Following on the Andrea Yates case, TV3, a nationwide free-to-air channel, was running a story on post-natal distress for its *20/20* program, and had come to Sara for advice. After the producer mentioned post-natal depression and puerperal psychosis, Sara had recommended that the article should also cover postpartum PTSD. After the producers agreed to this, she had then called people whom she had previously treated for those conditions: would they be kind enough to be interviewed for the show?

Sue received the call at a critical time. With her second daughter having settled into school, she was reviewing her options; was there anything more to be done with TABS? After a little thought, she agreed to Sara's request, and not long afterwards was interviewed for the program. Though Sue's time on air was less than 5 minutes, it aroused considerable interest. The involvement in the program of Sara, a respected figure in maternal mental illness practice, lent credibility to the inclusion of PTSD, at the same time giving the message its widest yet level of exposure.

Marcé

In September 2001, TABS presented at the Marcé Society Biennial Conference in Christchurch. Representing TABS were Sue and Rob, the husband of a mother who had come to TABS, who was to speak from a man's perspective. The keynote speaker at the Conference was Professor Cheryl Beck, from the University of Connecticut, USA. During her address, she referred to the different types of post-natal mental distress. In doing so, she mentioned PTSD, but added that she was aware that there was to be a consumer presentation about it, and said that she was looking forward to the presentation.

A highly appreciative audience of leading mental health specialists heard Sue's and Rob's presentations. After the presentations, Professor Beck (from now on, referred to as Cheryl) approached Sue directly. In the course of the conversation, Cheryl said how much she appreciated the presentation, and said that she would like to work with TABS on research into postpartum PTSD. Sue agreed to this. After the conference, Cheryl and Sue remained in contact by email, with Cheryl including TABS in her plans for a trip to Australia in September 2002.

The Marcé Conference was a turning point for TABS. Its credibility had been growing, as the invitation to the Marcé Conference showed. However, while most presentations led at most to an exchange of emails, and perhaps the contribution of an article to the website, Cheryl has since worked closely with TABS on a number of research projects that have resulted in published articles.

Structure

Although working well and efficiently, in legal terms TABS was only a group of individuals, and had had no independent legal status. Therefore it could not apply for financial assistance from Trusts and corporate donors that would only assist officially registered bodies. Under New Zealand law, registering as a Charitable Trust is one way, very common in the voluntary sector, for a not-for-profit organization to operate as a legal entity in its own right. The women decided to make TABS a Charitable Trust, and with the help of a lawyer, the Trauma and Birth Stress Charitable Trust was set up, and registered with the Registrar of Charitable Trusts on 18 January 2002. The Trust Deed provided for and named five Trustees: Narelle, Toni, Sue, Carolyn and Ralph, Sue's husband.

Now a legally recognized organization, TABS applied for funding from a wide range of other Charities and Donors. Donations received covered the cost of publications, presentations and administration. TABS could be more ambitious in its programs, particularly in paying travel costs of Trustees when they traveled to present, and now had the financial resources to commit with assurance to hiring venues for its presentations.

Apart from the establishment of the Trust, how TABS worked was also changing. The differing abilities and contributions of each Trustee had become more apparent, and as time passed their availability for TABS work changed. It had long been obvious that Sue, the Chairperson, networked effectively with other groups and agencies, as well as being an able administrator and a capable presenter. For these reasons, the other Trustees left a greater part of the work to her. Nonetheless, the Trust Deed required the Trustees to meet three times yearly. These meetings came to be concerned with reporting and governance, rather than operational and practical issues.

2002 Study Day

After the Marcé Conference, Cheryl accepted an invitation from TABS to present the results of her research in New Zealand while on her way to Australia in September 2002. The first announcement of the presentation was in the December 2001 Newsletter. The Trustees anticipated considerable interest in the event, with more attending than at previous TABS presentations. As a location, they chose the Waipuna Hotel, a venue in suburban Auckland that offered technical support for large-scale presentations as well as catering for meals. This was a big step up from the previous Study Day, but the Trustees were sure that the event warranted this scale of commitment.

The program was wide-ranging. With Debbie Hagar, a well-known women's issues advocate chairing proceedings, Cheryl was given the lead billing, to report on her current study of "The impact of Post Traumatic Stress Disorder on mothers and families in the post natal period." Sara Weeks and Nimisha Waller followed with major presentations. Also involved was Dereck Souter, a local obstetrician. This established a balance, avoiding reliance on overseas speakers who could be perceived as being out of touch with local conditions, and likewise not relying solely on local expertise; although the latter was strong enough for the Trustees to be challenged as to why it was necessary to have an overseas speaker at all.

The latter part of the program included a panel established for a symposium discussion. The panel would be able to explore issues more broadly, to reflect on the concerns and specific interests of the audience, and to respond to queries that arose from the presentations.

TABS publicized the event widely. Over 140 participants registered, making it the largest TABS event to date, and, as it has since turned out, the largest ever attendance for a TABS event. Registrations came from midwives, counselors, social workers and a number of mothers, women whom TABS had helped and who were keen to know more.

On the day, 23 September 2002, the event ran smoothly. The morning sessions were well received and Cheryl's presentation was particularly valued; while invited because of her interest in postpartum PTSD, the Trustees had not known about how prominent she was in maternal mental health studies, until a participant casually marveled at her participation. The panel discussion in the afternoon was lively, and elicited a diverse range of points of view. Following the main event, Cheryl spoke in the evening to the TABS mothers who had attended the Study Day, and shared from a more pastoral and less technical perspective.

The September 2002 Study Day marked the beginning of a new phase of activity for TABS. While, until then, its presentations had been well received, the participation of Cheryl lent TABS a new level of respect and greater acceptance in the obstetric and mental health communities. It also gave TABS greater confidence to set up and promote Study Days—lessons learnt in the events featuring Judy Crompton and Cheryl helped to refine the format for future Study Days.

Website

TABS was receiving many requests to publish a website. It was selling the booklets, and sharing resources, but the information was still not circulating as widely as it might have been. There was no single place where a sufferer or caregiver could find information easily and quickly. Other support groups had websites; why could TABS not have one also?

The Trustees found that setting a website was quite achievable. Sue engaged an acquaintance who built websites on a part-time basis to build and publish a website for TABS. Working with Ralph, he copied articles from CDs and floppy disks onto web pages, and on 31 March 2003, the completed website was published.

Ralph then took over the updating and promotion of the site, while Sue told all TABS's contacts about the website. The statistics from the web-hosting company showed steady growth in visits, with most visitors coming from sites based in New Zealand, the United States, the United Kingdom, Australia and other English-speaking countries. Visitors also came from almost all European nations as well as many in Asia and some in Africa.

Many updates followed, initially in place of the newsletters. These updates listed new articles and features added to the website. However, the growing availability of information and new material about postpartum PTSD made these updates less vital. Other updates listed additional helping organizations, both in New Zealand and overseas.

The influence of the site was quite evident; Internet searches for new material repeatedly turned up sites where the description of PTSD and its symptoms closely resembled the content on the TABS website. Generally, the sites acknowledged this indebtedness, but the Trustees still felt it necessary to publish a notice on the site asking people using TABS material for their own purposes to inform TABS.

The website also increasingly featured studies done in cooperation with Cheryl. The format and content changed also. Finally, in June 2011, TABS contact details were removed from the website; listed counselors took the place of the Trustees as sources of help and support.

A Balancing Act

TABS had always sought to be balanced in presenting its message. It was wary in case its message seemed to be an attack on the medical profession's care for women's health, which had been under close scrutiny since an earlier controversy around the treatment of cervical cancer in 1986 and 1987. Its goal was to inform, not to blame or discredit. Not taking sides was most important. Fortunately, the participation of recognized specialists in obstetrics and psychiatry who supported the message of TABS established a level of credence and comfort that encouraged other practitioners to consider postpartum PTSD in their practice.

TABS had strong support in the midwifery profession. One supporter was Joan Donley, a leading figure in the reinvigoration of the homebirth movement, who contributed an article to the website. Other professions also offered help in postpartum health care. Psychologists, psychotherapists and counselors sought to learn more and offer help. With the effects of postpartum PTSD often becoming obvious only after obstetric care ends, screening for it needs to extend far beyond the context of the birth event.

Other treatment providers also stepped forward. For many sufferers, homoeopathy, naturopathy and acupuncture, to take three such examples, have proved helpful. Without making any firm endorsement, TABS provided information on these options. One vendor of such products has sponsored TABS, and has presented at Study Days on the type of treatment that it offers.

TABS declined to list others who made contact, such as practitioners offering services that appeared fanciful or far-fetched. TABS would not publicize treatments that had no widespread acceptance, or were not anchored in a coherent scientific discipline of some kind.

Overall, TABS succeeded in maintaining contacts and support across a wide range of interest groups and professional communities. Voices questioning the validity of PTSD as an explanation for postpartum maternal distress were heard less often, and the diagnosis of postpartum PTSD became widely accepted as valid.

Study Days Continuing and Accredited

TABS continued to hold Study Days, including in places outside Auckland— in Hamilton, Napier, New Plymouth, Wellington, Christchurch and Dunedin. This made the information more accessible to health professionals unable to travel to Auckland. It also enabled TABS to invite qualified people from those areas to speak, thus anchoring the event more firmly in the local community, rather than being a "roadshow."

A core team of presenters emerged. Sue and Nimisha Waller combined with two others: Glenda Stimpson, a vastly experienced midwife nearing retirement who talked about how women could come to terms with the official records of their experiences, and Chérie Moran, a midwife and counselor with her own passion for women's well-being. These joined with locally based contributors to provide a consistent informative program.

It became apparent that the events would have more appeal for midwives, if they had Midwifery Council accreditation to count as part of the on-going professional development of midwives. Such development had become mandatory for midwives, who now had to complete courses and other activities with a total value of 50 points in each three-year recertification cycle. Accreditation would increase the reach of the message.

With this in mind, TABS applied in May 2005 to the New Zealand Midwifery Council for accreditation of the Study Days. This application was successful; the Midwifery Council accredited the course and assessed it being worth 10 points. This approval formalized a relationship between TABS and the midwifery profession. It was also a further recognition of TABS, while a consumer group, as a valuable contributor to professional education in this segment of the health sector.

Professional Bodies

TABS was in contact with many professional bodies. Its insights had won and gained the confidence and support of a number of professional bodies. TABS was a welcome contributor at the conferences of midwives and of the obstetricians and gynecologists, as well as presenting frequently at gatherings of mental health workers. Also welcoming its contributions were the counseling and social work professions, as well as other groups, such as SANDS, whose members' experiences frequently included traumatic experiences and subsequent PTSD. It is not common for an interest group in New Zealand to have such a wide audience.

Articles/Authorship

Following the 2001 Marcé Conference, Cheryl discussed with Sue a proposal for a study on posttraumatic stress after childbirth. She asked permission to recruit women for this study through TABS; TABS would publicize the study in New Zealand, and women interested in participating could contact Cheryl directly. The Trustees agreed to this proposal, and advertised the study in subsequent TABS Newsletters. Cheryl received survey responses from 38 women, 22 of whom lived in New Zealand, the others through contacts of TABS in Australia and Great Britain, and through Cheryl's networks in USA.

This response provided the basis for two articles, which *Nursing Research* journal accepted for publication. The first, published in the January/February 2004 issue, was "Birth Trauma—In the Eye of the Beholder," a study of the participants' experiences focusing on their perceptions of what happened to them. The conclusion was that the events that traumatized the women were often viewed as routine by the clinicians who attended them. This reflected what TABS had found in its support efforts, that there was often a vast gulf between how mothers and professional caregivers perceived and responded to what had happened, that even the most routine and apparently uneventful procedures could be a source of substantial trauma for mothers.

In the May/June 2004 issue, *Nursing Research* journal published a further article, "Post-Traumatic Stress Disorder—The Aftermath." This study was about the impact of postpartum PTSD on the lives of those who were affected by it. The article examined the ordeal undergone by sufferers, and advocated further investigation of means by which this suffering could be reduced. This article came from the experiences of the group of women surveyed for the first article, and showed a wider interest in the condition of postpartum PTSD as a separate field of study in its own right.

The November/December 2006 issue of *Nursing Research* contained an article about how postpartum PTSD sufferers experience anniversaries of their trauma. The study revealed a range of variously positive and negative experiences. It also identified similarities between these experiences and the anniversary of deaths, in particular the feeling that "failure to rescue" by clinicians and others was an integral part of trauma, and a cause for distress. The resulting conclusion was the need for both the physical and psychosocial needs of women at the time of birth to be addressed.

In 2006, Cheryl invited Sue to work with her. This brought the involvement of Sue under the umbrella of the University of Connecticut, requiring her to complete the University's ethics training. Her co-operation with Cheryl continued, first as a co-researcher, and later as a co-author. Out of this collaboration came a further study on the impact of birth trauma on breastfeeding. The study highlighted two alternative outcomes, one positive, the other negative. It challenged caregivers to take into account possible trauma when working with mothers about beginning and continuing to breastfeed.

Joan Donley had died in December 2005. To commemorate her contribution to the profession, the College of Midwives initiated a biennial symposium for midwifery-related studies to be presented, with an award for the best presentation. TABS found that it could take part, even though it was a consumer group. By then, a further study had produced clear and useful findings. TABS entered the event, and in September 2007, Sue made a presentation. The presentation was not only well received, but was a joint winner of the award.

The award was very welcome, but also signified more. The TABS presentation was the first by a consumer group. There was growing acceptance of contributions from such groups. It also showed that consumer groups, rather than simply being gatherings of individuals impacted by or interested in a given condition, were increasingly recognized as having a role in advancing knowledge and the treatment of those conditions.

Another study was into the impact postpartum PTSD had on a mother's attitude towards having another baby. For some, the thought of "going through it all again" put them off "trying again," while for others a subsequent pregnancy would give them the opportunity to "get it right." The research recognized the breadth of experience. Tokophobia (fear of death) was also a powerful factor where death had been a possible outcome of the mother's previous crisis. The study pointed to the opportunity for caregivers to use the whole process of pregnancy and childbirth to facilitate healing, but also sounded a note of caution for the treatment of women who had previously suffered postpartum PTSD.

At the time of writing, two further studies are continuing. One covers the experience of EMDR, a common treatment for PTSD, and the other examines the experiences of men in their support of and relationship with women who are suffering.

Movements

In late 2005, the composition of TABS had changed. Narelle had been diagnosed as having a brain tumour. While treatment brought some relief, the illness returned, and in April 2005, Narelle died. Since the Trust Deed required five Trustees, a vacancy had to be filled. After lengthy consideration, the Trustees decided against this. They had combined for a specific purpose, and had a common ethos. While they were aware of some worthy candidates, the Trustees decided to ensure the integrity of the ethos that had brought them together and guided them—they did not want "fresh blood" possibly pulling in a new direction, no matter how commendable that direction might be. Accordingly, they amended the Trust Deed, reducing the number of Trustees to four.

Stepping Back

In 2010, the Trustees considered the future of TABS. Much of what they had sought had eventuated. Postpartum PTSD was available as a diagnosis for post-natal distress. Many obstetricians, midwives, psychiatrists, psychologists and counselors were familiar with its characteristics. Study Days were still being scheduled, though requests for them were less frequent. While some health professionals still attempted to refer clients to TABS, as if TABS were a service provider, many more supported their clients by providing appropriate diagnosis and advice.

Women were continuing to send emails to the email addresses listed on the website; however, these contacts were fewer than in previous years. TABS had never claimed to have a monopoly on supporting sufferers. That appropriate help was available and being received was the main concern. The Trustees decided to review the future of TABS again in 2011, with a view to deciding on a way forward.

After a further Study Day in November 2010, the Trustees decided in June 2011 to scale back the operations of TABS. The website from then on would be the only support provided by TABS, serving as a resource for support and information about postpartum PTSD. The website would refer visitors to approved support providers. Further website updates would be infrequent, and for "housekeeping" only. TABS would no longer offer Study Days.

By 1 July 2011, the website reflected these decisions. While current research and writing projects continued, TABS stepped back from direct involvement in support and education. TABS had closed its "shop-front"; the "sign on the window" now referred visitors to the wide range of sources where postpartum PTSD support and information are available.

17 Secondary Traumatic Stress

Now that mothers' and fathers' experiences regarding traumatic childbirth have been addressed in this book, we turn our gaze in this chapter to the impact that being present at traumatic births can have on nurses and other clinicians. The following sections are addressed in this chapter: definition of secondary traumatic stress, research on secondary traumatic stress in clinicians, instruments available to screen health care providers, and interventions for secondary traumatic stress reported in the literature. Labor and delivery nurses' perspectives on traumatic childbirth are considered towards the end of the chapter. Experiences of five obstetrical nurses who were selected from a mixed methods research study Cheryl conducted on secondary traumatic stress in labor and delivery nurses are presented (Beck & Gable, 2012).

Persons can be traumatized either directly or indirectly. According to the DSM-IV criteria for PTSD (APA, 2000, p. 463):

> The essential feature of Posttraumatic Stress Disorder is the development of characteristic symptoms following exposure to an extreme traumatic stressor involving direct personal experience of an event that involves actual or threatened death or serious injury, or other threat to one's physical integrity or witnessing an event that involves death, injury, or a threat to the physical integrity of another person.

An understudied aspect of PTSD is secondary traumatic stress. In 1989, Figley wrote about the "cost of caring" for supporters of traumatized victims. Figley defined secondary traumatic stress as "the natural, consequent behaviors and emotions resulting from knowledge about a traumatizing event experience by a significant other. It is the stress resulting from helping or wanting to help a traumatized or suffering person" (1995, p. 10). Figley suggests using the term compassion fatigue as a substitute for secondary traumatic stress.

Figley (1995) proposes that secondary traumatic stress disorder is a natural consequence of caring between one person who has been traumatized initially and another person who is affected by the first person's trauma. Empathy and exposure are the two central concepts of compassion fatigue. Figley lists four reasons why professionals caring for trauma victims are at risk of compassion fatigue.

1   Empathy is a major resource for trauma workers to help the traumatized (Figley, 1995, p. 20).
2   Many trauma workers have experienced some type of traumatic event in their lives (Figley, 1995, p. 21).
3   Unresolved trauma of the worker will be activated by reports of similar trauma in clients (Figley, 1995, p. 21).
4   Children's trauma is also provocative for caregivers (Figley, 1995, p. 21).

Thomas and Wilson (2004) identified that empathy and exposure are two key risk factors for secondary traumatic stress. Leinweber and Rowe (2010) drew attention to the fact that heightened empathic identification in midwives' relationships with women during labor and delivery is a distinguishing characteristic of midwifery which also renders them vulnerable to secondary traumatic stress.

Secondary traumatic stress is different than burnout. Secondary traumatic stress can develop suddenly and with not much warning. Burnout, on the other hand, develops gradually, and results from emotional exhaustion. Symptoms of secondary posttraumatic stress can include a sense of helplessness/confusion and feeling isolated from supporters. These symptoms often are not connected to real causes (Figley, 1995).

Secondary traumatic stress has been reported in genetic counselors (Benoit, Veach, & LeRoy, 2007), mental health professionals (Buchanan, Anderson, Uhlemann, & Horwitz, 2006), child protection workers (Conrad & Kellar-Guenther, 2006), clergy (Roberts, Flannelly, Weaver, & Figley, 2003), social workers (Choi, 2011), domestic violence advocates (Slattery & Goodman, 2009), and pediatric health care providers (Meadows, Lamson, Swanson, White, & Sira, 2009–10). Focusing on the nursing profession, secondary traumatic stress has been investigated in emergency department nurses (Hooper et al., 2010; von Rueden et al., 2010), oncology nurses (Potter et al., 2010), sexual assault nurse examiners (Townsend & Campbell, 2009), pediatric nurses (Maytum, Heiman, & Garwick, 2004; Czaja, Moss, & Mealer, 2012), home care nurses (Yoder, 2010), and obstetrical nurses (Goldbort, Knepp, Mueller, & Pyron, 2011; Beck & Gable, 2012).

Goldbort et al. (2011) investigated nine intrapartum nurses' experiences in a traumatic birthing process. Using Colaizzi's (1978) phenomenological method to analyze the nurses' narratives one overarching theme, "From Behind Closed Doors," emerged. The following six subthemes provided a glimpse into what had occurred behind those closed doors of a delivery room: (1) Feeling the chaos; (2) Expect the unexpected; (3) It's hard to forget; (4) All hands on deck; (5) Becoming; and (6) For the love of OB.

In a mixed methods study Beck and Gable (2012) studied secondary traumatic stress in a random sample of 464 labor and delivery nurses. Nurses completed the Secondary Traumatic Stress Scale (STSS; Bride et al., 2004) and in the qualitative strand of the study described their experiences of being present at a traumatic childbirth. In this sample 35% of the labor and delivery nurses reported moderate to severe levels of secondary traumatic stress on the STSS. Using Bride's (2007) algorithm for the STSS, 26% of the sample met all the diagnostic criteria for screening positive for PTSD due to exposure to their traumatized patients. Content analysis of the obstetrical nurses' descriptions of their experiences of being present at traumatic births revealed six themes: (1) Magnifying the exposure to traumatic births; (2) Struggling to maintain a professional role while with traumatized patients; (3) Agonizing over what should have been; (4) Mitigating the aftermath of exposure to traumatic births; (5) Haunted by secondary traumatic stress symptoms; and (6) Considering forgoing careers in labor and delivery to survive. The narratives of five of the participants in this mixed methods study are presented later in this chapter.

The paucity of research on secondary traumatic stress in obstetrical health care providers is readily apparent with only these two studies to date having been conducted. The section that now follows describes instruments that are available to screen clinicians for secondary traumatic stress symptoms.

Instruments

Professional Quality of Life Scale (ProQOL)

This measures both positive and negative effects on clinicians working with persons who have experienced extremely stressful events (Stamm, 2010). It is a 30-item Likert scale. This instrument was originally called the Compassion Fatigue Self Test (CFST; Figley, 1995). Stamm (2002) added the concept of compassion satisfaction to the CFST and renamed the scale the Compassion Satisfaction and Fatigue test. Years later the name was again changed to the ProQOL (Stamm, 2010).

The ProQOL measures compassion satisfaction which is the pleasure one gets from being able to do your work well. Compassion fatigue, the second aspect assessed by the ProQOL, incorporates the two concepts of burnout and secondary traumatic stress. Stamm (2010, p. 13) defines burnout as

> feelings of hopelessness and difficulties in dealing with work or in doing your job effectively. These negative feelings usually have a gradual onset. They can reflect the feeling that our efforts make no difference, or they can be associated with a very high workload or a non-supportive work environment.

Secondary traumatic stress usually has a rapid onset and "is work-related, to secondary exposure to people who have experienced extremely or traumatically stressful events. The negative effects of secondary traumatic stress may include fear, sleep difficulties, intrusive images, or avoiding reminders of the person's traumatic experiences" (Stamm, 2010, p. 13).

Secondary Traumatic Stress Scale (STSS)

The STSS is a 17-item, Likert scale developed to measure posttraumatic stress symptoms associated with exposure to working with traumatized populations (Bride, Robinson, Yegidis, & Figley, 2004; Table 17.1). Each of the STSS items corresponds to one of the 17 posttraumatic stress disorder symptoms listed in the DSM-IV-TR (APA, 2000). Persons rate how frequently they have experienced the symptoms in the past 7 days ranging from never to very often. The STSS is

Table 17.1 Secondary Traumatic Stress Scale

The following is a list of statements made by persons who have been impacted by their work with traumatized patients. Read each statement, then indicate how frequently the statement was true for you in the past *seven (7) days* by circling the corresponding number next to the statement.

	Never	Rarely	Occasionally	Often	Very Often
1. I felt emotionally numb	1	2	3	4	5
2. My heart started pounding when I thought about my work with patients.	1	2	3	4	5
3. It seemed as if I was reliving the trauma(s) experienced by my patient(s).	1	2	3	4	5
4. I had trouble sleeping.	1	2	3	4	5
5. I felt discouraged about the future.	1	2	3	4	5
6. Reminders of my work with patients upsets me.	1	2	3	4	5
7. I had little interest in being around others.	1	2	3	4	5
8. I felt jumpy.	1	2	3	4	5
9. I was less active than usual.	1	2	3	4	5
10. I thought about my work with patients when I didn't intend to.	1	2	3	4	5
11. I had trouble concentrating.	1	2	3	4	5
12. I avoided people, places, or things that reminded me of my work with patients.	1	2	3	4	5
13. I had disturbing dreams about my work with patients.	1	2	3	4	5
14. I wanted to avoid working with some patients.	1	2	3	4	5
15. I was easily annoyed.	1	2	3	4	5
16. I expected something bad to happen.	1	2	3	4	5
17. I noticed gaps in my memory about patient sessions.	1	2	3	4	5

Source: Reprinted with permission from Bride et al. (2004, p. 33).

comprised of three subscales: Intrusion, Avoidance, and Arousal. The STSS differs from other instruments assessing posttraumatic stress symptoms in that the items on the STSS were created such that the traumatic stressor was exposure to patients/clients. Bride et al. (2004) assessed the psychometrics of the STSS with a sample of 287 social workers. In developing the STSS (Bride et al., 2004) reported Cronbach's alpha coefficients for the full STSS as r = .93, for Intrusion subscale as r = .80, for Avoidance subscale as r = .87, and for the Arousal subscale as r = .83. Confirmatory factor analysis of the STSS confirmed the data adequately fit the *a priori* hypothesized three factor model (Intrusion, Avoidance, and Arousal). The Goodness of Fit Index was .90, the Comparative Fit Index was .94, the Incremental Fit Index was .94, and the root mean square error of approximation was .069 (Bride et al., 2004).

Perron and Hiltz (2006) reported an alpha reliability coefficient of .92 for the STSS in their study of secondary trauma in 58 forensic interviewers of abused children.

Confirmatory factor analysis of the STSS was conducted on data from 275 social workers (Ting, Jacobson, Sanders, Bride, & Harrington, 2005). Analysis revealed the three factor model proposed by Bride et al. (2004) (Intrusion, Avoidance, and Arousal) adequately fitted the data but high factor correlations suggested a unidimensional scale.

Interventions

Crumpton (2010) proposed mindfulness training as a possible method to help prevent secondary traumatic stress in clinicians. She suggested a mindfulness-based stress reduction (MBSR) course as a low-cost educational program. Short periods of self-reflection and MBSR on a daily basis may be beneficial for clinicians who work with traumatized patients. Phillips (2011) suggested hardiness training for health care providers as a deterrent to secondary traumatic stress.

The Woman's Hospital of Texas now offers clinicians a "compassion fatigue" program which is primarily a self-care program (Coe, 2010). A lecture is given on the definition and symptoms of compassion fatigue. The focus of the program is on self-awareness of any symptoms of compassion fatigue such as irritability with patients and with co-workers. Clinicians are asked to promise to care for themselves. Staff members are encouraged to do something for themselves each day such as taking a walk once they get home from work.

Professional caregivers suffering from compassion fatigue need to restore balance in their lives and acknowledge their own personal needs (Showalter, 2010). Clinicians also need to learn to nourish their mind–body–spirit. Showalter encourages caregivers to find some personal healing ways and give themselves permission to rest so they can replenish their physical, emotional, and spiritual levels. Here is Showalter's compassion fatigue "do list" (2010, p. 241):

- Spend some quiet time: learning mindfulness is an excellent way to connect with you and achieve inner balance. Be still.

- Recharge, renew daily: a regular exercise program, a walk, prayer, meditation, committing to eat better, and feed your spirit and soul.
- Have one meaningful conversation each day: time with family, friends, or a spiritual advisor.
- Understand that your pain is normal, the work you do is intense.
- Get enough restful sleep.
- Develop and nurture interests outside of your work arena.
- Take some time off.
- Identify what is really important to you.
- Take one thing at a time.
- Laugh out loud.
- Follow a familiar routine.
- Maintain a healthy, regular diet.
- Create a safe place to escape into your imagination.
- Expect to be upset by upsetting events.
- Find a good therapist.
- Honor yourself.

As Showalter (2010, p. 42) concluded:

> The best gift a professional caregiver can give himself or herself is the time to sit with it and be still. It is in these quiet moments that reflection and balance will be one. It is then that one will learn to use the tools necessary to develop warrior traits of mindfulness, focus, and self-care. This will ultimately allow the professional to enhance their provision of care for others while balancing their life and life's work, thereby reducing signs and symptoms of compassion fatigue.

In the residency program for new oncology nurses at University of Carolina healthcare a 4-hour workshop on compassion fatigue is included (Walton & Alvarez, 2010). The first part of this workshop includes a discussion of the risks of compassion fatigue and its sequelae. Alvarez teaches the new nurses how to be mindful and present during the clinical day. In the second part of the workshop an experience of how to let go of some of one's compassion fatigue is presented. The participants are taken to the hospital chapel with soft lights and music and they are asked to center themselves in a private, sacred space for a few moments. Next Alvarez leads an oil-cleansing ritual to assist the new nurses to connect with themselves, release fatigue, and become grounded again.

The Resilience Alliance Project is another intervention that has been developed to prevent the effects of secondary traumatic stress in professional caregivers (Collins, 2009). This project focuses on reducing stress by means of increasing both resilience skills and social support. Chemtob (as cited in Collins, 2009, p. 12) said: "our intervention seeks to provide skills that have the effect of a 'psychological Hazmat suit'" to help clinicians who are exposed to toxic levels of traumatic circumstances.

In the last part of this chapter, labor and delivery nurses' perspectives on traumatic childbirth are considered. Experiences of five obstetrical nurses were selected from a mixed methods research study Cheryl conducted on secondary traumatic stress in labor and delivery nurses (Beck & Gable, 2012). These stories focus on cesarean birth without anesthesia, fetal demise, maternal death, postpartum hemorrhage, and witnessing a "gang rape."

Cesarean Birth Without Anesthesia

Approximately 2 years ago on a Sunday we had a crash c-section for a cord prolapse while I was charge nurse. Another RN rode the bed holding baby's head off the cord manually to OR. Got to the OR in approximately 2–3 minutes with obstetrician, pediatrician, tech, several RNs but no anesthesia. Despite fetal heart tones in the 120s and numerous pages for anesthesiology, the MD injected lidocaine/xylocaine and cut while patient screamed. We got word anesthesia was in a case and back-up on the way. MD continued for several minutes to inject local anesthetic and cut, inject and cut while patient felt everything. Anesthesiologist walked in the room and gave patient general anesthesia the same minute the baby was born. Despite the baby having good apgars and arterial gas within normal limits, 6 other staff members came to my home after work (birth occurred about 1400 and shift ended about 1930) to process the experience. There were at least 8–10 other staff who did not accept the offer to process with us that night or who worked in other capacities and did not attend, i.e., post-partum RNs who heard the screaming, the MDs (OB, Pedi, Anesthesia). We pieced together our separate views and consoled each other regarding the positive outcome. We all reported varying levels of intrusive thoughts, dreams, flashbacks, guilt, anger and sadness over the next few weeks. Some did not want to talk about it and others couldn't stop discussing it. At least one staff member sought out management staff and chaplain services. I had to force myself to be charge nurse in the future and I still get nervous, distracted, or angry when there is any delay in anesthesia, i.e., no one to do epidurals when c-sections are going on, anytime we go quickly to the OR and anesthesia is not actively seeming to hurry or show up in OR with us, etc. I find I need to tell the story frequently at work especially to new staff. I get very upset when anyone refers to any past experience in OR as "the worst" because I feel our experience was the worst. But I am most afraid of something awful happening again because I felt so totally, utterly, completely HELPLESS. I get livid when I think that there could be other awful things occur that I never ever thought possible. The prolapse I felt prepared for because I knew it could occur but *I NEVER EVER ENTERTAINED THE POSSIBILITY OF ANYONE GOING THROUGH MAJOR SURGERY WITHOUT PAIN RELIEF! I just did not know such a thing could happen. What else is possible that I know nothing about? How many more times will I be unable to evoke positive change for a patient?*

If I am this traumatized by the incident, what must the poor patient be enduring? I couldn't sleep and didn't feel like doing anything. I kept seeing how she looked and replaying that in my mind. I couldn't turn it off. I still have an overwhelming memory of this traumatic delivery and I can still see it when I close my eyes. I can't get her screaming out of my head. I feel like I will never get these sounds/images out of my head. It takes only a small thing to bring up these experiences.

Fetal Demise

At shift change, a 19-year-old G1P0 had come in for a 38-week labor check. Fetal heart tones could not be found, and the MD came in to declare an IUFD (intrauterine fetal death) within the hour. The patient and family responded appropriately—cycling through the phases of grief throughout the labor. Around 5 or 6 a.m. she started changing very quickly and began pushing at 06.30. The last few hours had gone well—several therapeutic conversations and even a smile or two were shared. I learned about her and her boyfriend, her family, the pregnancy—we really bonded. Then, when it was time for her to push, the whole energy shifted. It was as though the whole experience became real to her. She didn't complain, or act dramatic—she just pushed. She pushed with everything she had, and cried silently in between. The overwhelming despair on her face—and her strength in spite of it will stick with me forever. After the baby was born, she and her boyfriend sobbed. I remember her begging her baby to move, saying "Please, David, please move. Mommy loves you so much—please be okay!" It was horrible. I couldn't sleep all day—kept waking up hearing her scream. It still seems like yesterday when I care for a patient with an IUFD. Even now writing this I'm filled with sadness when I think of their loss. I cried for several days. It still haunts me. I have bad nightmares about dead patients and fetal demises.

Maternal Death

I had a mom being induced; she was delivering a stillborn at 38 weeks. The mom was 5 cms and requested her epidural. When the Dr. bolused the epidural, the patient went into respiratory distress, i.e., violent coughing, sats down to 70s. The anesthesiologist calmly programed her pump while I brainstormed the problem. B/P down? No. Spinal? No. I put O_2 on her, and then turned her to the side. The epidural doc left. Meanwhile her sats (oxygen saturation) were dropping. I paged him back to the room. He blessed me out—said it wasn't an anesthesia problem. I called the obstetrician who was on the unit to the room. He was highly annoyed that I called him but she wasn't ready to deliver. He did auscultate breath sounds and had to give her Terb and Phenergan as she was now vomiting and coughing up bloody fluid. He left the room. The patient continued to rally and then get worse for the next hour and a half. She would relax a bit, but would then sit straight up, breathing very rapidly and shallowly with her O_2 on. She kept telling me: "I don't want to die . . . I don't want to die." She tried to tell me about her 10-year-old autistic son she couldn't leave. I called the obstetrician back to the room when her sats were in the 50s and her resp (respirations) were 72/minute. The Dr. asked me: "What do you expect me to do for her?" I said: "Come in and watch her with me." He saw how bad she looked and ordered Lasix and a specialist. The specialist ordered some meds, anticipating a PE (pulmonary embolism). I put nitro paste on her and hung unfamiliar drugs. She got to 10 cm. She wanted to put lipstick on before she pushed. She pushed one time. I told her to push again and nothing happened. I remember feeling a little annoyed with her that she didn't push. Then I looked at her face and I knew she was dead. We coded her for an hour. It was two days before we knew it was an amniotic fluid embolism. Took her 4 hours to die. Then I had to prepare her body—never done this before—and do all the grief stuff for the baby. *Very hard.* I vividly remember the details of the events that transpired.

I couldn't walk past LDR #8 for a long time without getting teary. Finally I took a patient in that room. When she got her epidural, she stopped breathing. High spinal. I called for help, then I went and hid and fell apart. (I'd killed another one!) She was ultimately fine.

They had a special support group meeting for me. My boss kept saying: "Why don't you understand this isn't your fault? You need to get past this." It took a *long time.* A few years later I was packing up supplies from an obstetrical skills fair and came across the grief box I made that awful night. It contained handprints and plaster foot prints and a little blood-stained gown. I started shaking and got pretty teary. The family had never picked up these things. Was such a painful thing—I have never felt so *alone.*

Postpartum Hemorrhage

I was in recovery, having circulated a cesarean section on my original patient when the Team Leader told me another nurse was going to drop off her patient for me to recover, a common practice on the unit. I begin the second patient's recovery, just jotting vital signs and other information down while I make sure that everything is done for my original patient. In the back of my mind, I'm thinking, "You're breaking your basic rule— don't get behind in your charting." The report on my new patient includes the information that she did have a lot of bleeding during surgery, her uterus kept getting "boggy." She's good now, fundus firm and lochia scant. I finish the first patient's recovery, call report, and Transport. While I continue to just jot down the vital signs, I am diligent in the fundal checks, still no problems. As the hour comes to a close, I do a vigorous fundal massage. Satisfied everything is OK, I clean her up and place a clean obstetrical pad on her. I get her a cup of ice and she begins talking on her cell phone. A couple more quick tasks, and I return to her to remove the monitors. As I step closer, she just doesn't seem right. I touch her shoulder, "Are you OK?" She is getting more pale by the second. I shake her shoulder, "HEY!" Suddenly the cup of ice in her hand is crushed as she jerks her wrists inward, her head is thrust backwards, and she makes a sickening snoring sound. My brain screams, "OMG! NO, YOU DON'T!" I remember my mom talking of vigorous sternal rub. I do this and get no response. Gross, I see that yellow-waxy color. I've seen that before and I know what it means. A mili-second of panic before, thankfully, autopilot kicks in. The filed-away bits come to mind as if I had done this a hundred times. Pull the call light out of the wall, lower the head of the bed, get a blood pressure. My awesome peers immediately respond to the emergency light and come to help. It is then that I notice the pool of blood on the patient's covers. I know I had every drop of blood cleaned up less than 10 minutes ago. I relate this to the physician assessing the situation. A large clot, accompanied by a saturated Chux pad, is seen between her legs as the covers are pulled back. Fundal massage stops the tide after just a couple of minutes. She is conscious again, pleading for the fundal massage to stop. Transport has not come for the original patient, so someone is assigned to get her out of the room. We all realize that no blood pressure has been taken. The machine is prompted again. After several attempts, $^{70}/_{30}$ shows up. No one wants to say that we know that reading must be an improvement. With help, she is cleaned up again. For a split second, I reflect on the growing jumble of notes to be charted. Suddenly, there is another gush of blood—as much as before. I alert the physicians, still milling around. More fundal massage, more pleading from her to stop. Cytotec is administered. A second IV is started. Fluid boluses given. Again, the tide is stopped. She's cleaned up again, the linens are changed, and a fresh pad placed. The mood relaxes a bit. We are all shocked when the hemorrhage occurs for the third time. Now, the staffs of OB and anesthesia are in the room. The decision is clear: she must go back to the OR. I had never done a hysterectomy, but at this point, I am relieved to simply circulate a procedure allowing this woman to live to see her newborn. After all this, a hysterectomy doesn't seem scary at all. An uneventful hysterectomy is done and the patient is transferred to the PACU downstairs to recover. Examination of the removed uterus reveals a quarter-size hole in the back of her uterus, as well as a large hematoma on her left broad ligament. Mercifully, my team leader doesn't assign me another patient yet. I spend an emotional 30 minutes decompressing with my closest peers before getting down to the business of charting and properly documenting the most horrible experience of my licensed career.

Witnessing a Gang Rape

An emergency delivery of a young Indian woman: the emergency pager went off indicating a bradycardia. We readied the delivery room. A team assembled (4RNs, 2 med students, 3 anesthesiologists, 3 obstetricians). Her bed was rolled into the room and her eyes were wide open—she looked terrified.

The heart tones were low (60s–80s) and everyone in the room yelled for her to push. Screaming—no words could be heard. Fingers pulled/ripped the bottom of her vagina—people held her down like a gang rape. I tried to talk calmly to the woman and the doctors but I couldn't change the tone of the birth. The energy level was too high. Her legs were pulled back and a vacuum was shoved in her—it popped off twice and blood sprayed all of us who were "assaulting" her. The baby seemed stuck. The doctor was frantic and scared—this feeling spread and we were all afraid.

We had been in that situation many times before . . . things had been just fine. But this time the energy was different. The screaming made us crazy and forceful and frantic. The baby was ripped thru her vagina and blood was everywhere. Her tissue was torn through her rectum and looked awful.

I felt we had committed a crime. Guilt, sadness overwhelmed me as I looked at the vigorous infant. He was fine. We were wrong to let the fear take over the room. The woman would not look at her baby—she stared at the ceiling telling her husband to stop sobbing. He cried so loud. It was all we could hear. He thought we had saved his wife and baby—he thanked us, but he should have shot us. We traumatized her and assaulted her. This birth impacted me so profoundly—I've never been a part of such violence. I think of her eyes often. I still feel guilt, sadness and shame. I feel like I witnessed a gang rape. In the 13 years of labor and delivery I have worked, I've never been involved in something this horrible. I often feel I have to emotionally distance myself from patients because to become emotionally involved, and experience their labor and birth, would completely empty me of emotion and life.

Implications

Implications of the research to date for clinicians working with traumatized women begin with education about their vulnerability to secondary traumatic stress when caring for traumatized or suffering patients. Continuing education programs can focus on secondary traumatic stress symptoms and factors that can increase clinicians' resilience to this type of stress. Workplace resources to counter secondary traumatic stress need to be instituted. One such example comes from ambulatory care gynecologic oncology nurses (Absolon & Krueger, 2009). These nurses formed a support group which met monthly for an hour before work. A social worker led the support group to help the nurses learn about strategies to counteract the effects of secondary traumatic stress in their lives. It is hoped that as more research is conducted on secondary traumatic stress in providers, health care systems will design and implement mental health strategies for their staff.

References

Absolon, P., & Krueger, C. (2009). Compassion fatigue nursing support group in ambulatory/oncology nursing. *Journal of Gynecologic Oncology Nursing, 19*, 16–19.

American Psychiatric Association (2000). *Diagnostic and statistical manual of mental disorders: Text revision* (4th ed.) Washington, DC: American Psychiatric Association.

Beck, C. T., & Gable, R. K. (2012). Secondary traumatic stress in labor and delivery nurses: A mixed methods study. *Journal of Obstetric, Gynecologic, and Neonatal Nursing, 41*, 747–760.

Benoit, L. G., Veach, P. M., & LeRoy, B. S. (2007). When you care enough to do your very best: Genetic counselor experiences of compassion fatigue. *Journal of Genetic Counseling, 16*, 299–312.

Bride, B. E. (2007). Prevalence of secondary traumatic stress among social workers. *Social Work, 52*, 63–70.

Bride, B. E., Robinson, M. M., Yegidis, B., & Figley, C. R. (2004). Development and validation of the *Secondary Traumatic Stress Scale. Research on Social Work Practice, 14*, 27–35.

Buchanan, M., Anderson, J.O., Uhlemann, M. R., & Horwitz, E. (2006). Secondary traumatic stress: An investigation of Canadian mental health workers. *Traumatology, 12*, 272–281.

Choi, G. Y. (2011). Secondary traumatic stress of service providers who practice with survivors of family or sexual violence: A national survey of social workers. *Smith College Studies in Social Work, 81*, 101–119.

Coe, B. G. (2010). Program aims to combat compassion fatigue. *Healthcare Benchmarks and Quality Improvement, August*, 88–89.

Colaizzi, P. (1978). Psychological research as the phenomenologist views it. In R. S. Valle, & M. King (Eds.). *Existential phenomenological alternatives for psychology* (pp. 48–71). New York: Oxford University Press.

Collins, J. (2009). Addressing secondary traumatic stress: Emerging approaches in child welfare. *Children's Voice, March/April*, 10–14.

Conrad, D., & Kellar-Guenther, Y. (2006). Compassion fatigue, burnout, and compassion satisfaction among Colorado child protection workers. *Child Abuse & Neglect, 30*, 1071–1080.

Crumpton, N. M. (2010). Secondary traumatic stress and mindfulness training. *Journal of Emergency Nursing, 36*, 3–4.

Czaja, A. S., Moss, M., & Mealer, M. (2012). Symptoms of posttraumatic stress disorder among pediatric acute care nurses. *Journal of Pediatric Nursing, 27*, 357–365.

Figley, C. R. (1989). *Helping traumatized families*. San Francisco: Jossey-Bass.

—— (Ed.). (1995). *Compassion fatigue: Coping with secondary traumatic stress disorder in those who treat the traumatized*. New York: Brunner/Mazel.

Goldbort, J., Knepp, A., Mueller, C., & Pyron, M. (2011). Intrapartum nurses' lived experience in a traumatic birthing process. *MCN: American Journal of Maternal Child Nursing, 36*, 373–380.

Hooper, C., Craig, J., Janvrin, D. R., Wetsel, M. A., & Reimels. E. (2010). Compassion satisfaction, burnout, and compassion fatigue among emergency nurses compared with nurses in other selected inpatient specialties. *Journal of Emergency Nursing, 36*, 420–427.

Leinweber, J., & Rowe, H. J. (2010). The costs of 'being with the woman': Secondary traumatic stress in midwifery. *Midwifery, 26*, 76–87.

Maytum, J. C., Heiman, M. B., & Garwick, A. W. (2004). Compassion fatigue and burnout in nurses who work with children with chronic conditions and their families. *Journal of Pediatric Health Care, 18,* 171–179.

Meadows, P., Lamson, A., Swanson, M., White, M., & Sira, N. (2009–10). Secondary traumatization in pediatric healthcare providers: Compassion fatigue, burnout, and secondary traumatic stress. *Omega, 60,* 103–128.

Perron, B.B., & Hiltz, B.S. (2006). Burnout and secondary trauma among forensic interviews of abused children. *Child and Adolescent Social Work Journal, 23,* 216–234.

Phillips, J. (2011). Hardiness as a defense against compassion fatigue and burnout. *Journal of Emergency Nursing, 37,* 125.

Potter, P., Deshields, T., Divanbeigi, J., Berger, J., Cipriano, D., Norris, L., & Olsen, S. (2010). Compassion fatigue and burnout: Prevalence among oncology nurses. *Clinical Journal of Oncology Nursing, 14,* E56–E62.

Roberts, S. B., Flannelly, K. J., Weaver, A. J., & Figley, C. R. (2003). Compassion fatigue among chaplains, clergy and other respondents after September 11th. *Journal of Nervous and Mental Disease, 191,* 756–758.

Showalter, S. E. (2010). Compassion fatigue: What is it? Why does it matter? Recognizing symptoms, acknowledging the impact, developing the tools to prevent compassion fatigue, and strengthen the professional already suffering from the effects. *American Journal of Hospice & Palliative Medicine, 27,* 239–242.

Slattery, S. M., & Goodman, L. A. (2009). Secondary traumatic stress among domestic violence advocates: Workplace risk and protective factors. *Violence Against Women, 15,* 1358–1379.

Stamm, B. H. (2002). Measuring compassion satisfaction as well as fatigue: Developmental history of the Compassion Satisfaction and Fatigue Test. In C. R. Figley (Ed.). *Treating compassion fatigue* (pp. 107–19). New York: Brunner-Routledge.

—— (2010). *The concise ProQOL manual* (2nd ed.). Pocatello, ID: ProQOL.org.

Thomas, R., & Wilson, J. (2004). Issues and controversies in the understanding and diagnosis of compassion fatigue, vicarious traumatisation and secondary traumatic stress disorder. *International Journal of Emergency Mental Health, 6,* 81–92.

Ting, L., Jacobson, J. M., Sanders, S., Bride, B. E., & Harrington, D. (2005). The *Secondary Traumatic Stress Scale (STSS)*: Confirmatory factor analysis with a national sample of mental health social workers. *Journal of Woman Behavior in the Social Environment, 11,* 177–194.

Townsend, S. M., & Campbell, R. (2009). Organizational correlates of secondary traumatic stress and burnout among sexual assault nurse examiners. *Journal of Forensic Nursing, 5,* 97–106.

Von Rueden, K. T., Hinderer, K. A., McQuillan, K. A., Murray, M., Logan, T., Kramer, B., Gilmore, R., & Friedmann, E. (2010). Secondary traumatic stress in trauma nurses: Prevalence and exposure, coping and personal/environmental characteristics. *Journal of Trauma Nursing, 17,* 191–200.

Walton, A. M. L., & Alvarez, M. (2010). Imagine: Compassion fatigue training for nurses. *Heart of Oncology Nursing, 14,* 399–400.

Yoder, E. A. (2010). Compassion fatigue in nurses. *Applied Nursing Research, 23,* 191–197.

18 Epilogue

This book has been a compilation of research, clinical practice, and survivor response. Its purpose is to raise the level of awareness of health care practitioners with regard to assessment and identification of women who are living with posttraumatic stress related to birth trauma. We have presented the women's narratives, the qualitative data, the clinician's response, and the mother's response (a survivor of PTSD). Our hope is that you will want to learn more as the research continues to present itself in the literature and women continue to speak their voices.

As we have learned, 33–45% of women perceive their birth experiences as traumatic. Women have graciously and courageously shared with us their stories and their journeys through these experiences: the experiences as perceived by them and how they felt they were treated and/or cared for. The pervasive theme that the authors heard was that in so many ways the PTSD could have been, if not prevented, minimized. So many women shared with us how they felt invisible, not part of the process and yet it was their body. They often described the birth as "rape like," which brings forth a very different experiential sensation.

So much of these experiences had to do with lack of caring and respect and faulty or altered communication systems: women did not feel included; husbands/partners/lovers did not feel they were even considered as part of the picture, even though they had the most intimate relationship with the women in the room. They were rarely, if ever, asked for their input or their feelings after the birth experience. As you heard from some of the men, they suffered in silence, went on to support their partner in her becoming a mother while they vividly recalled their personal reality of having to have imagined their life without her and left with a newborn baby.

What is also striking is the intact memory of the women regarding the experience regardless of the years that had gone by between the event and the telling of the story. This speaks to the impact on the embedded memory in the brain. Yet, we know that most women who have birthed babies can recall the experience in detail even with a "normal" birth experience. Simpkin (2011) reminds us that the birth experience is a long-term memory. Positive memories of birthing depend on the process in which mothers are cared for and respected. This shows the power of the birth experience on the mind, body, and soul of a woman. What happens that we forget that this is such a powerful experience and we lose sight of what is "good" care? We know that bad things happen; the biggest dilemma is that at a birth when bad things happen there are usually people around to witness and experience the crisis. So why does the mother feel so all alone? Whose job is it to take care of her? Why does she feel abandoned and often betrayed?

We know that each woman brings into her pregnancy and her birth experience her history, her lived life. She comes into the experience with her own individualized coping strategies (good or bad) as a result of her lived life. She comes with her own preconceived notions and thoughts regarding what she thinks will happen to her based on her reading, interaction with others, previous birth experiences, and her hopes and fantasies. She has control over very little about the experience with the exception of how she takes it in, understands, makes sense, and integrates it. This is the important role of debriefing and what many of us have encouraged for years, for her to write down all her memories of the experience and keep a journal. Becoming a mother is a process that only begins with pregnancy. It continues forever as life happens and the child grows and develops.

So what can we do to prevent and/or minimize posttraumatic stress disorder secondary to birth trauma? The basic and fundamental principle is to *care* and to *communicate*: establish rapport with the patient, stay connected, treat the woman with respect and protect her dignity, and care for the patient. Now in today's technological world, this is in many ways harder in that many women have shared with us that the computer console was who they felt the nurse/doctor really communicated with. They felt that much of the checkup had to do with making sure the Doppler was in the right place so that the tracings were making sense. Right away, technology becomes a gift and a curse. Indeed the fetal monitor has significant value in the assessment of fetal well-being during contractions but it is how the computer console is treated that leads to maternal feelings of disconnection. Is she part of the process or part of the problem? Some women feel a bit infantilized as they are continually told to "lie still" and not move . . . More work needs to be done to get her out of bed so she can ambulate with a telemetry set up for fetal monitoring. We know that being in the bed, lying prone is not an ideal birthing position as it goes against gravity.

We are in an era where the use of the vacuum suction apparatus to facilitate delivery, forceps, fetal monitoring, intravenous lines, patient-assisted analgesia machines, computer consoles, etc. are the norm. Sadly communication is assumed rather than considered as a skill that needs to be constantly paid attention to. We assume that we know what people are thinking or how they are feeling often without asking them how they feel at all. Remember, PTSD is often the result of how an individual perceives an event; it is a very personal perceptive reality. So we cannot assume that we know what anyone is thinking or feeling without asking them to tell us their personal experience. This assumptive thinking often leads to inconclusive results and misinformation.

We have talked about the woman who is entering your system of health delivery to have her baby. She comes with her own lived experience and her fears and concerns. What often seems to happen is that we the care providers, who have complete comfort in our work settings, forget that she and her partner are basically "strangers in a strange land" and she is experiencing a once-in-a-lifetime episode, whether this is her first child or her tenth. She is asked to meet strangers and give over her trust to them without any relationship development prior to this encounter. She is asked to put on the clothes of the hospital and her partner is often invited in and out of the room based on what is going on with her and for periods that can be extensive if the staff forgets to invite him back. So when things are going smoothly, she and her partner feel a bit in control although their fear and anxiety are often masked and they are coping as hard as they can. When things go wrong and the focus is on "getting the baby out," the mother and her partner are often metaphorically pushed out of the room. The focus is on the baby and the mechanisms of assisted birth: vacuum, forceps, surgery. As we have read in the women's and the partners' stories, they did not know what to do and were left with their own mental images and projected realities. Who is there to care for them? They are living their own terror and in many ways so are the staff. Each person is in a "fight or flight" biological state and communication often stops at this time. It feels as if there is no room or time for caring, empathic connection and communication and this is the most important time. How can we change the reality of this experience? Is there a way that when the crisis occurs, a crisis team steps in? What would it be like if, when there is an emergency, there is a policy and protocol for one nurse to assume the role of primary care of the mother: to move right away into the position at the head of the bed? The nurse would be there to care for the mother and her partner through this crisis/emergency to the best of all their abilities. We would probably not prevent posttraumatic stress episodes or disorders but we could minimize the effects of the experience. So often we heard the women say in their narratives that no one paid attention to them. They felt invisible. They were stripped of their dignity.

High level nursing care for a woman in labor, in delivery, and in the postpartum setting includes caring, respecting, facilitating, encouraging, supporting, nurturing, and in many ways protecting the woman, her partner, and her baby from the potential of harm. A nursing care plan needs to be developed for each woman as she enters the birthing experience. This can begin at the admission phase as the nurse asks the woman her expectations, her hopes and dreams of the experience. Also the woman is asked about her personal experiences prior to the admission: any history of sexual, physical and/or emotional abuse (Simpkin & Klaus, 2004); any history of mood and or anxiety issues; any family history of mood and/or anxiety issues. Asking her how she feels and allowing her to truly describe those feelings are important. One word answers often signal much more underneath, so encourage her to verbalize how she feels at this moment in time. Develop a caring relationship and empathic connection. Stay with her and her partner as much as you can so that they feel cared for and are not left alone with their own fears and anxieties. Remember, giving birth is a lived experience and is not at all like the television shows or other people's experiences. This is unique to the mother and our goal as health care providers is to help her have the best experience she can within the given parameters of the experience.

The propensity to develop PTSD has to do with how the women felt they were treated in labor, whether they felt in control, whether they panicked or felt angry during labor, whether they dissociated, and whether they suffered "mental defeat," that is, they gave up, feeling overwhelmed, hopeless, as if they could not go on (Ayers, 2007; Czarnocka & Slade, 2000). Remember that as health care providers we can help to provide the "holding" in this scary, anxious time to allow women to feel in control, to the best of their ability. Encourage the conversation so that women do not feel worked on as opposed to being worked with. We cannot stress enough the need for caring and active communication with validation and clarity. Do not assume that anyone knows anything about having a baby or about being in the hospital and/or a birthing center. Remember that this is the woman and her partner/husband/lover's experience and they do not have any level of comfort. It is NOT their place of work and a place they will only be for a few days. They will, however, take home the psychological impact of their experience of labor, delivery, and postpartum.

We have learned in this book that many health care providers suffer from vicarious traumatization. It would be really interesting to have psychiatric/ mental health resources for the staff in hospitals that have labor/delivery and postpartum units. A person who could run regular support groups for the staff, to process the emergencies, the responses, the feelings/thoughts/concerns. Perhaps that would lessen some of the secondary traumatization of the staff and lead to a more consistent provision of psychosocial care to the laboring/birthing woman and her family. Would it decrease the amount of burnout and PTSD for the staff? It does seem as though there is a fair amount of "moving on" and compartmentalizing of feelings and concerns. Often we hear the expression if you don't take good care of the mother, no one is happy. It also applies to the nursing staff. If their mental health is not considered important and part of the culture of the hospital system, then what do we expect from them? Physicians have mental health needs too that need to be addressed and met. Otherwise, critical health providers are continuously suppressing and compartmentalizing their thoughts and feelings.

Many of the narratives shared by the women in this book spoke about how there were times when the nurse seemed to disagree with the midwife or the physician but did not speak out loud but rather spoke to the patient. It is a form of passive aggressive behavior that is pushed on to the woman/patient and she has not the power in her mind to act on the information. What were these nurses afraid of? Or is this their way of dealing with their own secondary traumatic victimization? Nurses need to trust their intuitive voice and speak up for the patient. What message is there in keeping silent? Nurses have amazing experiential backgrounds and many have years of clinical practice in monitoring, facilitating and encouraging birthing women, yet they do not trust that experience. How do we again promote healthy communication among the professionals? How do we help them to be able to bring up different opinions with rationale and experience and the expectation that a mature conversation will follow, not anger or acting out? We are hoping this book will raise the level of awareness in the professionals so that PTSD related to birth trauma may be minimized, yet many of the providers are also living with PTSD secondary to their clinical practice. We now conclude this book with some recommendations.

Recommendations

Assessment of vulnerability of the mother

- Know who your patient is . . . what history does she bring to the experience?
- Ask her what she expects, what is her fantasy birth versus reality; what does she need? Encourage the conversation.
- Get to know her as a person, not just as a woman having a baby.

Assessment of vulnerability of the partner

- An under-recognized part of pain during childbirth is the effect it can have on partners witnessing the laboring woman in pain (Simpkin, 2011).

Failure to rescue: The need to promote respect, dignity, and caring for women.

- Communication.
- Caring.
- Prevent talking over and around the mother/woman and her family.
- Facilitate a sense of control.
- Treat every woman with care as though she were a survivor of a previous traumatic experience (Crompton, 2003).

Impact of a traumatic birth on the mother–infant relationship

- Assessment of infant–maternal interaction/relationship.
- Assessment of breastfeeding interactions.
- Referrals to maternal–infant mental health providers if there appears to be a problem. Do not just assume it will go away when they go home as it often does not.

The invisibility of the traumatic experience: Anniversary reactions

- This traumatic event does not just go away. There is a grief reaction and a continual re-triggered time: the birthday of the baby.

- Keep the date and note highlighted on the woman's chart so that you will acknowledge and ask how she is doing regularly. Do not ignore or pretend that nothing happened. That is sadly the predominant way the world deals with sad/scary/not so nice occurrences: pretending that everything is okay is not a type of psychosocial care at all. For many women it is felt as devaluing and feeling invisible in their pain.
- Pediatricians and family practitioners: keep a highlighted note on the chart so that at each well child visit, the mother is acknowledged and her experience validated.

How to help women recover their souls

- Tell me about your birth experience: allow the patient to verbalize perceptions of the experience.
- Early recognition of precursors to PTSD: acute stress reaction (ASR): appearing dazed, experiencing reduced levels of consciousness or agitation and withdrawal.
- How did this experience compare with what you had expected (Stone, 2009)?
- Referral to psychosocial services during postpartum stay and give names of specialty practitioners (psychiatric/mental health) in the community.
- If baby is in the NICU: regular meetings with social worker or psychiatric-mental health liaison professional (nurse/psychiatrist).
- Screening for posttraumatic stress symptoms at follow-up visits with the nurse midwife and physicians.

The cost of caring for clinicians

- Nurses need to stop silencing their voices and speak up for the patient and not be intimidated by other health providers. Remember the quote from Eleanor Roosevelt, "No one can make you feel inferior unless you let them." Do not let anyone treat you with disrespect.
- Nurses need to trust their intuitive sense of reality. Many of the nurses in the labor/delivery/postpartum units are nurse experts based on years of clinical practice. They need to take a stand and trust this expert knowledge and realize that they play a major role in the holistic care of this woman, her baby, and her partner and/or family.

Facilitation of growth as a result of PTSD

- Facilitate the process of healing, encouraging the ability to change how women internalize. Help women make sense of the experience.
- Help to make subsequent birth experiences a corrective experience and healing for the woman and her family.

References

Ayers, S. (2007). Thoughts and emotions during traumatic birth: A qualitative study. *Birth, 34,* 253–263.

Crompton, J. (2003). Posttraumatic stress disorder and childbirth. *Childbirth Educators New Zealand Education Effects, Summer,* 25–31.

Czarnocka, J., & Slade, P. (2000). Prevalence and predictors of post-traumatic stress symptoms following childbirth. *British Journal of Clinical Psychology, 39 (Pt.1),* 35–51.

Simpkin, P. (2011). Pain, suffering, and trauma in labor and prevention of subsequent posttraumatic stress disorder. *Journal of Perinatal Education, 20,* 166–176.

Simpkin, P., & Klaus, P. (2004). *When survivors give birth: Understanding and healing from the effects of early sexual abuse on childbearing women.* Seattle, WA: Classic Day Publishing.

Stone, H. L. (2009). Post-Traumatic Stress Disorder in postpartum patients: What nurses can do. *Nursing for Women's Health, August,* 284–291.

Index